PROMOTING HEALTH
A Practical Guide

To all those working to reduce inequalities in health

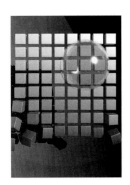

PROMOTING HEALTH
A Practical Guide

Linda Ewles MSc BSc SRD
Bristol, UK

Ina Simnett MA (Oxon) DPhil CertEd
Bristol, UK

FOURTH EDITION

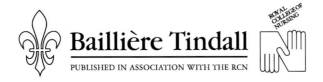

Baillière Tindall

PUBLISHED IN ASSOCIATION WITH THE RCN

EDINBURGH LONDON NEW YORK PHILADELPHIA SYDNEY TORONTO 1999

Baillière Tindall
An imprint of Harcourt Publishers Limited

First edition 1985 Wiley
Second edition 1992 Scutari Press
Third edition 1995 Scutari Press
    Reprinted 1996 Baillière Tindall
Fourth edition 1999 Harcourt Brace & Company Limited
    Reprinted 1999
    Reprinted 2001

ISBN 0 7020 2308 6

British Library Cataloguing in Publication Data

A catalogue record for this book is available from the British Library

Printed and bound in Great Britain

Linda Ewles MSc BSc SRD

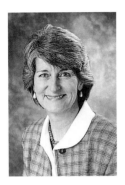

Linda Ewles is the Health Promotion Commissioning Manager for Avon Health Authority, responsible for the strategic development of health promotion. This includes local implementation of national health promotion strategy, developing health promotion collaboratively with local authorities and other agencies, and commissioning health promotion services and programmes from NHS trusts and other organizations.

She started her career as a dietitian, working in hospital and community dietetics in England and Bermuda, and then held health education officer posts in Bristol and East Sussex for several years in the 1970s. Afterwards she was Senior Lecturer in Health Education at Bristol Polytechnic for 5 years, directing the postgraduate Diploma in Health Education, and teaching health education, nutrition and communication to students on health visiting and nursing courses.

In 1985 she moved from teaching to practice as the District Health Promotion Officer for Bristol and Weston Health Authority for 6 years. During this time, as head of the District's growing Health Promotion Department, she gained much practical experience of planning and managing health promotion, often in collaboration with statutory and voluntary agencies. She was also actively involved in planning and teaching health promotion on in-service training courses for health and allied professionals. In 1991, following the NHS reforms, she became one of the first health authority 'purchasers' for health promotion, a role which she has retained and developed through subsequent local health service reorganizations in the Bristol area.

She participates in many national and local conferences, and is a member of the Society of Health Education and Health Promotion Specialists, the Association for Public Health, and the Institute of Health Services Management.

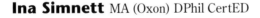

Ina Simnett MA (Oxon) DPhil CertED

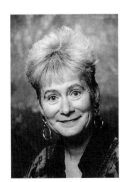

Dr Ina Simnett works as a freelance trainer and health promotion consultant. Her current activities include contributing to a project to generate learning and resource materials for hospital doctors in the West Midlands which will support them in their role in prevention and health promotion. She recently contributed to research and development work on interventions and alliances to promote physical activity, commissioned by the Health Education Authority and based in the Centre for Health Planning and Management, Keele University.

She previously managed an Open Learning Centre for Health Service managers participating in the Managing Health Services programme. She has contributed to a number of open learning materials in health promotion and is the author of *Managing Health Promotion* – a practical guide to the management of health promotion activities. She started her career as a research physiologist, then worked in health promotion for 12 years, including managing the Northumberland Health Education Department for 5 years, and later as a Training Consultant with the National Health Service Training Authority and in management training for health service managers. She has extensive experience of planning and teaching health promotion to health professionals, teachers and social services staff in the UK, and has recently undertaken health promotion consultancy in Australia.

Contents

Preface

The aim of this book is to provide an easy-to-read, practical guide for all those who practise health promotion in their everyday work. These people include health professionals such as health education/promotion specialists; hospital and community nurses, health visitors and midwives; hospital doctors and general practitioners; dentists and dental hygienists; pharmacists; health service managers; and the professions allied to medicine, for example dietitians and chiropodists. We also include a very wide range of statutory and non-statutory agents and agencies, for example local authority staff such as environmental health officers, planners, housing officers, social services staff, and recreation and leisure services; voluntary organizations and charities; pressure groups and self-help groups; youth and community workers; teachers in schools, colleges and institutions of higher education; probation officers and police officers.

For all these people, whether they are students in basic or post-basic training, or individuals with years of experience who wish to take a fresh look at the health promotion aspects of their work, this book will encourage the establishment of sound principles on which to base their own practice and improve their competence in a variety of health promotion methods.

The book is designed to be used as a self-teaching aid and as a source of material and ideas for group teaching by course tutors. We have included exercises, case-studies, quizzes, questionnaires and cartoons to make learning stimulating, relevant and enjoyable.

The first, second and third editions of this book were welcomed by students and tutors on many courses, such as courses training health visitors, teachers and district nurses; postgraduate courses in health education and health promotion; Health Education Certificate courses and Foundation courses; and by many other health promoters, for three main reasons. One is that health promotion is an applied field of study rather than an established discipline in its own right. As a result, it is difficult for health promoters to locate relevant and understandable material, which is scattered throughout a wide range of sources. Secondly, health promotion is receiving greater emphasis in the training and practice of an ever-widening range of disciplines and professions. Thirdly, the general public is increasingly interested in health issues, and is expressing a need for more heath promotion.

Since the publication of the third edition, there have been important developments in health promotion, some relating to the context in which health promoters work, and some to the content of the work. We have incorporated these developments in the fourth edition, so that it remains an up-to-date resource for health promoters. Importantly, there is an ever-growing body of published research which should underpin sound health promotion practice. New data, both from within the UK and internationally, have provided more information about the causes of inequalities in health. Evidence of growing inequalities in health in the UK shows that they have not yet been satisfactorily addressed. There are now well-informed proposals suggesting how this could be tackled.

The Labour government, elected in 1997, is pledged to tackle the root causes of illness and reduce inequalities in health. We hope that this will, indeed, be a turning point. We welcome the appointment of a Minister for Public Health to lead the way. The national strategy for health is being re-launched as *Our Healthier Nation*. Government commitment to take account of the impact of all policies on health is also welcomed. Other notable developments are the upsurge of interest in environmental and ecological issues and the emergence of local authority initiatives aiming to ensure a sustainable future. Also, there is increased emphasis on using public money wisely for activities which are affordable, effective and provide value for money. Finally, we now have agreed national occupational standards for health promotion and we have indicated where these relate to the different sections of the book.

We hope that this fourth edition will be useful both to those who have used the previous editions, and to the increasing number of people who are getting actively involved in improving the health status of the population, through empowering themselves and others to take more control over aspects of their lives which affect their health. We hope that this book will challenge, inform and contribute to the spread of good practice in health promotion.

Linda Ewles, Ina Simnett
1998

Acknowledgements

We are indebted to numerous people who have shared with us their health promotion experience and ideas. They include tutors and students on Health Education Diploma and Certificate courses, basic training courses for a range of health professionals, and professional development courses for teachers, youth workers, environmental health officers, police, social services staff and others. Wherever possible, the exercises contained in the book have been tested with one or more of these groups of students, and without their involvement it would have been impossible to produce a book which is, it is hoped, relevant to the real needs and concerns of all health promoters.

We would also like to acknowledge the contribution of all those people who have influenced the development of our own learning and ideas throughout the years of our health promotion experience and writing. Special thanks are due to Stella Mountford, Keith Hazeltine, Alan Beattie, Sue Habeshaw, Trevor Habeshaw, Stewart Greenwell, Roger Silver, Jane Randell, John Heron, Hazel Johns, Donna Brandes, Bob Ticktum, Martin Evans, Linda Wright, Peter Allen, Ian Fairfax and all the health promotion officers in the Bristol & Weston Health Promotion Department.

We are grateful to many people for giving us ideas for exercises included in this book, but especially to Sue Habeshaw and Penny Mares.

We would like to thank Peter England, Iain Harkess, Sue Steel and Kathy Weare for reading draft chapters and offering support and critical comment which helped us to produce the second edition. Students on the Health Education Certificate Course at Brunel Technical College, Bristol, 1989/90 and 1990/91 and the MA in health education at Southampton University 1990/91 were particularly helpful with comments, new teaching ideas and exercises and as fruitful sources of case studies and illustrative examples. Many thanks, too, to Elizabeth Williams for comments which have helped us to incorporate revisions into the third and fourth editions.

Many other people have helped in different ways. We appreciate and thank Jan Smithies for producing the foundation material for Chapter 15, 'Working with Communities', Sylvia Tilford for ideas and material incorporated into Chapter 1 of the fourth edition, Liz Rolls for helping us to get to grips with the new Occupational Standards for health promotion, and Christopher Flook for ideas and skill in producing the cartoons. Many people in Avon Health Authority and its predecessors have given help and support, and we thank especially Ian Baker, Clive Baish, Kieran Morgan and Jane Villa.

Finally, for their practical and moral support we thank our husbands, Jack Humphreys and Jim Pimpernell, and our editors, Patrick West for the first and second editions, Jim McCarthy for the third edition and Jacqueline Curthoys for the fourth edition. Special acknowledgements are due to Jacqueline for her suggestions and advice throughout writing the fourth edition and for helping us to bring to life her vision of the fourth edition.

Linda Ewles, Ina Simnett
1998

This poem has been pinned above the desk of one of us (LE) for many years, and we wanted to share it with readers. When it was first published in this book, we were unable to trace its source, and we asked readers to contact us if they knew who wrote it and where it came from.

We are grateful to Jean Hall and Pam Cooper, readers from Teeside, who found out that the author is Maline, and the poem was first published in 1953 in the Journal of Soil Association 7 (4) p 24. It came to light again in 1980, in the Proceedings of the British Student Health Association, where it was quoted in an article by Walter Yellowlees, a general practitioner from Aberfeldy. It seems to have been part of health promotion folklore for decades.

How disturbing that we still feel it's relevant even though the poem is 46 years old, the NHS is over 50, and the world is preparing for the next millennium.

The Ambulance in the Valley

T'was a dangerous cliff, as they freely confessed
Though to walk near its crest was so pleasant;
But over its terrible edge there had slipped
A duke and full many a peasant.

The people said something would have to be done
But their projects did not at all tally
Some said 'put a fence around the edge of the cliff'
Some 'an ambulance down in the valley'

The lament of the crowd was profound and was loud
As their hearts overflowed with their pity,
But the cry for the ambulance carried the day
As it spread through the neighbouring city.

A collection was made to accumulate aid
And dwellers in high-rise and alley
Gave pounds or pence, not to furnish a fence,
But an ambulance down in the valley.

For the cliff is quite safe, if you're careful they said,
'And if people should slip and are dropping –
It isn't the slipping that hurts them so much
As the shock down below when they're stopping.'

So for years we have heard as these mishaps occurred,
Quick forth would the rescuers sally.
To pick up the victims who fell from the cliff
With the ambulance down in the valley.

Said one as his plea 'It's amazing to me
That you'd give so much greater attention
To repairing the results than to curing the cause,
You had much better aim at prevention.

'For the mischief of course, should be stopped at its source –
Come, neighbours and friends, let us rally.
It is far better sense to rely on a fence
Than an ambulance down in the valley.'

'He's daft in the head' the majority said.
'He would end all our earnest endeavour.
He's a man who would shirk this responsible work
But we will support it forever.'

'Aren't we picking up all, just as fast as they fall.
And giving them care liberally?
A superfluous fence is of no consequence
If the ambulance works in the valley.'

Note on Terminology

We have tried to practise non-sexist writing throughout this book, using the principles and ideas we discuss in the paragraphs on non-sexist writing in Chapter 11. We have not always succeeded, and there are times when, for the sake of clarity, we have needed to refer to a health promoter or a client as 'he' or 'she'. In these instances, we have chosen to refer to the health promoter as 'she' and to the recipient of health promotion as 'he'. This is not, of course, intended to imply that all health promoters are female, nor that people receiving or using health promotion are always male. It is simply to avoid confusion and clumsy repetition of 'he/she' and 'himself/herself'.

Also, we have often referred to the people health promoters are working with as 'patients', 'consumers', 'users' or 'clients'. This does not imply, for example, that where we have referred to patients the text is irrelevant to healthy clients or vice-versa. It is solely to avoid the use of awkward terms such as 'patient or client'.

Introduction to the Fourth Edition

This book is addressed to all health promoters – everyone who practises health promotion as all or part of their everyday work.

Health promotion in the UK today encompasses a wide variety of activities with the common purpose of improving the health status of individuals and communities. This book is concerned with the what, why, who and how of health promotion. It aims to help you to explore important questions such as:

- What is health?
- What affects health?
- What is health promotion and what is health education?
- Who are the agents and agencies of health promotion?
- Who needs health promotion and what are these needs? How can priorities be set?
- How can health promotion be planned, managed, and evaluated?
- How can health promoters best carry out health promotion? What are the competencies they require? How do you actually *do* it?
- What are the key issues currently facing health promotion?

The range of health 'topics' is clearly enormous, and different professions and disciplines will all have their own areas of expert knowledge. They will also have specialist skills, for example in treatment, therapy, or technical tests. We do not aim to discuss these topics or specialist areas of knowledge and skills, but to focus on the theories, principles and competencies which you need to consider whatever your background.

As in previous editions, we have organized the book into three sections. *Part 1 Thinking about Health and Health Promotion* deals with basic ideas of what health, health promotion and health education are about, the different approaches and ethical issues which need to be considered, and identifies the agencies and people who have a part to play in promoting health.

Part 2 Planning and Managing for Effective Practice looks at planning and evaluation at the level of a health promoter's daily work and starts by introducing you to a basic planning and evaluation framework. It continues with a discussion of how you can identify and assess needs and priorities, and develop skills to manage yourself and your work effectively.

Part 3 Developing Competence in Health Promotion looks at how you can develop your competence in carrying out a range of activities including helping people to learn in one-to-one and group settings, helping people towards healthier living, working with communities and changing policies and practices. The fundamentals of communication and of using communication tools are also addressed.

Our book was first published in 1985, and we have produced each subsequent edition to take account of rising demand and rapid change in the world of health promotion. In the second edition in 1992, we incorporated a number of important changes:

- Health education had become subsumed in a broader approach to promoting health, encompassing both efforts to change socioeconomic and environmental conditions and health education aimed at individuals, groups and communities.
- The World Health Organization had emphasized the importance of targets for health promotion, both nationally and locally, and cities, towns and communities were increasingly adopting a strategic approach to health promotion.
- There was an increased emphasis on the management, planning and evaluation of health promotion.
- We defined and addressed the core competencies needed to practise health promotion. These included not only traditional health education competencies in communicating and educating, but also in managing, researching, planning, evaluating, marketing, facilitating, networking, and influencing policies and practices.
- We paid more attention to the views of users and receivers of health promotion, and to the concept of working in partnership with the public through personal and community empowerment, so that people can have more control over aspects of their lives which affect their health.
- We took account of the major changes in the way national and local services were organized and delivered. More emphasis was also placed on international developments such as the emerging influence of the European Community, and global factors, such as the importance of the environment and ecosystems for human health and well-being.

In the third edition in 1995, we continued to take account of all these developments. Additionally, we incorporated material which reflected important developments in health promotion:

- Organizational changes within the NHS, brought about by the 1990 NHS and Community Care Act, which meant that many health promoters now worked in NHS Trusts or Health Authorities with new 'purchasing' functions. Changes in GP contracts and the advent of GP fundholding were also having an impact on health promotion undertaken in GP practices.
- The national strategy for health in England *The Health of the Nation* (1992) and its equivalent strategies in Scotland, Wales and Northern Ireland, gave new impetus to health promotion work.
- Changes within local authorities, with resource constraints and policies of contracting out services affecting the way in which local authority staff approached health promotion.
- An ever-growing body of published research to underpin sound health promotion practice.

This fourth edition for 1998 has a livelier and more colourful presentation, so that it is easier and more fun for you to use. We have revised the content so that it will take you into the millennium understanding recent developments, especially the following:

- New reports and findings about the effects of inequality on health.
- The upsurge of interest both nationally and internationally in environmental and ecological issues, including Local Agenda 21 initiatives focusing on meeting the needs of the present without compromising the ability of future generations to meet their own needs.

- The increased attention to the *outcomes* of health promotion activities, especially towards identifying which interventions are most effective, affordable and provide best value for money.
- The change of government in 1997, followed by the appointment of a Minister for Public Health and a pledge to tackle the root causes of illness and reduce inequalities in health. Also government commitment to an integrated approach across all government departments and to a revised health strategy '*Our Healthier Nation*'.
- The development of National Occupational Standards for health promotion work.

We have retained the 'user-friendly' approach adopted in the previous editions. We aim to keep you involved, so that studying this book will be an active educational experience.

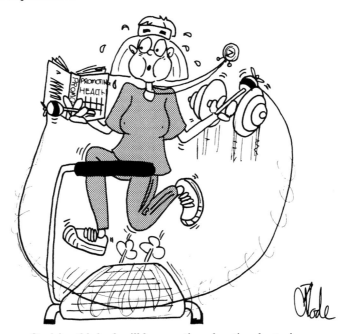

Studying this book will be an active educational experience.

We have included exercises to do as an individual or in a group, and examples and case studies which we hope will help you to apply ideas to your own situation. Often the exercises are designed to stimulate thought and discussion, and as there may be no 'right' answers, we do not provide them. Some readers may find this frustrating or uncomfortable. If so, we ask you to think it through, talk it over and work it out for yourself. In this way the 'answers' will have personal meaning and application. This is an example of how education can play a part in personal empowerment, and models the sort of approach we advocate in health promotion.

1 THINKING ABOUT HEALTH AND HEALTH PROMOTION

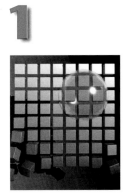

Part 1 has three purposes:

1. It sets the context for the whole book, by introducing key concepts, principles and ideas, and providing you with a shared language in which to communicate about health promotion.
2. It provides an introduction to the dimensions and scope of health and health promotion, which enables you to focus on the wide range of activities and approaches and on the diverse agents and agencies involved.
3. It highlights important philosophical and ethical issues which are explored in a practical context later in the book.

Health is an extremely difficult word to define but it is clearly important that you know what you mean by it. We discuss this in Chapter 1, along with a description of the major influences on health, inequalities in health, and approaches to addressing the determinants of health.

In Chapter 2 we explore the scope of health promotion and demonstrate that it encompasses a wide range of activities. We offer a framework for classifying the major areas of health promotion activity, and outline the national occupational standards for professional activity in health promotion, launched in 1997.

In Chapter 3 we analyze the aims and values associated with different approaches to health promotion, explore a number of ethical dilemmas, and provide guidance on how to make ethical decisions.

In Chapter 4 we identify the agents and agencies of health promotion and provide you with help in clarifying your own health promotion role.

1   What is Health?

SUMMARY

We start by looking at what 'being healthy' means to you and reviewing the wide variation in people's concepts of health. In the next section we identify dimensions of health (physical, mental, emotional, social, spiritual and societal) and discuss a holistic concept. We then look at factors which affect health, and include a discussion on the role of medicine and the issue of widening inequalities in health. A case study focuses on what shapes the health of people in widely differing circumstances. In the final section we review how the fundamental determinants of health are being addressed, and the contribution of global and national movements towards better health in the last quarter of the 20th century.

What Does 'Being Healthy' Mean to You?

'Being healthy' means different things to different people. Much has been researched and written about people's varying concepts of health.[1] More important than academic discussion, though, is the need for all health promoters to explore and define for yourselves what being healthy means to you and may mean to your clients.

Exercise 1.1 generally shows that different people identify different aspects of 'being healthy' as important for them. What you choose is often a reflection of your particular circumstances at the time. For example, if you are feeling stressed at work you are likely to identify 'enjoying my work without too much stress' as important, but if you have just given up smoking you are likely to identify 'never smoking'. As circumstances change, your idea of what 'being healthy' means to you is likely to change too.

Lay and Professional Concepts of Health

To the general public, being healthy may just mean 'not being ill'. Health is taken for granted, only considered when illness or health problems are interfering with people's everyday lives. This may be summed up as 'you don't think about your health until you've lost it'.

There are perhaps some more positive ways in which the general public thinks of health. The first is reflected in phrases like 'building up strength' and having 'resistance' to infection. This implies that health means strength and robustness, and having reserves which can be called on to fight illness and cope with stress and fatigue. Secondly, people talk about being 'off-colour' or 'out of sorts' or, conversely, being 'in good form'. In this way, health may be closely associated with moods and feelings, and a sense of balance and equilibrium.[3]

Exercise 1.1   What does 'being healthy' mean to you?[2]

In Column 1, tick any of the statements which seem to you to be important aspects of your health. Tick as many as you like.

For me, being healthy involves:	Column 1	Column 2	Column 3
1. Enjoying being with my family and friends			
2. Living to a ripe old age			
3. Feeling happy most of the time			
4. Having a job			
5. Hardly ever taking tablets or medicines			
6. Being the ideal weight for my height			
7. Taking regular exercise			
8. Feeling at peace with myself			
9. Never smoking			
10. Never suffering from anything more serious than a mild cold, flu or stomach upset			
11. Not getting things confused or out of proportion – assessing situations realistically			
12. Being able to adapt easily to big changes in my life such as moving house or a new job			
13. Drinking only moderate amounts of alcohol or none at all			
14. Enjoying my work without too much stress			
15. Having all the parts of my body in good working condition			
16. Getting on well with other people most of the time			
17. Eating the 'right' foods			
18. Enjoying some form of relaxation or recreation			

In Column 2, tick the six statements which are the *most important* aspects of 'being healthy' to you.

Then in Column 3, rank these six in the order of importance – put 1 by the most important, 2 by the next most important and so on down to 6.

If you are working in a group, compare your list with other people's. Look at the similarities and differences, and discuss the reasons for your choices.

Researchers in different settings have found a wealth of complex notions about health. For example:

- mothers of small children in Wales said that having the capacity to cope and function as expected was an important aspect of 'health' for them, and they also associated positive health with being cheerful and enthusiastic;[4]
- people may see health and illness as moral categories: some socially disadvantaged women in a Scottish study thought of illness in terms of spiritual or moral malaise;[5]
- elderly Scottish people saw three major dimensions of health: the absence of illness and disease, a dimension of strength–weakness, and being fit to do the jobs expected;[6]
- Australian men responded to the question 'what does it mean to be a healthy person?' in terms of functional capacity, psychological well-being, absence of illness and physical fitness;[7]
- some South Asians in Britain have been found to hold a theory of health as a consequence of the bodily balance between 'hot' and 'cold'[8].

Exploration of children's concepts of health is another area of study. Studies have shown that British children's ideas of being healthy and what makes them healthy are strongly tied up with being physically active and eating 'healthy' foods such as fruit and vegetables.[9] Children link smoking, the environment and 'unhealthy' food and drinks (such as sweets, crisps and fizzy drinks) with being unhealthy.[10]

Concepts of health are linked with people's social and cultural situations. Thus, to the mothers of small children in the Welsh study, coping with the family was their key concern. Middle class women are more likely to identify aspects of emotional or mental well-being as part of their idea of health than working class women, who more frequently concentrate on being physically fit.[11] 'Folk knowledge' of illness, prevention and treatment can also be powerful in shaping people's concept of health. Such knowledge may be part of a cultural heritage, passed on through generations.[12]

Standards of what may be considered 'healthy' also vary. An elderly person may say she is in good health on a day when her chronic bronchitis and arthritis have eased up enough to enable her to hobble down to the shops. A smoker may not report his early-morning cough as a symptom of ill-health, because to him it is normal. People assess their own health subjectively, according to their own norms and expectations.

People may also 'trade-off' different aspects of health.[13] A common example is that people may accept the physical health damage from smoking as the price they pay for the emotional benefit: 'I know smoking is bad for me but it calms me down and I'd be in a worse state if I didn't'.

Because of this variety and complexity of the ways in which people think about health, it is difficult to measure health (as opposed to measuring illness).[14]

To summarize, then, people's ideas of 'health' and 'being healthy' vary widely. They are shaped by their experiences, knowledge, values and expectations, as well as their view of what they are expected to do in their everyday lives, and the fitness they need to fulfil that role.

To professionals in the field, 'health' may be viewed more objectively as freedom from medically-defined disease and disability. But there may be a world

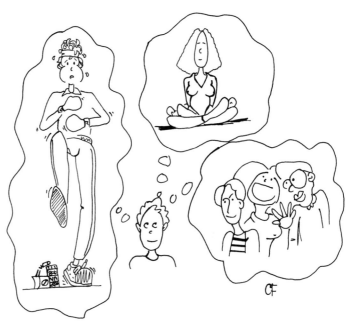

People's ideas of being healthy very widely

of difference between a lay and professional person's perception of what 'counts' as illness or disability, what causes it and what to do about it.[15] There will also be differences between health workers themselves, who may have widely varied concepts of health. For example, practitioners of alternative medicine hold to a range of beliefs about what health is, with different concepts of how health can be restored or improved.[16]

Towards a Holistic Concept of Health

Half a century ago, the World Health Organization (WHO) defined health as 'a state of complete physical, mental and social well-being, and not merely the absence of disease and infirmity.'[17] In its time, this was quite an innovatory statement, since it encompassed the three aspects of physical, mental and social well-being. In the 19th and earlier 20th century, as medical discoveries were made and medical practice developed, there had been a preoccupation with a mechanistic view of the body and consequently with physical health. Before that, of course, there had been centuries of many philosophies of health across the world in different civilizations, such as Greek and Chinese.

The 1948 WHO statement is still extensively quoted, although WHO has developed its view considerably since that time.[18] This historic definition has been heavily criticized, mainly on two grounds. One is that it is totally unrealistic and idealistic (how often does anyone truly feel in a state of 'complete ... well-being'?). The other criticism is that it implies a static position, whereas life and living are anything but static. The idea that health means having the ability to adapt continually to constantly changing demands, expectations and stimuli can be seen to be preferable.

Another criticism of the WHO definition is that it appears to assume that someone, somewhere, has the ability and right to define a state of health, whereas we have seen that people define their own state of health in a myriad of different ways. On the other hand, the definition can be defended on the grounds that it embraces the notion of positive health and acknowledges the central place of social and mental well-being.

Exercise 1.1 'What does being healthy mean to you?' involved you in identifying a number of different dimensions in the concept of health. These may be classified as follows.

Physical health. This is, perhaps, the most obvious dimension of health, and is concerned with the mechanistic functioning of the body.

Mental health. By mental health, we mean the ability to think clearly and coherently. We distinguish this from emotional and social health, although there is a close association between the three.[19]

Emotional health. This means the ability to recognize emotions such as fear, joy, grief and anger and to express such emotions appropriately. Emotional, or 'affective' health also means coping with stress, tension, depression and anxiety.

Social health. Social health means the ability to make and maintain relationships with other people.

Spiritual health. For some people, spiritual health is connected with religious beliefs and practices; for other people it is do with personal creeds, principles of behaviour and ways of achieving peace of mind and being at peace with oneself.

Societal health. So far, we have considered health at the level of the individual, but a person's health is inextricably related to everything surrounding that person. It is impossible to be healthy in a 'sick' society which does not provide the resources for basic physical and emotional needs. For example, people obviously cannot be healthy if they cannot afford necessities for food, clothing and shelter, but neither can they be healthy in countries of extreme political oppression where basic human rights are denied. Women cannot be healthy when their contribution to society is undervalued, and neither black nor white can be healthy in a racist society where racism undermines human worth, self-esteem and social relationships. Unemployed people cannot be healthy in a society which only values people in paid employment, and it is very unlikely that anyone can be healthy if they live in an area which lacks basic services and facilities such as health care, transport and recreation. Michael Wilson puts this graphically when he says that health cannot be possessed. 'It can only be shared. There is no health for me without my brother. There is no health for Britain without Bangladesh'.[20]

The Holistic View

The identification of these different aspects of health is a useful exercise in raising awareness of the complexity of the concept of health. But in practice, it is obvious that dividing people's lives into categories such as 'physical' and 'mental' often imposes artificial divisions and unhelpful distortions of a situation. Sexual health, for example, crosses all these boundaries. All aspects of health are interrelated and interdependent, and we subscribe to the view that a holistic view of health is of greater value to you and the people you work with.

Exercise 1.2   Dimensions of Health

1. Go back to your answers in Exercise 1.1 'What does being healthy mean to you'? Tick if any of the following dimensions of health are reflected in the statements you ticked in Column 1:

    Physical   Emotional

    Mental   Spiritual

    Social   Societal

**Is any one of these dimensions more important to you that the others?
How do they relate to each other?**

2. **Has your idea of 'health' changed since childhood? If so, how and why? How do you think your idea of health may change as you grow older?**
3. **If you have had professional training in health or a related area of work, what difference has this made to your idea of health?**
4. **What do you think 'being healthy' may mean to someone who:**
    - **has learning difficulties?**
    - **has a permanent physical disability such as deafness or paralysis?**
    - **has an illness or infection for which there is currently no known cure such as diabetes, arthritis, HIV, schizophrenia?**
    - **lives in poverty?**
5. Identify three or four key points you have learnt from this exercise about your own ideas of 'being healthy'.

Other writers have provided useful analyses of what 'health' means from the viewpoint of a philosopher and a sociologist, and these are recommended for further study.[21]

The first of these (Seedhouse) proposes the idea of health as the foundation for achieving a person's realistic potential: enabling people to fulfil their own potential. It is about empowering people: enabling them to become all that they are capable of becoming.[22] Working for health is thus linked closely with improving people's quality of life.

This notion of health as the foundation for achieving human potential has much to offer the health worker. It recognizes that health is a dynamic state, that each person's potential is different, that each person's health needs are different. Working for health is both an individual and a societal responsibility, and involves empowering people to improve their quality of life.

WHO also identify key aspects of 'health' which encompass these notions. WHO propose:

a conception of health as the extent to which an individual or group is able, on the one hand, to realize aspirations and satisfy needs; and, on the other hand, to change or cope with the environment. Health is, therefore, seen as a resource for everyday life, not the objective of living; it is a positive concept emphasizing social and personal resources, as well as physical capacities.[23]

This is a rich definition, worth considering carefully. It encompasses ideas of:

- personal growth and development ('realize aspirations');
- meeting personal basic needs ('satisfy needs');
- ability to adapt to environmental changes ('change or cope with the environment');
- a means to an end not an end in itself ('a resource for everyday life, not the objective of living');
- not just 'absence of disease' (a 'positive concept');
- a holistic concept ('social and personal resources … physical capacities').

This discussion of 'what is health' leads on to thinking about what affects people's health.

What Affects Health?

Being healthy is rarely, if ever, the result of chance or luck. A state of health or ill-health, however defined, is the result of a combination of factors having a particular effect on a particular individual at any one time. In order to work towards better health, it is necessary to identify these influential factors. We suggest that you begin by identifying factors which influence your own health, using the following exercise (1.3).

Exercise 1.3 will have identified a huge range of factors which affect health. They are likely to include genetic make-up, gender, family, religion, culture, friends, income, advertising, social life, social class, race, age, employment status, working conditions, health services, self-esteem, self-confidence, access to leisure facilities and shops, housing, education, national food policy, environmental pollution and many more.

The Role of Medicine

There has been much debate since the early 1970s about the relative importance of these many and varied determinants of health. One of the central concerns has been an increasing awareness that medicine, as a professional practice, has had surprisingly, and disappointingly, little effect on the nation's health. The National Health Service has evolved as a treatment and care service for people who are ill (a 'National Illness Service'), not as the major means of improving public health.[25] Only about 5% of deaths in the UK today are preventable through good medical treatment. Cancers and heart disease, for example, are the most significant causes of death, but medical care has little impact on the overall death rate from them.[26]

Some people have taken this argument further and claimed that the practice of Western medicine has, in fact, done considerable harm. The side-effects of treatment, complications which set in after surgery, and dependence on prescribed

Exercise 1.3   What affects your health?

The aim of this radiating circle exercise[24] is to identify factors which affect your health. The exercise can be done:

- individually;
- individually, followed by comparing results with other people;
- as a group, pooling your ideas about what influences your health.

You are at the centre of the rings:
In the inner ring, write in factors which influence your health *which are to do with yourself as an individual.*
In the second ring, write in factors which influence your health *which are to do with your immediate social and physical environment.*
In the outer ring, write in factors which influence your health *which are to do with your wider social, physical or political environment.*

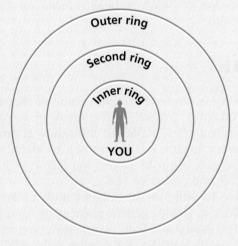

How do these factors influence your health – positively or negatively?
Which factors do you think are the most important?
Are there factors which you have not identified for yourself, but which may be important for other people?

drugs are all examples of this. But more important, perhaps, is that control over health and illness has been taken away from people themselves, who become dependent on doctors and medicines, expecting a cure for every ill and losing their own ability to cope with sickness, disability and death. Aspects of life which may be difficult, such as adolescence, pregnancy, the menopause and old age have been increasingly labelled 'medical', and the onus of responsibility shifted from the lay public to the medical profession. These arguments that medicine is, at best, a treatment and care service for the ill, and at worst, a means of undermining people's competence and confidence to improve their health, probably reached a peak around 1980.[27]

Inequalities in Health

Alongside this discussion on the role of medicine, concern emerged about differences in the health status of different groups of people. This concern grew in the 1970s, with a government working group on inequalities in health leading to the publication of *The Black Report*, in 1980. This showed that, for almost every kind of illness and disability, people in the upper socioeconomic classes had a greater chance of avoiding illness and staying healthy than those in the lower classes. It also showed differences in the risks to men compared with those to women, and variations in the apparent 'healthiness' of living in different parts of the country.

All this pointed to the fact that the major determinants of health were concerned with social class, occupation, economic conditions, geographical location and gender. Further evidence towards the end of the 1980s and in the 1990s shows that these inequalities are continuing to grow. This means that while overall health may have improved, the rate of improvement is not equal across all sections of society. The gap between the health status of the lower social classes compared with the higher social classes continues to become wider because of social and economic disadvantage, which in turn is associated with poorer housing, unemployment, stress, poorer nutrition and less social support.[28]

More recent work comparing data across different countries has shown a new slant on the issue of inequalities.[29] It is not the richest societies which have the best health, but those that have the smallest income differences between rich and poor. It is the *relative* difference in income levels which is crucial. The reason seems to be that small income differences across society mean an egalitarian society which has a strong community life and better quality of life in terms of strong social networks, less social stress, higher self-esteem, less depression and anxiety and more sense of control. All of this adds up to better health.

It poses the challenge of improving health by building *social capital*. Social capital is the term used to describe investment in the social fabric of society, so that communities have characteristics such as high levels of trust, and many networks for the exchange of information, ideas and practical help.[30] Social capital is produced when, for example, there are neighbourhood schemes of childcare and crime prevention, community groups and social activities which engage a wide range of interests and people.

Other work shows that differences in health experience (often also called 'variations' in health) are not just about differences in social class. There are also important differences in rates of illness and death between ethnic groups, which may be related to differences in income, education and living conditions, cultural factors or genetic make-up.[31]

There are also differences associated with age, sex, occupation, and where people live.[32]

Addressing the distribution of wealth in society, reducing the gap between rich and poor, and tackling socioeconomic disadvantage are clearly political issues. The evidence of increasing inequalities in health shows that they have not yet been satisfactorily addressed. There are well-informed proposals for action,[33] and we wait to see if the millennium will be a turning point in reducing inequalities in health.

Case studies 1.1 and 1.2 — What shapes people's health and health beliefs?

Case 1.1 – Salma

This case study is taken from a research study of 16 Asian women in Bristol who had suffered from depression. The women were interviewed in depth in their own language.[34]

Salma had been widowed twice, and now believed that people were plotting against her. At the same time, she was in desperate straits, living with her four children in a small, crumbling, two-bedroomed terraced house. She had no money for repairs, and no husband to support her or help put things right. She says:

'When we moved here – from one pit to another – I left all my furniture behind. We live like animals here.'

There was little wallpaper in any of the rooms. The geyser was broken and there was only cold water in the bathroom. To have a bath, Salma had to heat water on the cooker downstairs and carry it up. The plumbing needed repair, and there was no water in the cold water tap of the washbasin. Salma slept with her daughter in one of the bedrooms and her three sons slept in the other. One of the downstairs rooms could not be used because it needed replastering, and the floor boards were dangerous in another.

'Yes, we've applied for a repair grant, but that was about a year and a half ago. They came and took pictures and didn't do anything about it. You know what these people are like, they just see us and turn away. I don't understand it. We've also applied for a council house, but they say it will take a long time.

'You ask about my health, where do I start? There's nothing wrong with me, just nerves … I feel like my life is being squeezed out of me.'

Then there was worry about her children. They could not play outside or go to the park *'because the English children fought with them'*, and the house was too small and dangerous to play in.

- What affects the health of Salma and her children?

- What is Salma's own view about her health?
- What should be done to improve and promote the health of Salma and her children?

Case 1.2: – Tracy and Catherine

This case study is based on a feature headlined 'generation gap' in the *Independent* newspaper, although we have changed the names.[35]

Tracy is 6 months pregnant and smokes 10 a day.

'My great-grandma smoked stronger fags than I do, and more than me. She lived to be 91 and everyone says I'm just like her. If you're going to die, you're going to die. I started smoking ages ago, when I was 13, and I smoked at home. I used to stick my clothes along the crack at the bottom of my bedroom door and smoke out of the window.

'You're not meant to smoke when you're pregnant but people do and have bright children. It doesn't damage the children's lungs – they just manage with a bit less oxygen. The doctors just say the birthweight will be a bit lighter. My friend smoked all the time and her three kids are really bright.

'My mum is hypocritical. She used to smoke. Every time she tells me not to I want to smoke more. She makes me conscious of it. If she wasn't here, I wouldn't be smoking. I'd be watching the tele.

'If you're going to get cancer, you'll get it anyway. Lots of our family died of cancer. Roy Castle died of cancer and he never smoked. I think passive smoking is more dangerous. That way, the smoke reaching the baby isn't filtered, but my cigarettes are filtered. My lungs are healthy. I did that smoking test where you blow into a bag, and my lungs are really healthy. My baby is kicking because it's healthy.

'I'd give up just like that, but Mike can't; his job's too stressful. What's the point of me giving up if I'll be doing passive smoking from his? I could be worse – I could be taking drugs, but I don't because it makes me feel funny. And I don't drink, because drinking makes you feel bad about yourself, and that will make the baby feel bad. But all cigarettes do is calm me down, I could be hit by a bus tomorrow and I might as well die unstressed.'

Catherine is Tracy's mother. This is what she says:

'Tracy's grandparents both died very young of smoke-related illnesses – throat cancer and lung cancer – and so my children never knew those grandparents.

'You're given a beautiful child that you love and nurture for however many years, then she does this to herself. Her eyes are dull, her hair loses its sheen, her skin grows sallow. The smell is repulsive – her clothes reek.

'I stopped 25 years ago when I was first pregnant. My husband was a heavy smoker but he gave up completely before the children were born because I made him. We tried to set a good example. We never let anyone smoke at home when they were little.

'But Tracy has never seen anyone die – someone with bronchitis, then emphysema like her uncle. He can't breathe without a nebuliser. She's never seen anyone die because they couldn't breathe at all.

'She was so health-conscious when she was younger. She wrote a poem about not testing cosmetics on rabbits and here she is harming her own baby. I thought she'd have more sense. Also, cigarettes are an appetite suppressant and she wants to stay looking like a stick insect while she's pregnant.

'I'm worried about the baby. She knows that if she smokes, there is more likelihood of a cot death, or the baby being stillborn. If it's born alive, it'll weigh less, have more chest infections and be less intelligent. If it's any less intelligent than Tracy, it will probably start smoking itself. Her baby is kicking because it's fighting for breath.'

- What does Tracy believe about smoking and health – her own health, and her baby's? What influences her beliefs?
- What does Catherine believe about smoking and health – her own health, Tracy's and Tracy's baby? What influences her beliefs?
- What has influenced Tracy's attitude and behaviour about smoking?
- What has influenced Catherine's attitude and behaviour about smoking?
- Should the health workers seeing Tracy in her pregnancy and afterwards address the question of Tracy's smoking? If so, how do you think they should approach it?
- Should anything else be done about Tracy's smoking and the smoking habits of others like her?

Addressing the Determinants of Health

So far, we have seen that 'health' is a complex concept, which means different things to different people. We have also seen that the degree of 'healthiness' is linked up with people's ability to reach their full potential. This, in turn, is affected by a wide range of factors which may be broadly classified as lifestyle factors to do with individual health behaviour, and broader social, economic and environmental factors such as whether people live in an egalitarian society, what social support networks are available, and how they live in terms of employment, income and housing.

The emphasis of health promotion work – whether it is on individual health behaviour or socioeconomic factors – has changed over the last few decades. Early public health work in the first half of this century concentrated on environmental reforms such as slum clearance, improved sanitation and clean air. Then in the 1950s and 1960s the focus shifted towards the need for changes in individual health behaviour about, for example, family planning, venereal disease, accident prevention, immunization, cervical smear checks, weight control, alcohol consumption and smoking. This emphasis on the 'lifestyle approach' meant a concentration of effort on health education.[36]

During the 1970s, this emphasis became heavily criticized, because it distracted attention from the social and economic determinants of health, and tended to blame individuals for their own ill-health. For example, people with heart disease could be blamed for it because they were overweight and smoked, but the reasons for being overweight and smoking were ignored. (Reasons may have included lack of education, no help available to stop smoking, eating and smoking used a way of coping with stresses such as poor housing or unemployment, lack of availability of cheap nutritious foods, and so on.)[37] This was known as 'victim-blaming'.

So in the 1980s, the pendulum swung again, and there emerged the broader approach of health promotion we now see in the 1990s which encompasses health education but also addresses the need for political and social action and, importantly, grass-roots involvement of people themselves in shaping their own health destiny.

See Chapter 2.

The World Health Organization (WHO) has taken a leading role in action for health promotion in the 1980s and 1990s. WHO stated in 1977, at the Thirtieth World Health Assembly, that 'The main social target of governments and WHO in the coming decades should be the attainment of all citizens of the world by the year 2000 of a level of health that will permit them to lead a socially and economically productive life'.[38] This was the beginning of what has come to be known as the *Health For All* movement which led to the development of a Regional Strategy for the WHO European Region in 1980.[39]

This regional strategy called for fundamental changes in the health policy of member countries, including a much higher priority for health promotion and disease prevention. It called not only for health services but for all public sectors with a potential impact on health to take positive steps to maintain and improve it. Specific regional targets were set and published in 1985 which emphasized the following themes, which are widely quoted as '*Health For All* principles':

- reducing inequalities in health;
- positive health through health promotion and disease prevention;
- community participation;
- cooperation between health authorities, local authorities and others with an impact on health;
- a focus on primary health care as the main basis of the health care system.

A further milestone was the publication in 1986 of what became known as the *Ottawa Charter*[40] (because it was launched at a World Health Organization international conference on health promotion held in Ottawa, Canada). This identified five key themes for health promotion:

- building a healthy public policy;
- creating supportive environments;
- developing personal skills through information and education in health and life skills;
- strengthening community action;
- reorienting health services towards prevention and health promotion.

Like the *Health For All* principles, the emphasis was on developing health promoting policies and environments and working with communities, not just focusing on individual health behaviour. This 'new public health', as it became known in the late 1980s, has found expression in different ways.[41] Some examples are given below:

1. The Faculty of Community Medicine published a 'Charter for Action' which outlined ways in which the United Kingdom could work towards the achievement of 'health for all by year 2000' in the UK.[42]
2. The Public Health Alliance was formed in 1987 as an independent voluntary association bringing together individuals and organizations to campaign for better public health.[43]
3. The Association for Public Health was founded in 1992 as a multidisciplinary organization drawing members from the NHS, local government, the voluntary sector and academic institutions to promote public health policy at national and local levels.[44]
4. WHO set up the 'Healthy Cities' project, which focuses on action for health promotion at city level, aiming to place health high on the agenda of political decision-makers, key groups in the city and the population at large.[45]
5. An increasing number of community health projects was set up, as a response to the failure of traditional health education to reach the most needy people. They are also a response to the challenge of involving lay people at the 'grass roots' in identifying the health issues which they set at the top of their agendas, and acting on those issues.

See Chapter 15.

6. An upsurge of interest in environmental and ecological health issues, including Local Agenda 21 initiatives, with their focus on 'sustainable development': meeting the needs of the present without compromising the ability of future generations to meet their own needs.[46]

See Chapter 16, p. 305.

7. Growing analysis and awareness of the impact of social issues and policies outside the health arena on the health of the population, such as transport, housing, food, unemployment and poverty.[47]

An important development in the early 1990s was the advent of national strategies for health: *The Health of the Nation* in England, and comparable strategies for Wales, Scotland, and Northern Ireland.[48] These were welcome, as they were the first national strategies to focus on health and health gain, rather than illness and health services. The extent to which they looked broadly at the fundamental determinants of health varied. *The Health of the Nation* took the narrowest approach. It scarcely acknowledged the socioeconomic determinants of health and emphasized individual lifestyle change as the focus for action. However, there was a proposal to add a new area about the environment in 1996.[49] The Welsh, Scottish and Northern Ireland strategies took a rather broader approach, with more emphasis on environmental and social factors.

Further developments took place in 1997. In Northern Ireland, a new strategy *Health and Wellbeing: into the Millennium* was published.[50] In Wales, new guidance was issued on the development of local strategies for health.[51] In England and Scotland, their national strategies *The Health of the Nation* and *Scotland's health: a challenge to us all*, were reviewed by the Labour government. Consultation ('green') papers were published in early 1998: the 'green' paper for England was called *Our Healthier Nation*, and for Scotland, *Working Together for a Healthier*

See also Chapter 7.

Scotland.[52] Following consultation, new strategies ('white' papers) will be produced.

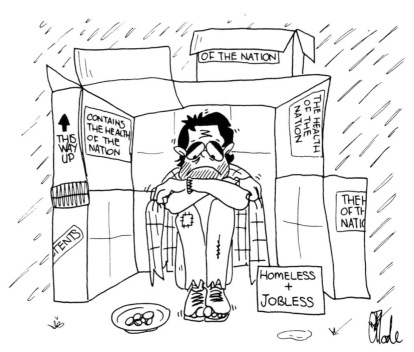

The Health of the Nation *scarcely acknowledged the socioeconomic determinants of health*

So by the late 1990s, we have developed considerable understanding about what affects people's health, and we have national strategies for health. The reality, however, is growing inequality in health status, and glaring problems of poverty, unemployment and homelessness. This raises questions about the distribution of wealth in society and social and economic policies, and demonstrates the extent to which health is a political issue. The change of government in 1997 heralds new directions again, with more emphasis on addressing inequalities in health and the socioeconomic factors which affect people's health.[53] The Minister for Public Health said, soon after the Labour government was elected in 1997: 'We want to attack the underlying causes of ill-health and to break the cycle of social and economic deprivation and social exclusion. This signals a major change in the nation's policies, to maximize good health, as well as treating sickness. You might call it being tough on the causes of ill-health.'[54] We wait to see whether this aspiration is turned into reality.

This chapter has discussed what 'health' is, what affects health, and the ways in which health issues have been addressed over the last few decades. Against this background, we look in the next chapter at what is meant by 'health promotion' and the principles and activities it encompasses.

- 'Health' and 'being healthy' mean different things to different people, and you need to explore and understand what they mean to you and to your clients.

- A wide range of factors at many levels influence and determine people's health.

- There are wide *inequalities* or *variations* in the health of different groups of people: people from different social classes, ethnic groups, age groups, sexes, and people who live in different places.

- Improving people's health means addressing the social, environmental and economic factors which affect their health, as well as individual health behaviour and lifestyle.

- International and national strategies and movements have emerged to tackle the socioeconomic and environmental determinants of health, and to reduce inequalities in health.

Recommended Reading

On Concepts of Health and Illness
A key text from WHO:
➤ World Health Organization (1984) Health Promotion: a WHO discussion document on the concepts and principles. Reprinted in: *Journal of the Institute of Health Education* **23** (1), 1985.

A classic text with an international perspective:
➤ Wilson M (1976) *Health is for People*. London: Darton, Longman and Todd.

About health belief systems (biomedical, alternative and non-western) and people's responses to illness:
➤ Jones L (1994) *The Social Context of Health and Health Work*. Chapter 10, Health beliefs and health action. Basingstoke: Macmillan.

About concepts of health and influences on health:
➤ Katz J & Peberdy A (1997) *Promoting Health: Knowledge and Practice*. Chapter 2, What is health? and Chapter 3, Behavioural and environmental influences on health. Basingstoke: Macmillan, in association with the Open University Press.

On concepts of health and illness among ethnic minority groups in Britain:

➤ Mares P, Henley A & Baxter C (1985) *Health Care in Multiracial Britain*. Cambridge: National Extension College.
➤ Dickinson R & Bhatt A (1994) Ethnicity, health and control: results from an exploratory study of ethnic minority communities' attitudes to health. *Health Education Journal*, **53**, 421–429.
➤ Smaje C (1995) *Health, 'Race' and Ethnicity – making sense of the evidence*. Chapter 6, section on Health beliefs and knowledge. London: King's Fund Institute.

A philosopher's perspective on the concept of 'health':
➤ Seedhouse D (1986) *Health: The Foundations for Achievement*. Chichester: Wiley.

A sociological perspective on the concept of 'health':
➤ Aggleton P (1990) *Health*. London: Routledge and Kegan Paul.

Historically significant texts on how we have arrived at our current understanding of the determinants of health, especially the role of medicine and health services:
➤ Cochrane A L (1972) *Effectiveness and Efficiency – Random Reflections on Health Services*. Nuffield Provincial Hospital Trust

➤ McKeown T (1979) *The Role of Medicine: Dream, Mirage or Nemesis*. Oxford: Blackwell.

➤ Illich I (1977) *Limits to Medicine – Medical Nemesis: the Expropriation of Health*. Harmondsworth: Pelican Books.

On inequalities in health:
➤ Townsend P, Whitehead M & Davidson N (1992) *Inequalities in Health*. Harmondsworth: Penguin Books. (This volume contains *The Black Report* by Townsend & Davidson (first published in 1982) and *The Health Divide* (2nd edition) by Whitehead (first published in 1992) together in one volume.)

For a graphic exposition of how family health is affected by the unequal distribution of resources in society:
➤ Graham H (1993) *Hardship and Health in Women's Lives*. Hemel Hempstead: Harvester Wheatsheaf.

For research-based argument that classic lifestyle factors (smoking, alcohol, diet and exercise) are important for health, but that social circumstances are more important than lifestyle habits:
➤ Blaxter M (1990) *Health and Lifestyles*. London: Tavistock Publications.

Explores the role of health promotion in opposing the impact of race and racial discrimination and discusses lessons learnt from health promotion work in Smethwick and Sandwell:
➤ Douglas J (1997) Developing health promotion strategies with Black and minority ethic communities which address social inequalities. Chapter 27 in Sidell M, Jones L, Katz J & Peberdy A (1997) (eds) *Debates and Dilemmas in Promoting Health*. Basingstoke: Macmillan/Open University Press.

A research report which reviews qualitative research into the relationships between health behaviour, health promotion and social variations, and considers the implications for health promotion when dealing with health inequalities:
➤ Rogers A, Popay J, Williams G & Latham M (1997) *Inequalities in health and health promotion: insights from the qualitative research literature*. London: Health Education Authority.

On what should be done to tackle inequalities in health:
➤ Benzeval M, Judge K & Whitehead M (1995) *Tackling Inequalities in Health: an agenda for action*. London: King's Fund. (Summary available from The King's Fund, 2 Palace Court, London W2 4HS.)

Notes and References

1   See suggestions in *Recommended Reading* and:

Helman C G (1990) *Culture, Health and Illness*, 2nd edn. Guildford, Surrey: Wright.

Payer L (1990) *Medicine and Culture*. London: Gollancz. (Looks at the different philosophies of health in Britain, USA, France and West Germany.)

Four books from the Health Education Authority on how people view health and health issues:

Prout A (1996) *Families, cultural bias and health promotion*. London: Health Education Authority. (A survey on health perception in 12 households, including case studies and implications for targeting health promotion messages to families.)

Hogg C, Barker R & McGuire C (1996) Health promotion and the family: messages from four research studies. London: Health Education Authority. (Looks at the main health concerns of parents and their families, how they communicate and respond to health promotion.)

Holland J, Mauthner M & Sharpe S (1996) *Family matters: communicating health messages to the family*. London: Health Education Authority. (Explores communication about health within the family.)

Brynin M & Scott J (1996) Young people, health and the family. London: Health Education Authority. (Attitudes of young people towards major health issues.)

Research Unit in Health and Behavioural Change, University of Edinburgh (1989) *Changing the Public Health*. Chapter 3. Chichester: Wiley. (A review with particular emphasis on research methodology and theoretical problems of research on concepts of health.)

2   This exercise is adapted with kind permission, from:

The Open University (1980) *The Good Health Guide*, p. 16. Harmondsworth: Pan Books. (First published by Harper and Row.)

3   The idea for this analysis is based on the findings of an early French study on lay people's concept of health:

Herzlich C (1973) *Health and Illness*. European Monographs in Social Psychology. London: Academic Press.

4   Pill R and Stott N (1982) Concepts of illness causation and responsibility; some preliminary data from a sample of working class mothers. *Social Science and Medicine* **16** 43–52.

5   Blaxter M and Patterson L (1982) *Mothers and Daughters: a Three Generation Study of Health Attitudes and Behaviour*. London: Heinemann Educational Books.

6   Williams R (1983) Concepts of Health: An Analysis of Lay Logic. *Sociology* **17** 185–204.

     For another study on the health beliefs of older people:

     Victor C R (1990) What is health? A study of the health beliefs of older people *Journal of the Institute of Health Education* **28** (1), 10–15.

7   Paxton SJ, Sculthorpe A & Gibbons K (1994) Concepts of health in Australian men: a qualitative study. *Health Education Journal* **53**, 430–438.

8   Donovan J (1986) *We Don't Buy Sickness, It Just Comes*. Aldershot: Gower. Quoted on p. 101 of Smaje C (1995) *Health, 'Race' and Ethnicity – Making sense of the evidence*. London: King's Fund Institute.

9   Backett K & Alexander H (1991) Talking to Young Children about Health: methods and findings. *Health Education Journal* **50** (1), 34–38.

     Pridmore P & Bendelow G (1995) Images of health: exploring beliefs of children using the 'draw-and-write' technique. *Health Education Journal* **54** (4), 473–488.

10   Pridmore P & Bendelow G (1995) Images of health: exploring beliefs of children using the 'draw-and-write' technique. *Health Education Journal* **54** (4), 473–488.

     Oakley A *et al.* (1995) Health and cancer prevention: knowledge and beliefs of children and young people. *British Medical Journal*, April 22, 1029–1033. (Study of 9–10 year-olds and 15–16 year-olds about knowledge of different types of cancer; beliefs about health; sources of information. Smoking, pollution and other environmental factors were seen as the dominant causes of cancer; television and media were the most important sources of information.)

11   Calnan M (1987) *Health and Illness – The Lay Perspective*. Chapter 2. London: Tavistock Publications.

12   Calnan M (1987) *Health and Illness – The Lay Perspective* London: Tavistock Publications.

13   Backett K *et al.* (1994) Lay evaluation of health and healthy lifestyles: evidence from three studies. *British Journal of General Practice*, June, 277–280.

14   On the difficult issue of measuring health status, see:

     Bowling A (1997) *Measuring Health: a review of quality of life measurement scales*, 2nd edn. Buckingham: Open University Press.

     Fallowfield L (1990) *The Quality of Life: The Missing Measurement in Health Care*. London: Souvenir Press.

     Teeling Smith G (1988) *Measuring Health: A Practical Approach*. Chichester: Wiley.

15   The issues of different lay and professional perceptions of health and illness, what causes illness and what should be done about it is dealt with extensively in literature on the sociology of health and illness. For example, see:

     Backett K *et al.* (1994) Lay evaluation of health and healthy lifestyles: evidence from three studies. *British Journal of General Practice*, June, 277–280. (Draws on three qualitative social research projects and analyses some of the ways in which lay people make sense of health and illness. Lay understanding of evidence about health and illness drew on a wide variety of perceived influences, not only behaviour but social, political and economic factors; the environment, and luck, chance or fate. Lay people often drew on different frames of reference and relevance from those of medical practitioners, health educators and health researchers.)

     Davey B & Seale C (eds) (1996) *Experiencing and explaining disease*. Revised and updated edition. Buckingham: Open University Press. (A multi-disciplinary account of the factors influencing how states of wellness or illness are experienced by lay people and explained by professionals.)

     Morgan M, Calnan M & Manning N (1985) *Sociological Approaches to Health and Medicine*. London: Croom Helm.

     Fitzpatrick R, Hinton J, Newnan S, Scambler G & Thompson J (1984) *The Experience of Illness*. London: Tavistock Publications.

     Milburn K (1996) The importance of lay theorising for health promotion research and practice. *Health Promotion International* **11** (1), 41–46. (This paper argues that we should take more notice of lay people's thinking which underpins their everyday health-relevant behaviour.)

16   Aakster C (1993) Concepts in Alternative Medicine. Chapter 9 in Beattie A, Gott M, Jones L & Sidell M (eds) *Health and Wellbeing – a reader*. Basingstoke: Macmillan.

17   World Health Organization (1948) Constitution.

18   World Health Organization (1984) Health Promotion: a WHO discussion document on the concepts and principles. Reprinted in: *Journal of the Institute of Health Education* **23** (1), 1985.

19   Defining 'mental health', and the relationship between social, emotional and mental health, is a

controversial area. For an in-depth look at this and the whole subject of mental health promotion, see:

Tudor K (1996) *Mental Health Promotion: Paradigms and Practice*. London: Routledge.

A helpful framework for mental health promotion, which includes a section on 'what is mental health?' is set out in:

Health Education Authority (1997) *Mental health promotion: a quality framework*. London: Health Education Authority.

20   Wilson M (1976) Health is for People, p. 117. London: Darton, Longman and Todd.

21   Seedhouse D (1986) *Health: The Foundations for Achievement*. Chichester: Wiley.

Aggleton P (1990) *Health*. London: Routledge.

22   Mansfield K (1977) *Letters and Journals*. London: Pelican Books.

(Mansfield discusses health in terms of becoming all that she is capable of becoming, which has become a much-quoted phrase.)

23   World Health Organization (1984) *Health Promotion*: a WHO discussion document on the concepts and principles. Reprinted in: *Journal of the Institute of Health Education* **23** (1), 1985.

24   The 'radiating circle' model is taken from:

Burkitt A (1982) Providing Education about Health. *Nursing*, June, 29–30. (Reproduced by kind permission of Medical Education (International) Ltd.)

25   For early significant analyses of the determinants of health, including the role of health services, see:

Cochrane A L (1972) *Effectiveness and Efficiency – Random Reflections on Health Services*. Nuffield Provincial Hospital Trust

McKeown T (1979) *The Role of Medicine: Dream, Mirage or Nemesis*. Oxford: Blackwell.

26   Jacobson B, Smith A & Whitehead M (eds) (1991) *The Nation's Health: A Strategy for the 1990s*, revised edition, p. 114. London: King Edward's Hospital Fund.

27   For further study of this critique of medicine, see:
Illich I (1977) *Limits to Medicine – Medical Nemesis: the Expropriation of Health*. Harmondsworth: Pelican Books.

Horrobin D F (1978) *Medical Hubris*. Edinburgh: Churchill Livingstone. (Horrobin's book is a reply to Illich's arguments in *Limits to Medicine*.)

Inglis B (1981) *Diseases of Civilisation*. London: Hodder & Stoughton.

Kennedy I (1981) *The Unmasking of Medicine*. London: George Allen and Unwin.

28   For review and discussion of inequalities in health, see:

Townsend P, Whitehead M & Davidson N (1992) *Inequalities in Health*. Harmondsworth: Penguin Books. (This book contains *The Black Report* by Townsend & Davidson (first published in 1982) and *The Health Divide* (2nd edn) by Whitehead (first published in 1992) together in one volume.)

Davey Smith G, Bartley M & Blane D (1990) The Black Report on Socioeconomic Inequalities in Health 10 Years On. *British Medical Journal* **301**, 373–377.

Wilkinson R G (ed.) (1986) *Class and Health*. London: Tavistock.

Jacobson B, Smith A & Whitehead M (eds) (1991) *The Nation's Health: A Strategy for the 1990's*, revised edn, Chapter 8. London: King Edward's Hospital Fund.

Whitehead M (1991) The Concepts and Principles of Equity and Health. *Health Promotion International* **6** (3), 217–228.

Judge K (1994) Why are Some People Healthy and Others Not? The Determinants of Health of Populations. *British Medical Journal* **309**, 1454.

Department of Health (1995) *Health of the Nation: Variations in Health – what can the Department of Health and the NHS do?* London: Department of Health.

Blane D, Brunner E & Wilkinson R (eds) (1996) *Health and Social Organization*. London: Routledge.

Lawson R (1997) *Bills of Health*. Abingdon: Radcliffe Medical Press.

29   Wilkinson R (1996) *Unhealthy Societies: the affliction of inequality*. London: Routledge.

30   Wilkinson R (1996) *Unhealthy Societies: the affliction of inequality*. Chapter 11 London: Routledge.

Gillies P (1997) Social capital: recognising the value of society. *Healthlines* **45** September 1997, 15–17.

31   Balarajan R & Soni Raleigh V (1993) *Ethnicity and Health: a guide for the NHS*. London: Department of Health.

Health Education Authority (1994) *Black and Minority Ethnic Groups in England: health and lifestyles*. London: Health Education Authority.

Smaje C (1995) *Health, 'Race' and Ethnicity – making sense of the evidence*. London: Kings Fund Institute.

32   Department of Health (1995) *Health of the Nation: Variations in Health – what can the Department of Health and the NHS do*? London: Department of Health. (On differences by social class, sex, region and ethnicity.)

Dennehy A, Smith L & Harker P (1997) *Not To Be Ignored: young people, poverty and health*. London: Child Poverty Action Group (On the connection between poverty and the health of young people.)

33   Benzeval M, Judge K & Whitehead M (eds) (1995) *Tackling Inequalities in Health: an agenda for action*. London: The King's Fund.

Association for Public Health (1996) *Policy Statement on Poverty and Health*. London: APH.

Dennehy A, Smith L & Harker P (1997) *Not To Be Ignored: young people, poverty and health*. London: Child Poverty Action Group.

34   Commission for Racial Equality (1993) *The Sorrow In My Heart. Sixteen Asian women speak about depression*. London: CRE. (Reproduced by kind permission of the CRE.)

35   The Independent Tabloid Monday 21.10.96 *Generation Gap: Pregnant Daughter, Smoking Gun*. (Reproduced by kind permission of The Independent.)

36   The first major government statement on health education clearly reflects the 'lifestyle approach':

Department of Health and Social Security (1976) *Prevention and Health – Everybody's Business*. London: HMSO.

37   For discussion and illustration of the individualistic 'victim-blaming' approach, see: Rodmell S & Watt A (eds) (1986) *The Politics of Health Education – Raising the Issues* London: Routledge and Kegan Paul. (Especially Chapters 1 and 2.)

For research-based argument that classic lifestyle factors (smoking, alcohol, diet and exercise) are important for health, but that social circumstances are more important than lifestyle habits, see:

Blaxter M (1990) *Health and Lifestyles* London: Tavistock.

38   WHO resolution WHO30.43, quoted in:

WHO Regional Office for Europe (1985) *Targets for Health For All*, p. 1. Geneva: World Health Organization.

39   WHO Regional Office for Europe (1985) *Targets for Health For All*. Geneva: World Health Organization.

For further reading on how health strategies have developed in different countries, see:

Nutbeam D & Wise M (1996) Planning for Health for All: international experience in setting health goals and targets. *Health Promotion International* **12** (1), 9–19.

40   World Health Organization (1986) *The Ottawa Charter for Health Promotion*. Geneva: WHO.

The Ottawa Charter is reproduced in full as an Appendix in:

Dines A & Cribb A (eds) (1993) *Health Promotion – Concepts and Practice*. Oxford: Blackwell.

41   For further reading on the 'new public health', see:

Ashton J & Seymour H (1988) *The New Public Health*. Oxford: University Press.

Martin C & McQueen D (eds) (1989) *Readings for a New Public Health*. Edinburgh: University Press.

42   Faculty of Community Medicine (1986) *Health For All By The Year 2000: Charter for Action*. London: Faculty of Community Medicine, Royal College of Physicians.

43   Public Health Alliance, 138 Digbeth, Birmingham B5 6DR. Tel. 0121 643 7628.

44   Association for Public Health, Trevelyan House, 30 Great Peter Street, London SW1P 2HU Tel. 0171 413 1896.

45   For more information on the WHO 'Healthy Cities' movement, see:

Kickbush I (1989) Healthy Cities: a working project and a growing movement. *Health Promotion*, **42**, 77.

Ashton J (ed.) (1992) *Healthy Cities*. Buckingham: Open University Press. (Background to Healthy Cities movement and progress in urban areas in general and cities in Europe (including Liverpool and Sheffield), North America, New Zealand and Australia.)

Davies J K & Kelly M P (1993) *Healthy Cities: research and practice*. London: Routledge.

Tsouros A D (1995) The WHO Healthy Cities Project: state of the art and future plans. *Health Promotion International* **10** (2), 133–141.

46   Examples of a new focus on environmental and ecological issues include:

J Button (1989) *How to be Green*, pp. 148–170. London: Century Hutchinson.

Grey M & Keeble B (1989) *Greening the NHS* (Letter), *British Medical Journal* **299**(1), 4–5.

Friends of the Earth (1995) *Prescription for change: health and the environment*. London: Friends of the Earth. (Rationale and proposals for improving the environment in the areas of air, water, waste, transport, the built environment, radiation, ozone depletion and food, by a national charity which campaigns for environmental improvement.)

Crombie H (1995) *Sustainable Development and Health*. Birmingham: Public Health Alliance. (Available from Public Health Alliance, 138 Digbeth, Birmingham B5 6DR.)

Fearn H (1996) Positive planetary aspects bode well for health. *Healthlines*, Issue 37, pp. 14–16. (Examples of local action for sustainable developments as part of the Local Agenda 21 strategy.)

47   For example, see:

On homelessness:

*Davies E (1993) The Health of the Homeless

On transport:

*Hillman M (1993) Social Goals for Transport Policy

*Hunt S (1993) The Public Health Implications of Private Cars

*In Beattie A, Gott M, Jones L & Sidell M (1993) *Health and Wellbeing – a reader*. Basingstoke: Macmillan, in association with the Open University Press.

On food and poverty:

Lobstein T (1997) *Myths about food and low income*. London: National Food Alliance.

Save the Children (1997) *Out of the frying pan: the true cost of feeding a family on a low income*. London: Save the Children.

Department of Health (1996) *Low Income, Food, Nutrition and Health: strategies for improvement*. London: Department of Health.

On unemployment:

Kammerling R M & O'Connor S (1993) Unemployment rate as a predictor of rate of psychiatric admission. *British Medical Journal* **11**, 1536–1539.

Wilson S H & Walker G M (1993) Unemployment and health: a review. *Public Health* **107** (3), 153–162.

On poverty:

Association for Public Health (1996) *Policy Statement on Poverty and Health*. London: APH.

48   Secretary of State for Health (1992) *The Health of the Nation: A Strategy for Health in England*. London: HMSO.

Welsh Office (1989) *Strategic Intent and Direction for the NHS in Wales*. Welsh Office NHS Directorate: The Welsh Health Planning Forum.

Scottish Office (1992) *Scotland's health: a challenge to us all*. Edinburgh: HMSO.

Department of Health and Social Services (1991) *A Regional Strategy for the Northern Ireland Health & Personal Social Services 1992–1997*. London: HMSO.

49   Department of Health & Department of the Environment (1996) *Health of the Nation Consultation Document: The Environment and Health*. London: Department of Health.

50   Department of Health and Social Services (1997) *Health and Wellbeing: into the next millennium*. Belfast: DHSS.

51   Letter from the Welsh Office to health authorities, NHS trusts, local authorities and others, 11 June 1998, headed *New Strategic Plans*. Letter ref. DGM (97) 50

52   Secretary of State for Health (1998) *Our Healthier Nation: a contract for health. A consultation paper*. London: The Stationery Office.

Department of Health Scottish Office (1998) *Working Together for a Healthier Scotland: a consultation paper*. London: The Stationery Office.

53   Munro J & Rayner G (1997) Frank Talking on Health Inequality. *Health Matters*, Issue 29, pp 6–7.

Chalmers F (1997) New Labour: New Health of the Nation. *Healthlines*, June, 3–4.

Department of Health (1997) *Target: Our Healthier Nation*. Newsletter, Issue 25, July 1997.

54   Department of Health Press Release, 7 July 1997, headlined *Public health strategy launched to tackle root causes of ill health*.

2 What is Health Promotion?

SUMMARY

We start this chapter by discussing how to define the term 'health promotion', and outline the debate over the difference between the concepts of 'health promotion' and 'health education'. We continue with a discussion on the origins and meaning of the term 'health gain' and its links with health promotion. After this we discuss the scope of health promotion work and provide frameworks for activities for health gain and for health promotion. We then outline the broad areas of practice covered by professional health promoters, core competencies in health promotion, and the Key Roles which provide a framework for National Occupational Standards, indicating where each of these is discussed in later chapters. We end with an overview of the uses of National Occupational Standards. Exercises are included to help readers explore the range of health promotion activities, and the extent of their own health promotion work.

The previous chapter focused on health; we now move on to consider the meaning of health promotion.

Defining Health Promotion

Health promotion is about raising the health status of individuals and communities. Too often the word *promotion*, when used in the context of health promotion, is associated with sales and advertising, and taken to mean a propaganda approach dominated by use of the mass media. This is a misunderstanding. By *promotion* in the health context we mean improving health: advancing, supporting, encouraging and placing it higher on personal and public agendas.

We have seen that major determinants of health are social, economic and environmental, aspects which are often outside individual or even collective control. Therefore a fundamental aspect of health promotion is that it aims to empower people to have more control over aspects of their lives which affect their health.

These twin elements – improving health and having more control over it – are fundamental to the aims and processes of health promotion. The World Health Organization's definition of health promotion[1] neatly encompasses this:

> *Health promotion is the process of enabling people to increase control over, and to improve, their health.*

This definition has become widely adopted.[2]

As discussed in the previous chapter, WHO goes on to say:

This perspective is derived from a conception of 'health' as the extent to which an individual or group is able, on the one hand, to realize aspirations and satisfy needs; and, on the other hand, to change or cope with the environment. Health is, therefore, seen as resource for everyday life, not the objective of living; it is a positive concept emphasizing social and personal resources, as well as physical capacities.

Health Promotion or Health Education?

There has been much debate over the use of the terms health promotion and health education since the mid 1980s. The debate came into focus because the range of activities undertaken in the pursuit of better health widened from traditional health education, which was about giving information and working towards individual attitude and behaviour changes.

With rising criticism that this approach was too narrow, focused too much on individual lifestyle and could become 'victim-blaming', more work was done about wider issues. Examples are:

- political action to change social policies;
- putting employee health on the agenda of employers;
- engaging in community development work for health.

Such activities went beyond the scope of traditional health education, and health promotion became widely used as the umbrella term to encompass all these activities. Health education is seen as an important element in health promotion.

We subscribe to the view that using health promotion as an umbrella term for a range of activities is the most useful and practical way forward. However, to avoid misunderstandings and time-consuming arguments about the meaning of words, we need to identify clearly the range of activities which are included in health promotion. This is the subject of the section, 'The Scope of Health Promotion', later in this chapter.

Before moving on, though, it is important to appreciate that there is currently no clear, widely adopted consensus of what is meant by 'health promotion'. Some definitions focus on activities, others on values and aims. The WHO definition we have adopted defines health promotion as a *process* but implies an *aim* ('enabling people to increase control over, and improve, their health') with a clear philosophical basis of self-empowerment. Perhaps in the next century a consensus will emerge, but for the 1990s it is necessary to continue to question, research and clarify.

Linking Health Promotion to Health Gain

In the UK, the term 'health gain' emerged from the work of the Welsh Health Planning Forum.[3] In 1991, the World Health Organization Collaborative Centre for European Health Policy announced that the 1990s were 'the decade of health gain', and the first of a series of Health Gain Standing Conferences was held in Belfast. In 1992 the national health strategy *The Health of the Nation*[4] was published in England and the term health gain began to be widely used in relation to the debate about improving health. However, as with the term health promotion, the meaning of health gain continues to be a matter for much debate. One useful

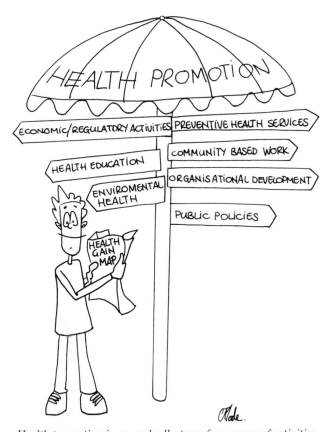

Labels in the image: HEALTH PROMOTION

ECONOMIC/REGULATORY ACTIVITIES | PREVENTIVE HEALTH SERVICES

COMMUNITY BASED WORK

HEALTH EDUCATION

ORGANISATIONAL DEVELOPMENT

ENVIROMENTAL HEALTH

PUBLIC POLICIES

HEALTH GAIN MAP

Health promotion is an umbrella term for a range of activities

definition of health gain has been developed by Peter Brambleby.[5] He says that health gain is:

> *A measurable improvement in health status, in an individual or population, attributable to earlier intervention.*

This is very similar to the definition used in the Introductory Guide to the National Occupational Standards for professional activity in health promotion and care (there is more about these later in this Chapter), which states that health gain is:[6]

> *A measurable improvement in the status of health and social well-being, in an individual or a population, which is attributable to an earlier intervention.*

It is now widely accepted that health gain is a useful concept. It focuses attention on the health outcomes and on how different choices or priorities can be compared by considering the extent to which they contribute to health gains for individuals or groups. However, it is also accepted that to achieve health gain the involvement of agencies outside the NHS is often crucial, and it is important to bear in mind that these agencies may not be familiar with the concept of health gain and associated burgeoning jargon!

Closely associated with the move towards focusing on health gain and outcomes is the pressure on all sectors of health and social care to demonstrate that interventions provide 'value for money' and 'prove' that they are efficient and effective. So the outcomes and costs of health promotion activities are being

See Chapter 7, p. 128. closely scrutinized. This is no easy task since health promotion is a complex multiagency process with outcomes which are often very long-term.

One important aspect of this is to gather knowledge on what are effective health promotion interventions, through reviewing the evidence provided by research. This, too, is a difficult task, partly because what counts as success will depend on the approach to health promotion being used (and the values underlying it). So, if you are using a self-empowerment approach, a smoker taking a 'free' choice to continue smoking could be considered to be a success. Using a medical approach, this would be a failure. In addition, all research is not good research, and it is See Chapter 7, p. 121. important that those appraising the research evidence have the skills to do so.

We now move on to more practical matters: how you can think about health promotion in a functional way, as activities you undertake.

The Scope of Health Promotion

The following exercise aims to start you thinking about the range of activities which may be included in health promotion.

| Exercise 2.1 | **Exploring the scope of health promotion** |

Consider each of the following statements, and decide whether you think each activity is or is not health promotion:

Yes   No

1. Using TV advertisements to encourage people to be more physically active
2. Campaigning for increased tax on tobacco
3. Explaining to patients how to carry out their doctor's advice
4. Setting up a self-help group for people who have been sexually abused as children
5. Providing 'lollipop' people to help children across the road outside schools
6. Raising awareness of how poverty affects health
7. Giving people information about the way their bodies work
8. Immunizing children against infectious diseases such as measles
9. Protesting about a breach in the voluntary code of practice for alcohol advertising
10. Running low-cost gentle exercise classes for older people at local leisure centres
11. Providing 'healthier' menu choices at workplace canteens
12. Teaching a programme of personal and social education in a secondary school
13. Providing support to people with learning disabilities living in the community

What were your reasons for saying 'yes' or 'no'? Can you identify the criteria you are using for deciding whether an activity is 'health promotion'?

The questions in the exercise give examples of the wide range of activities which may be classified as health promotion. Answering 'yes' to each one indicates a broad view of what may be included: mass media advertising, campaigning on health issues, patient education, self-help, environmental safety measures, public policy issues, health education about physical health, preventive and curative medical procedures, codes of practice on health issues, health-enhancing facilities in local communities, workplace health policies and social education for young people. Answering 'no' indicates that you identify criteria which exclude these activities from the realms of 'health promotion'. For example, you may have said 'no' to Question 2 because increasing tobacco taxation would place a heavier burden on smokers in poor financial circumstances thus putting their health even more at risk.

The many attempts to provide frameworks for classifying health promotion activities have helped to clarify the issues.[7] Drawing on these, we propose to start by focusing on identifying the activities which contribute to health gain (Fig. 2.1).

Fig 2.1   **Activities for health gain.**

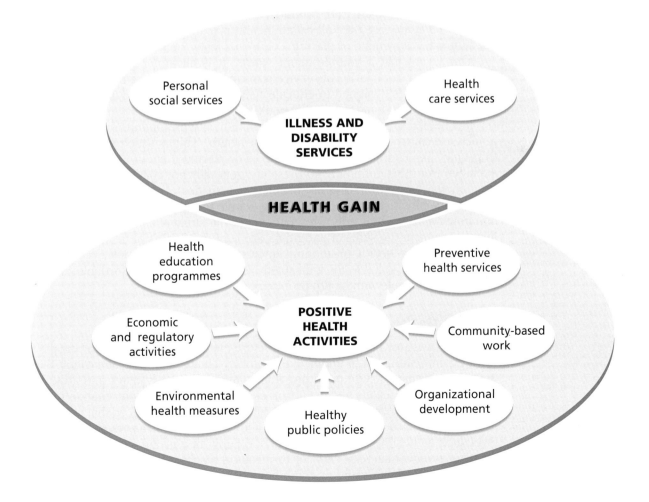

Figure 2.1 maps out all those activities which aim to improve people's health. The first point to note is that there are two sets of activities: those which are about providing services for the ill and disabled, and positive health activities which are about personal, social and environmental changes aiming to prevent ill-health and develop healthier living conditions and ways of life. These two sets of activities overlap, because they both contribute to health gain, and they are often closely related in practice. We identify nine categories of activities, comprised of two illness and disability services and seven types of positive health activities, as follows.

Illness and Disability Services

Personal social services. This includes all those social services which aim to address the needs of sick or disabled members of society whose health (in its widest sense) is improved by those services. This includes, for example, community care of mentally ill people and home help services.

Health care services. This includes the major work of the health services: treatment, cure and care in primary care and hospital settings.

We now need to address a difficult issue: if all effective illness and disability services improve health (i.e. produce varying amounts of health gain), which they obviously do, are they all called 'health promotion'? For example, is taking out someone's appendix, or placing a child in a foster home, 'health promotion'?

This is not just a quibble about words. It is an important question when considering the boundaries of service provision by health promotion agencies, of the many courses designed to educate health promoters in the necessary skills and knowledge, and, indeed, of this book.

It is helpful to go back to our definition of health promotion, 'enabling people to increase control over, and improve, their health'. Things which need to be done to people (like taking out their appendixes or placing them in foster homes) are excluded from this definition, so these are generally not considered to be health promotion activities (but they are health gain activities). But those aspects of care and treatment which are about enabling people to take control over their health and improve it, such as educating patients in the skills of self-care, or educating foster parents in the skills of parenting, are legitimate areas of health promotion. So is creating a health promoting environment by, for example, modifying a home to make it suitable for a disabled person or providing affordable housing for homeless people with health problems.

Positive Health Activities

Health education programmes. These are planned opportunities for people to learn about health, and to undertake voluntary changes in their behaviour. Such programmes may include providing information, exploring values and attitudes, making health decisions and acquiring skills to enable behaviour change to take place. They involve developing self-esteem and self-empowerment so that people are enabled to take action about their health. They can happen on a personal one-to-one level such as health visitor/client, teacher/pupil, in a group such as a smoking cessation group or exercise class, or by means of reaching large audiences through the mass media, health fairs or exhibitions.

See Chapters 10, 11, 12, 13 and 14.

As we have already discussed, health education programmes may also be a part of health care and personal social services, and because of this it is useful to understand the concept of primary, secondary and tertiary health education.

Primary health education is directed at healthy people, and aims to prevent ill-health arising in the first place. Most health education for children and young people falls into this category, dealing with such topics as hygiene, contraception, nutrition and social skills and personal relationships, and aiming to build up a positive sense of self-worth in children. Primary health education is concerned not merely with helping to prevent illness, but with positively improving the quality of health and thus the quality of life.

There is also often a major role for health education when people are ill. It may be possible to prevent ill-health moving to a chronic or irreversible stage, and to restore people to their former state of health. This is known as **secondary health education** – educating patients about their condition and what to do about it. Restoring good health may involve the patient in changing behaviour (such as stopping smoking) or in complying with a therapeutic regime and, possibly, learning about self-care and self-help. Clearly, health education of the patient is of great importance if treatment and therapy are to be effective and illness is not to recur.

But there are, of course, many patients whose ill-health has not been, or could not be, prevented and who cannot be completely cured. There are also people with permanent disabilities and handicaps. Tertiary health education is concerned with educating patients and their carers about how to make the most of the remaining potential for healthy living, and how to avoid unnecessary hardships, restrictions and complications. Rehabilitation programmes contain a considerable amount of tertiary health education.

However, it is not always easy to see where people fit into this primary, secondary or tertiary framework because, as we have already seen, a person's state of health is open to interpretation. For example, is educating an overweight person who appears to be perfectly well, despite being overweight, primary or secondary health education?

Preventive health services. These include medical services which aim to prevent ill-health such as immunization, family planning and personal health checks, as well as wider preventive health services such as child protection services for children at risk of child abuse.

Community-based work. This is a 'bottom-up' approach to health promotion, working with and for people, involving communities in health work such as local campaigns for better facilities. It includes community development, which is essentially about communities identifying their own health needs and taking action to address them. The sort of activities which may result could include forming self-help and pressure groups, and developing local health-enhancing facilities and services.

See Chapter 15.

Organizational development. This is about developing and implementing policies within organizations which promote the health of staff and customers. Examples include implementing policies on equal opportunities, providing healthy food choices in staff dining rooms and working with commercial organizations to develop and promote 'healthier' products, such as leaner meat, lower fat spreads and cheeses, low and non-alcoholic drinks and biodegradable packaging.

See Chapter 16.

Healthy public policies. Developing and implementing healthy public policies is what the 'new public health' is about. It involves statutory and voluntary agencies, professionals and the public working together to develop changes in the conditions of living. It is about seeing the implications for health in policies about, for example, equal opportunities, housing, employment, transport and leisure. Good public transport, for example, would improve health by reducing the number of cars on the road, lessening pollution, using less fuel and reducing the stress of the daily grind of travelling for commuters. It could also reduce isolation for those who do not own cars and enable people to have access to shopping and leisure facilities, all measures which improve well-being.

See Chapter 16.

Environmental health measures. This is about making the physical environment conducive to health, whether at home, at work or in public places. It includes traditional public health measures such as providing clean food and water and controlling pollution, as well as working on newer issues such as smoke free areas in pubs, and controlling the use of environmentally damaging chemicals.

See Chapter 16.

Economic and regulatory activities. This is political and educational activity directed at politicians, policy-makers and planners, involving lobbying for and implementing legislative changes such as food labelling regulations, pressing for voluntary codes of practice such as those which relate to alcohol advertising or advocating financial measures such as increases on tobacco taxation.

See Chapter 16.

A Framework for Health Promotion Activities

We now propose the framework in Fig. 2.2 for health promotion activities.

Fig 2.2   **A framework for health promotion activities.**

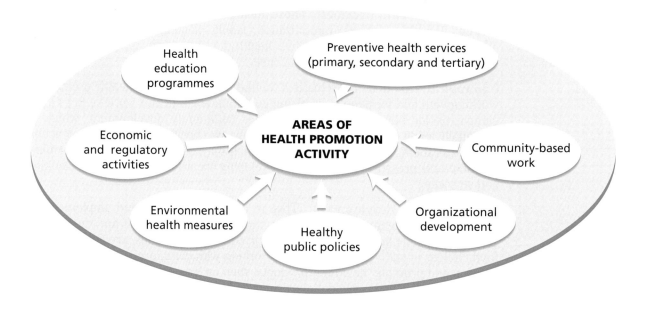

There are two important points to make about the use of this framework. The first is that activities do not always fall tidily into categories. For example, would a health visitor who was supporting a local women's health group be engaged in a health education programme because she provided health information to the group and set up stress management sessions, or community-based work because some members of the group had got together to lobby their local health services for better sexual health advice clinics for young people? Would an environmental health officer concerned about air pollution levels on a factory site be engaged in organizational development because she was working towards healthier working conditions for the staff, or environmental health measures because she aimed to achieve cleaner air for the local community?

Obviously, areas of activity overlap, but this is not important. What *is* important is to appreciate the range of activities encompassed by health promotion, and the many ways in which you can contribute to improvements in health status.

The second point about using this framework is to note that we are talking about planned, deliberate activities, and it is important to recognize that a great deal of health promotion happens informally and incidentally. For example, portrayal of damage caused by excessive drinking on a television soap opera, provision of low-cost exercise classes by a local entrepreneur and an advertising campaign to promote wholewheat breakfast cereals are all health promotion activities which are not likely to be planned with specific health promotion aims in mind. They may, however, be significant influences for change.

See Chapter 11, section on mass media.

The next exercise is designed to help you to identify your own contribution to health promotion.

Exercise 2.2	**Identifying your health promotion work**

Look at Fig. 2.2 again, which identifies seven major areas of health promotion activity. By each of the seven headings, note down any parts of your work which you think come into that category. (If you are not sure what each category includes, look back at the explanations.) Then think about each category again, and consider whether there is scope for developing your work within each category.

Developing Competence in Health Promotion

Having mapped out the activities the health promoter may be engaged in, we now look at the skills and methods used when those activities take place; in other words, we are considering the competencies which health promoters need to develop. By 'competencies' we mean the specific combination of knowledge, attitudes and skills needed to do a particular job.[8]

It is useful to think that there are broadly two aspects of your work to consider. One is the technical/specialist aspect: immunizing a child, taking a cervical smear test, recording blood pressure, undertaking microbiological tests for food hygiene purposes, enforcing legislation, building safer roads, interpreting welfare rights legislation or damp-proofing a home. All of these are the subject of specialist training, and outside the scope of this book.

The other aspect of your work is about working with people to promote health in many different situations with a variety of different aims. To do this, you need to have knowledge of particular methods and acquire special skills; in other words, to have health promotion competencies. First, we look at the range of competencies you need, and then at the National Occupational Standards which are being developed in health promotion.

Core Competencies in Health Promotion

We do not claim that these competencies are exclusive to health promotion work, but we suggest that they are the core competencies of health promotion. ('Core competence' is a term used to refer to those which are common to a number of different occupations.)

- *Managing, Planning, and Evaluating.* Managing resources for health promotion, including money, materials, oneself and other people, is crucial. Systematic planning is needed for effective and efficient health promotion. All health promotion work also requires evaluation, and different methods are appropriate for different approaches.

All these are addressed in Part 2: Planning and Managing for Effective Practice, Chapters 5,6,7,8 and 9

- *Communicating.* Health promotion is about people, so competence in communication is essential and fundamental. A high level of competence is needed in one-to-one communication and in working with groups in various ways, both formal and informal.

Communication is addressed in Chapters 8, 9, 10 and 11

- *Educating.* Educating about health requires good communication, but it also requires additional educational competence so that health educators can work in different settings such as formal lecturing or informal group work, and select and use appropriate strategies for different educational goals.

Educational competence is obviously used in health education programmes, but it is also used when undertaking other kinds of activities. For example, patient education is an integral part of preventive health services, education on policy implementation (such as a healthy food policy) is part of organizational development, public education is part of implementing an environmental health measure and educating members of statutory organisations may be a key part of political action for social change.

Education is addressed in Chapters 11, 12, 13 and 14

- *Marketing and Publicising.* This requires competence in, for example, marketing and advertising, using local radio and getting local press coverage of health issues. It may be used when undertaking any health promotion activities which would benefit from wider publicity.

Marketing and publicising are addressed in Chapter 11

- *Facilitating and Networking.* By this, we mean helping others to promote their own and other people's health, using various means such as sharing skills and information, and building up confidence and trust. These competencies are particularly important when working with communities. They are also vital for working with other agencies and forming alliances for health which cross barriers of organizations and disciplines.

Facilitating and networking are addressed in Chapters 9,13 and 15

- *Influencing Policy and Practice.* Health promoters are in the business of influencing policies and practices which affect health. (By 'policies' we mean broad plans of action, which set the direction for detailed planning.) These can be at any level, from national (such as policies set by government or political parties, about, for example, housing, transport and future directions for the NHS) to the level of day-to-day work of a health promoter (such as what sort of health promotion programmes will be run in a GP practice, or what resources will be devoted to specific health promotion activities in an environmental health department).

In order to influence policy and practice, you need to understand how power is distributed and exercised between people at any level, from a group of colleagues to those in positions of great authority or influence. You need to be able to use that knowledge to affect decisions. This includes working with statutory, voluntary and commercial organisations to influence them to develop health promoting policies for their staff and to produce health enhancing products and services. It also includes working for healthy public policies and economic and regulatory changes requiring lobbying and taking political action.

Influencing policy and practice is addressed in Chapter 16.

These six clusters of competencies are not exhaustive. As health promotion work grows and develops, and as it is practised in a variety of innovatory ways, there will be many more methods adopted and skills required. This is to be welcomed; what we aim to do here is to identify current core competencies and help you to acquire these.

It is clearly unrealistic to expect all health promoters to be highly competent in all aspects of health promotion. A practice nurse, for example, will work predominantly in health education and preventive health services, needing a high level of competence in communication and education. However, she also needs other competencies in order to plan and evaluate her work, market her health promotion programmes to her patients, facilitate change in her patients and be able to refer them to a network of helpful contacts. She will also need to be able to influence the development of health promotion policy in her practice.

All six competency areas we have identified are fundamental to health promotion activities, but you will probably find that you need some to a greater degree than others. They will be acquired in a variety of ways, including your life experience outside work, basic training, in-service training and work experience.

National Occupational Standards for Health Promotion

Cross reference to Chapter 3, section on values and principles of good practice.

National Occupational Standards for health promotion and care were launched in 1997 and these are now being used to improve the quality of health promotion work and to assist allocation of resources.[9] The national occupational standards describe performance – what people are expected to do in their jobs. They are derived from the values, ethics and principles on which good practice in the health and social care sector is based. They thus provide a specification, agreed nationally, of what should be achieved in health promotion and care work. The standards are grouped into three broad areas, each of which contains four Key Roles (key areas of work). These are set out below, along with an indication of where each Key Role is addressed in this book.

Box 2.1.	**Overview of the National Occupational Standards for Professional Activity in Health Promotion and Care**[10]

The Foundations of Professional Activity – area A

This includes four key roles:

Key role 0

The first **principles and values** on which practice is built – promoting and valuing the rights, responsibilites and diversity of people.

Key role 0 is addressed in Chapter 3.

Key role 1

Developing one's own and others' knowledge and practice – through planned development opportunities, the integration of research and development into one's own practice, and as a reflective practitioner.

Key role 1 is addressed throughout the book.

Key role 2

Promoting effective communication with people be they users of services, colleagues or the public at large.

Key role 2 is addressed in Chapters 8, 9, 10 and 11.

Key role 3

Building and sustaining relationships with and between practitioners and agencies be they working in the health and care sector or beyond.

Key role 3 is addressed in Chapters 4 and 9.

The context of professional activity – area B

This includes four key roles:

Key role 4

Influencing and developing policies to optimize health and social well-being – these policies may be specifically directed at the promotion of health and social well-being or have an impact on it.

Key role 4 is addressed in Chapter 16. Chapters 1 and 2 also contain fundamental knowledge essential for doing this.

Key role 5

Commissioning research to develop knowledge and practice about optimizing health and social well-being be this focused on development, implementation or evaluation.

How to use and review research is addressed in Chapter 7.

Key role 6

Commissioning a range of different means of optimizing health and social well-being – they may be services, projects or activities.

Key role 7

Managing processes whose purpose is to optimize health and social well-being – whether these are the services of health and social care providers or are projects and activities which are designed to promote health and social well-being.

The range of means of optimizing health is addressed in Part 2 and Part 3. Detailed processes of commissioning are beyond the scope of this book.

Key role 7 is addressed in Part 2.

The Range of Professional Activities – Area C

This includes four key roles:

Key role 8

Key role 8 is addressed in Part 2 and Part 3.

Creating and maintaining environments and practices which promote people's health and social well-being – the environments and practices may be community wide, within organizations or within health and social care services.

Key role 9

Key role 9 is addressed in Chapters 3, 4, 9 and Part 3.

Working in partnership with individuals, families, groups, communities and organizations to enable them to address issues which affect health and social well-being, using a range of models from community and personal development models through to awareness raising and health projects.

Key role 10

Key role 10 is addressed in Chapter 8, section on Managing Change, and Chapter 14. Specialist knowledge about disability is beyond the scope of this book.

Enabling people to manage disability and change throughout their lives and helping people to understand and manage effectively the changes and disabilities which other people are experiencing.

Key role 11

How to identify and assess health promotion needs is addressed in Chapter 6. How to assess and develop programmes of care is beyond the scope of this book.

Assessing individuals' needs and developing, monitoring and reviewing programmes of care to meet those needs.

There are some important points to note related to these occupational standards.

1. They cover the whole range of professional activities related to health gain, including health care services and personal social services (look back at the framework for health gain activities if you are unsure about this). This book is specifically about health promotion work, so some of the occupational standards are beyond its scope, as we indicate above. Also, this book is aimed at those who *provide* health promotion and the detailed processes of commissioning are beyond its scope.
2. You will need to choose which of the Key Roles are applicable to your job, and which part (called a Unit) of each Key Role is relevant to you.
3. Principles of good practice have been integrated into the occupational standards through the language used. So, for example, the word 'enable' has been used rather than 'help', to show that the health promoter should use approaches which give clients the opportunity to decide for themselves what should happen. You will need to think carefully about the meaning of the standards.

Ways in Which the Occupational Standards Can be Used

Broadly speaking there are three uses for the occupational standards.

1. Employers and managers can use the standards to improve the quality of the performance of their staff. The Key Roles and Units can enable an organization to map what it is trying to achieve and link this to its service specifications and thence to its management of human resources through job specifications, staff appraisal and performance review. The standards could also be used as the basis for auditing a service (checking whether it meets quality standards).

2. Individuals can use the standards to improve their competence through identifying their Key Roles, assessing their own performance, identifying their learning needs and defining the learning outcomes needed to meet the national standards.

3. Education and training providers may wish to look at the standards to see how they can modify their programmes to enable practitioners to achieve the standards, or use the standards as the basis of their programme design.

We discuss audit in more detail in Chapter 7.

For more about how to do this, see Chapter 12.

PRACTICE POINTS

- It is important for you to think about what *you* mean by health promotion, to identify the full scope of your health promotion work and to see how this fits with the work of your organization or employer.

- Health care services, personal social services and health promotion activities all make valuable contributions to improved health and well-being, so it is important that all these functions are linked together.

- The National Occupational Standards for professional activity in health promotion and care provide a map which can be used by organizations, managers, education and training providers and individuals to improve the quality of health promotion and care.

- You can use this book as a guide to your own health promotion development and to assist you in assessing how well you are doing.

Recommended Reading

On the historical development of health education and health promotion:

➤ Naidoo J and Wills J (1994) *Health Promotion: Foundations for Practice*. Chapter 4, The development of health education and health promotion. London: Baillière Tindall.

➤ Parish R (1995) Health promotion – rhetoric and reality. Chapter 2 in Bunton R, Nettleton S & Burrows R (eds) *The Sociology of Health Promotion*. London: Routledge.

➤ Katz J & Peberdy A (1997) *Promoting Health: Knowledge and Practice*. Chapter 4, The rise of health promotion and Chapter 10, Educating for health. Basingstoke: Macmillan in association with the Open University Press.

A discussion of what health promotion is and its relationship to the new public health:

➤ Bunton R & Macdonald G (eds) (1992) *Health Promotion: Disciplines and Diversity*. Chapter 1, Health promotion: discipline or disciplines? London: Routledge.

An analysis of the concept of health promotion and the implications for professional practice:

➤ Tones K (1996) in Scriven, A. and Orme, J. (eds) *Health Promotion: Professional Perspectives*. Chapter 1, The anatomy and ideology of health promotion: empowerment in context. Basingstoke: Macmillan/The Open University.

A critical discussion on the meaning of health promotion and a scrutiny of current models of health promotion:

➤ Seedhouse D (1997) *Health Promotion: Philosophy, Prejudice and Practice*. Chapters 1 and 2. Chichester: Wiley.

Notes and References

1 World Health Organization (1984) *Health Promotion: a WHO discussion document on the concepts and principles*. Reprinted in: *Journal of the Institute of Health Education*, 23(1), 1985.

2 See, for example:

Whitehead M (1989) *Swimming Upstream: trends and prospects in education for health*, p. 7. London: King's Fund Institute.

3 See:

Welsh Health Planning Forum (1989) *Strategic Intent and Direction for the NHS in Wales*. Cardiff: Welsh Office.

Welsh Health Planning Forum (1990) *Protocol for Investment in Health Gain – Cancers*. Cardiff: Welsh Office.

4 Secretary of State for Health (1992) *The Health of the Nation: a Strategy for Health in England*. London: HMSO.

5 Quoted in:

Simnett, I. (1995) *Managing Health Promotion: Developing Healthy Organisations and Communities*, p. 4. Chichester: Wiley.

6 Care Sector Consortium (1997) *National Occupational Standards for Professional Activity in Health Promotion and Care – Introductory Guide*. Glossary. London: Local Government Management Board.

7 Some of these are summarized in:

Naidoo J and Wills J (1994) *Health Promotion: Foundations for Practice*. Chapter 5. London: Baillière Tindall.

8 For a model of the different aspects of competence, see:

Mansfield B and Mitchell L (1996) *Towards a Competent Workforce*. London: Gower.

9 Care Sector Consortium (1997) *National Occupational Standards for Professional Activity in Health Promotion and Care – Introductory Guide*. London: Local Government Management Board.

10 These Key Roles are from:

Care Sector Consortium (1997) *National Occupational Standards for Professional Activity in Health Promotion and Care – Introductory Guide*. Sections 3.2, 3.3 and 3.4. London: Local Government Management Board. (Crown copyright is reproduced with the permission of the Controller of Her Majesty's Stationery Office.)

3   Aims and Values in Health Promotion

SUMMARY

In this chapter we identify and explore some key philosophical issues about aims and values in health promotion practice. We start with two fundamental questions about the aims of health promotion: whether we aim to change the individual or change society, and whether we aim to ensure compliance with a health promotion programme or to enable clients to make an informed choice. We provide a framework of five approaches to health promotion as a tool for analysing key aims and values, with two exercises and case studies. We discuss eight more ethical issues, set out a framework of questions to help health promoters to make ethical decisions, and an exercise on making ethical decisions. We finish with a discussion on the values base of Occupational Standards in health promotion, a sample code of practice in health promotion and two more exercises.

In this chapter, we tease out some of the key philosophical issues in health promotion. We encourage you to think deeply about why you are engaging in specific activities, what values are reflected in your work and what ethical dilemmas are presented. We consider guidelines on how to approach ethical decision-making and some key principles of practice.

Philosophical issues are important.[1] Health promotion work, if successful, will affect the lives of other people and it would be irresponsible to equip you with practical skills without also helping you to understand the values and ethics implicit in your work.

First, we look at the aims of health promotion.

Clarifying Health Promotion Aims

Aiming to change the individual or change society?

See section on Defining Health Promotion in Chapter 2

For more than a decade, there has been much debate over different approaches (often called 'models') of health education and health promotion[2].

Much of the debate centres around the aims of the work. A key question is: should it aim to change individual behaviour and lifestyles, or to change the socio-economic and physical environment?

As we discussed in Chapter 1, a great deal of traditional health education has aimed to change the behaviour of individuals towards healthier lifestyles. In other words, it aims to change people to fit the environment, and has done little to make the environment a healthier place to live in. It has also resulted in 'blaming the victims' for their own ill-health, which is an ethical issue health educators need to face. On the other hand, it can be argued that individuals often can do something to improve their own health, that they want to take responsibility for themselves and that health education is an essential tool in that process. It is also argued that sensitive health education can promote people's self-esteem and confidence, empowering them to take more control over their own health.

Proponents of the lifestyle change approach also argue that medical and health experts have the knowledge which enables them to know what is in the best interests of their patients and the public at large, and that it is their responsibility to persuade people to adopt the 'healthiest' measures. Furthermore, society has vested that responsibility with them, and people often seek advice and help in health matters; it is not necessarily a matter of persuading clients against their will. Sometimes, too, individuals may not be in a position to take responsibility for themselves, because they may be too young, too ill, or have severe learning difficulties.

There are several points to be taken into account if the lifestyle change aim is pursued.

- You cannot assume that lay people believe that 'experts' know best. The public perceives 'experts' to change their minds constantly. For example, whether jogging does more harm than good, whether eggs, chicken and beef are safe to eat or whether living near a nuclear power plant is hazardous to health. Sometimes the 'experts' are proved wrong.
- There is a danger of imposing alien values on a client. Frequently, this is the imposition of white middle-class values on working-class people. For example, a doctor may perceive that the most important thing for a patient is losing weight and lowering blood pressure, but drinking beer in the pub with friends may be far more important to the overweight, middle-aged, unemployed patient. Who is to say which set of values is 'right'? Whose life is it anyway?
- Linked to this, a health promoter advocating lifestyle changes can be seen as making a moral judgement on clients' failure to change, that it is 'their own fault' if, for example, the baby of a mother who smokes is born with low birthweight or dies from a cot death.
- Pushing a lifestyle change approach may produce negative and counter-productive feelings: of guilt for failing to comply, or rebelliousness and anger at being told what to do.
- We cannot assume that individual behaviour is the primary cause of ill-health. This a limited view, as we have seen when looking at determinants of health and inequalities in health in Chapter 1. There is a danger that focusing on the individual distracts attention from the more significant (and, of course, politically sensitive) determinants of health such as the socioeconomic factors of racism, relative deprivation, poverty, housing and unemployment.
- Finally, we also cannot assume that individuals have a genuine freedom to choose 'healthy' lifestyles. Freedom to choose is often very limited. Economic factors may affect the choice of food because, for example, fresh fruit and wholemeal bread are relatively more expensive than biscuits and white bread. Social factors are also important: there is very little real freedom of choice about smoking for adolescents whose parents and friends all smoke, and who risk ridicule if they do not. Also, how much freedom do people really have to

change other health-demoting factors such stressful working conditions and unemployment? It is easy to become 'victim-blaming': blaming people for their own ill-health when in fact they are the victims of their circumstances. In situations where resources of time, energy and income are limited, health choices become health compromises. What a health promoter may see as irresponsibility may actually be what the client sees as the most responsible action in the circumstances.[3] For example, chips are cheap, filling and enjoyed by children; if money for food is short, and cooking skills and facilities are limited, chips are a sensible choice for a mother with several hungry mouths to feed. Another example is the mother who smokes because it is the only way she knows of relieving her stress; it helps to stop her hitting her children when they drive her to breaking point.

Part 3 of this book on Developing Competence in Health Promotion addresses how you can promote health in a way which is sensitive to these issues, and Chapter 16 on Changing Policy and Practice looks particularly at what you can do to challenge and change health-related policies.

It is crucially important that everyone engaged in health promotion should be aware of these ethical issues and have an opportunity to consider them in relation to their own work, particularly if they are engaged in health education with the aim of changing individual lifestyles. The following exercise is designed to help you to think through the issues.

Exercise 3.1   Analysing your philosophy of health promotion[4]

Consider the following statements A and B.

> A.   The key aim of health promotion is to inform people about the ways in which their behaviour and lifestyle can affect their health, to ensure that the information is understood, to help them explore their values and attitudes, and (where appropriate) to help them to change their behaviour.

> B.   The key aim of health promotion is to raise awareness of the many socioeconomic policies at national and local level (e.g. employment, housing, food subsidies, advertising, transport and health service policies) which are not conducive to good health, and to work actively towards a change in those policies.

1.   Taking Statement A:
  • list arguments in support of this view;
  • list any points about the limitations of this view, and any arguments against it.
2.   Do the same with Statement B.
3.   **Do you think that the views in A and B are *complementary* or *incompatible*? Why?**
4.   Imagine these two views at either end of a spectrum:

   A | ..... | ..... | ..... | ..... | ..... | B
       1   2   3   4   5

Indicate the two positions on the scale of 1 to 5 which most closely reflect (a) *what you actually do* in practice and (b) *what you would like to do* if you were free to work exactly as you would wish to.

Aiming for Compliance or Informed Choice?

Another key question about the aims of health promotion centres on what you aim to do with or for the client (whether the client is a single individual, a community, or an organization). Is your aim to ensure that your client complies with your programme, using a mixture of education, publicity and persuasion as required? Or is it to enable your client to make an informed choice, and have the skills and confidence to carry that choice through into action, whatever that choice may be?

To take an example: supposing a health promoter is working with a client whose sexual behaviour is such that there is a serious risk of catching sexually transmitted diseases, and even HIV. If the aim is compliance it is more likely that the health promoter will be persuasive, will stress the risks to the client, and will consider the session a failure if the client does not choose to behave differently. If, on the other hand, the health promoter's aim is to enable the client to make an informed choice, the health promoter will ensure that the client understands the facts and the risks, will put a lot of effort into encouraging and supporting the client and accept that if the client chooses not to change behaviour, this choice will be respected. It would not be interpreted as a failure, because the client made an informed choice.

The same issues arise with health promotion work on a larger scale. For example, is the aim of a campaign to promote 'natural' food untouched by additives, chemical fertilisers and pesticides to persuade people to a particular point of view or to give them the information on which to make up their own minds?

This is a difficult question. Most health promoters are doing their jobs because they believe that the action they are advocating is in the best interests of individuals and society as whole. It raises questions about how far to go in imposing your own values and ideas of what is 'good' and 'right' on other people.

While considering this question, it is also worth noting that it raises the issue of defining 'success' in health promotion. In the first example about sexual health behaviour, if the aim is to change behaviour then success is likely to be measured in terms of rates of sexually transmitted disease and unplanned pregnancy. But if the aim is solely to educate, success will be measured in terms of changes in people's knowledge of health risks.

Analysing Your Aims and Values: Five Approaches

In our view, there is no one 'right' aim for health promotion, and no one 'right' approach or set of activities. We need to work out for ourselves which aim and which activities we use, in accordance with our own professional code of conduct (if there is one), our own carefully-considered values and our own assessment of our clients' needs.

Different models of health promotion and health education are a useful tool of analysis, which can help you to clarify your own aims and values. We identify a framework of five approaches to health promotion, and suggest some of the values implicit in any particular approach.

1. **The medical approach.** The aim is freedom from medically-defined disease and disability, such as infectious diseases, cancer and heart disease. The approach involves medical intervention to prevent or ameliorate ill-health, possibly using a persuasive or paternalistic method – for example, persuading parents to bring their children for immunization, women to use family planning clinics and middle-aged people to be screened for high blood pressure.

This approach values preventive medical procedures, and the medical profession's responsibility to ensure that patients comply with recommended procedures.

2. **The behaviour change approach.** The aim is to change people's individual attitude and behaviour, so that they adopt a 'healthy' lifestyle (as defined by you or your employing organization). Examples include teaching people how to stop smoking, education about 'sensible' drinking, encouraging people to be more physically active, look after their teeth, eat the 'right' foods and so on.

Those using this approach will be convinced that a 'healthy' lifestyle is in the best interests of the clients, and will see it as their responsibility to encourage as many people as possible to adopt the 'healthy' lifestyle they advocate.

3. **The educational approach.** The aim is to give information, ensure knowledge and understanding of health issues, and to enable well-informed decisions to be made. Information about health is presented, and people are helped to explore their values and attitudes, and make their own decisions. Help in carrying out those decisions and adopting new health practices may also be offered. School health education programmes, for example, emphasize helping pupils to learn the skills of healthy living, not merely to acquire knowledge.

Those favouring this approach will value the educational process, will respect the individual's right to choose their own health behaviour, and will see it as their responsibility to raise with clients the health issues which they think will be in the client's best interests.

4. **The client-centred approach.** The aim is to work with clients to help them identify what they want to know about and take action on, and make their own decisions and choices according to their own interests and values. The health promoter's role is to act as a facilitator, helping people to identify their concerns and gain the knowledge and skills they require to make changes happen. Self-empowerment of the client is seen as central.[5] Clients are valued as equals who have knowledge, skills and abilities to contribute, and who have an absolute right to control their own health destinies.

5. **The societal change approach.** The aim is to effect changes on the physical, social and economic environment, to make it more conducive to good health. The focus is on changing society, not on changing the behaviour of individuals.

Those using this approach will value their democratic right to change society, will be committed to putting health on the political agenda at all levels, and to the importance of shaping the health environment rather than shaping the individual lives of the people who live in it.

We have set out our **Five Approaches to Health Promotion** because it is a simple framework which helps health promoters to appreciate that there are many ways of tackling health promotion, and these different ways reflect

Table 3.1		Five Approaches to Health Promotion – Summary and Example		
	Aim	Health Promotion Activity	Important Values	Example – smoking
Medical	Freedom from medically-defined disease and disability	Promotion of medical intervention to prevent or ameliorate ill-health	Patient compliance with preventive medical procedures	*Aim* – freedom from lung disease, heart disease and other smoking-related disorders *Activity* – encourage people to seek early detection and treatment of smoking-related disorders
Behaviour change	Individual behaviour conducive to freedom from disease	Attitude and behaviour change to encourage adoption of 'healthier' lifestyle	Healthy lifestyle as defined by health promoter	*Aim* – behaviour changes from smoking to not smoking *Activity* – persuasive education to prevent non-smokers from starting and persuade smokers to stop
Educational	Individuals with knowledge and understanding enabling well-informed decisions to be made and acted upon	Information about cause and effects of health-demoting factors. Exploration of values and attitudes. Development of skills required for healthy living	Individual right of free choice. Health promoter's responsibility to identify educational content	*Aim* – clients will have understanding of the effects of smoking on health. They will make a decision whether or not to smoke and act on the decision *Activity* – giving information to clients about the effects of smoking. Helping them to explore their own values and attitudes and come to a decision. Helping them to learn how to stop smoking if they want to
Client-centred	Working with clients on the clients' own terms	Working with health issues, choices and actions which clients identify. Empowering the client	Clients as equals. Clients' right to set agenda. Self-empowerment of client	Anti-smoking issue is only considered if clients identify it as a concern. Clients identify what, if anything, they want to know and do about it
Societal change	Physical and social environment which enables choice of healthier lifestyle	Political/social action to change physical/social environment	Right and need to make environment health-enhancing	*Aim* – make smoking socially unacceptable, so it is easier not to smoke than to smoke *Activity* – no smoking policy in all public places. Cigarette sales less accessible, especially to children, promotion of non-smoking as social norm. Banning tobacco advertising and sports' sponsorship

---

Exercise 3.2   **Identifying your aims and values**

Select two or three specific health promotion activities you are engaged in, such as a group health education programme, a publicity campaign, a patient education scheme, an immunization programme, a one-to-one meeting with a client, a community activity or working on a health policy. Select different kinds of activities if you can.

With reference to the chart 'Five approaches to health promotion', identify which approach you are using for each activity (you may find that you will identify more than one approach).

For each activity, define the aim and the important values implicit in your work (you may find it helpful to look at the Case Studies 3.1 and 3.2.).

Discuss your findings with a partner or in a small group.

Case studies 3.1 and 3.2   **Approaches A and B**

Case study 3.1 Approach A

Jill is a hospital nurse running a programme of rehabilitation for patients who have had heart attacks. She decides that she is working with an educational approach, aiming for her patients to make informed decisions and have knowledge and skills about taking exercise, modifying their diet, etc. She accepts that some patients will choose not to do so. She thinks that sometimes she may be working in a behaviour change model, because she sincerely believes that her patients would be better off if they changed their behaviour and she finds that she sometimes really wants to persuade them. In the end, she decides that it is their choice and their life, and that she will not pressure them into doing what they do not want to do. Jill is aware, though, that some of her colleagues (who favour the behaviour change approach) think she should be tougher and shock the patients into complying by horror stories of what may happen to them if they do not.

Case study 3.2. Approach B

Terry is a community worker, based in a deprived housing estate. Facilities for recreation, exercise and buying good food (among other things) are poor. He decides that he is working with a mixture of client-centred and societal-change approaches, because people in the community have identified that they want a better diet, and he is helping them to set up a food cooperative and help each other to learn new cooking skills. He is also helping them to lobby their local councillor for better green spaces on the estate where the children can play.

---

differing viewpoints and values. Our framework has rightly been questioned and challenged, and this is part of a healthy debate as the theory and practice of health promotion continues to develop.[6] There are other well-known models.[7]

Some More Ethical Dilemmas

There are many more difficult questions for health promoters to get to grips with. The following are some of the commoner ones you are likely to encounter.

Bottom-up or Top-down?

There is a key issue of control and power at the heart of health promotion work: who decides what work will be done; who sets the agenda? Is it 'bottom-up', set by people themselves identifying issues they perceive as relevant, or is it 'top-down', set by health promoters who have the power and resources to make decisions and impose their own ideas of what should be done?

Put this way, it appears to be a straightforward polarized choice. In practice, of course, it is not simple. The issue can be considered at different levels.

At the level of individual health promoters there is a spectrum of possible positions which they could take: at one end, coercion or persuasion, then giving advice, then a more neutral position of giving the facts but leaving the client to decide. The position at the other end of the spectrum is the health promoter who listens, gives information when asked and supports the client but never offers advice or even an opinion.

The client, too, could be at any point along the spectrum. Ideally, the health promoter and client will adopt compatible positions: for example, with the health promoter giving information and the client happy to make up his own mind what to do about it. Problems can arise when positions are not compatible. An example is a client who wants to be told what to do and a health promoter who wants to empower him with information and confidence to make his own decision.

At a national level, governments identify certain health promotion priorities with the advice of professionals. These programmes are then imposed on the population who may or may not perceive them as relevant. But ultimately the decision to implement these programmes is that of the government elected by the people in a democratic society; so we come full circle.

There is also a danger that when the public is involved in health promotion at a local level, local people can be manipulated into changing their agenda to match that of the health promoters. Community development should be about empowering the public to work on their own agendas of health issues, even if these are radically different from the agendas of those working for health in a professional capacity. But health promoters have a responsibility to raise awareness of health issues, provide information about them and create demand for change: so where does this process differ from manipulating the community into wanting what the health promoters wanted in the first place?

Perhaps one way forward is to be aware of the necessity to be absolutely honest and open about your aims and the limitations of your freedom to act on other people's priorities.

Just Widening the Inequalities?

As discussed in Chapter 1, there are wide differences in the health status of different groups of people, and generally those in poorer social and economic conditions are the least healthy, with the gap between the health status of rich and poor becoming ever wider.

See discussion of inequalities in Chapter 1

There is danger that health promotion activities only reach the better-off, who have the time, money and education to make use of health information and take health action. Those who are trapped in poor financial circumstances and who

Some ways of working with those most in need, and often hardest to reach, are discussed in Chapter 15 on Working with Communities.

struggle to survive are less likely to be in a position to change their lifestyle or devote their energies to lobbying for social or political changes.[8] There is clearly a need to be sensitive to this.[9]

The Health Promoter: a Shining Example?

Consider the cases of an overweight dietitian, a nurse who smokes and an environmental health officer who does not use unleaded petrol. All three are in a position where they need to address these issues as part of their work and possibly be asked for advice which they clearly do not follow themselves.

Few health promoters would claim that they are perfect examples of healthy living, but we suggest that they have a responsibility to consider their own health, ways in which it could be improved, and ways in which they could contribute to a healthier environment. Health promoters are teaching by example, and the examples discussed above convey silent messages that it is okay to be overweight, to smoke, or to pollute the atmosphere with leaded petrol. It is probably best to be open and honest in situations where health promoters' own lifestyles are at odds with the health promoting ways they are advocating. Personal experience can also be turned to good advantage: for example, if the dietitian has a constant struggle to control her own weight, she can use that experience to develop a greater understanding of her clients' difficulties.

Facts, Fads or Fashions?

A common complaint from the public is that experts keep changing their minds, and there are many examples which illustrate this. Examples include controversy about the safety of beef in the light of 'scares' about 'mad cow disease', and changed guidelines about sensible drinking advice.[10] Health issues go in and out of the news, and the public may see them as fads or fashions with little solid foundation in fact and certainly low credibility.

A difficulty is that research continuously turns up new information, often controversial and not accepted as generally 'received wisdom' until it has been independently confirmed from new sources. This may take many years. But media attention focuses on the new and controversial, so the public becomes alerted to the debates.

At what point do you decide that the evidence is sufficiently convincing to begin publicizing a new message, or to campaign to change an aspect of health policy or legislation? If you have insufficient knowledge or experience to judge questions which may be medically or technically complex, on what basis do you make the decision? Or is it more appropriate to discuss the conflicting views openly and just air the debate more widely?

Health or Healthism?

In their enthusiasm for improving health, there is a danger that health promoters come to see health as the be-all and end-all: as an end in itself, not as a means to the end of enabling people to fulfil their own potential and live life to the full. This ideology of health as the ultimate goal incorporating all life is sometimes called 'healthism'.

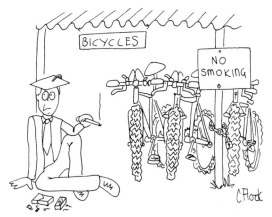

Few health promoters would claim that they are perfect examples of healthy living

The danger is that it may lead to a lack of acceptance that health means different things to different people, shaped by their various values and experiences. Health may become a stereotyped image of the health promoter's own idea of perfection, leading to a prescription of what people should and should not do. This is clearly contrary to the concept that health promotion is about enabling people to increase their own control over their health and improve it in ways they see fit.

Health Information: an Insensitive Blunderbuss?

All health promotion should be sensitive to the social, ethnic, economic and cultural background of the people it is working with and for. Sadly, this is often not the case. Because of insensitivity, ignorance or the need to produce materials on a large scale for economic reasons, health information, and indeed entire health promotion programmes, are frequently aimed at an 'average' person, or the largest client group. So they often, for example, portray only white people, are only available in English, or assume a level of income above the poverty line. Frequently it is those with greatest needs who are in the minorities and therefore ignored.

There is growing awareness of this issue, but there is still a long way to go before health promotion can truly claim to practise equal opportunities.

To Professionalize or Empower the People?

Health promotion requires special competencies, some of which are the subject of this book. It is a whole or part of the work of very many professions, including health, education and community work. As it becomes increasingly specialized, with its own body of knowledge based on research, and its own academic qualifications, there is a danger that health promotion 'experts' will exclude other workers and the public from the business of health promotion.

This would be a sad mistake. Health promotion, as we have said often, is about empowering people to take more control over their own health. Health promotion specialists therefore need to seek to share their knowledge and experience with lay people, to learn from them, and to see them and other workers as valued partners in health promotion.[11]

Health For Sale?

With scarce resources available for health promotion, and a climate of market economy and income generation, there is an increasing trend towards sponsorship for health promotion activities. One pitfall is the issue of perceived endorsement of products. For example, a health authority could be seen as advocating that patients should take vitamins if it accepted sponsorship of appointment cards printed with the name of the sponsoring vitamin manufacturer.

There is also a move to involve commercial companies in promoting products in a way which also promotes health. For example, food manufacturers may be involved in special promotions for lower fat products. There are dangers here, the most obvious one being that the interests of the company may not be in harmony with those of the health promoter, who will be perceived as endorsing the product. There is also a possibility that the independent credibility of the health promoter is compromised, with the public thinking 'they're just trying to sell me something' instead of perceiving an unbiased credible health message.

Another pitfall is that health promotion, which should be a fundamental part of the free national health service, is seen as a potential money-maker. Basic services, such as health information materials, health teaching, and giving advice to commercial companies on health promotion for employees, become subject to charges.

There is a clear need to develop policies and guidelines on these issues.[12]

Making Ethical Decisions

We have identified many areas of ethical concern, and raised difficult issues which do not present easy resolutions or 'right' answers. The following set of questions is designed to help you to think through some of the dilemmas you face, and to make decisions about ethical questions when faced with alternative courses of action.[13]

1. Questions Fundamental to Decisions About Health

- Will I be creating autonomy in my clients, enabling them to choose freely for themselves and direct their own lives?
- Will I be respecting the autonomy of my clients, whether or not I approve of what they are doing?
- Will I be respecting persons equally, without discrimination?
- Will I be serving basic needs before any other wants?

2. Questions About Duties and Principles

- Will I be doing good and preventing harm?
- Will I be telling the truth?
- Will I be minimizing harm in the long term?
- Will I be honouring promises and agreements?

3. Questions About Consequences

■ Will I be increasing individual good?
■ Will I be acting for the good of myself?
■ Will I be increasing the good of a particular group?
■ Will I be increasing the social good?

4. Questions About External Considerations

■ Am I putting resources to best use: what is the most effective and efficient thing to do?
■ What is the degree of risk involved?
■ Is there a professional code of practice which has a bearing on this?
■ How certain am I of the evidence for the facts of the matter?
■ Are there any disputed facts?
■ Are there legal implications, and if so, do I understand them?
■ What are the views and wishes of other relevant people?
■ Can I justify my actions in terms of the evidence I have before me?

These questions are tools to help clear thinking and moral reasoning. They are not substitutes for personal judgement, but they help you to think through the issue, weigh up the pros and cons and come to a reasoned decision. Not all the questions will be relevant, but they act as a useful checklist. Some questions may reveal that, on the surface, a 'wrong' action is being taken (such as not telling the truth or being discriminatory) but using the checklist ensures that careful consideration is given to it and that it is justified. For example, a painful truth may be withheld from a seriously ill patient, or it may be necessary to discriminate between working with one group of people as opposed to another because there are insufficient resources to work with both.

Towards a Code of Practice

Many professions have codes of practice which are broad principles and guidelines on how professionals should and should not act. They reflect the values accepted as underpinning sound professional practice. We suggest that readers make sure they are familiar with the code of practice of their own professional bodies.[14]

Health promotion values are identified in the National Occupational Standards for health promotion. The first (Key Role 0) is about the principles and values on which practice is built, and focuses on promoting and valuing the rights, responsibilities and diversity of people.[15] The values and principles of good practice on which they are based are set out in the box below.

The National Occupational Standards for health promotion are explained in Chapter 2.

Box 3.1.	**National Occupational Standards for Professional Activity in Health Promotion and Care. July 1997[16]**

Values and Principles of Good Practice

Professional standards from a number of different professional bodies were analysed to identify the values and principles on which the national occupational standards for professional activity in health promotion and care should be based. The *values* identified are respect for:

- the human condition and its complexity;
- our essential humanity;
- the wealth of human experience;
- the holistic nature of health and social well-being;
- diversity.

The National Occupational Standards for Professional Activity in Health Promotion and Care have been built on ten *Principles of Good Practice:*

1. Balancing people's rights with their responsibilities to others and to wider society and challenging those which affect the rights of others.
2. Promoting values of equality and diversity, acknowledging the personal beliefs and preferences of others and promoting anti-discriminatory practice.
3. Maintaining the confidentiality of information provided that this does not place others at risk.
4. Recognizing the effect of the wider social, political and economic context on health and social well-being and on people's development.
5. Enabling people to develop to their full potential, to be as autonomous and self-managing as possible and to have a voice and be heard.
6. Recognizing and promoting health and social well-being as a positive concept.
7. Balancing the needs of people who use services with the resources available and exercising financial probity.
8. Developing and maintaining effective relationships with people and maintaining the integrity of these relationships through setting appropriate role boundaries.
9. Developing oneself and one's own practice to improve the quality of services offered.
10. Working within statutory and organizational frameworks.

The following *Principles of Practice* have been produced by the Society of Health Education and Health Promotion Specialists (SHEPS). SHEPS intend them for use by Health Education/Promotion Specialists and others working in the fields of health education, health promotion and public health, as they cover areas which all health promoters may find helpful to consider. They consider similar issues to those in the National Occupational Standards, but focus more specifically on health promotion activities.

Box 3.2.	**Society of Health Education and Health Promotion Specialists Principles of Practice. July 1997**[17]

Relationship to Client/Recipient

1. Adequate needs assessment, consultation with and involvement of the client or target group is essential to the effective planning, implementation and reviewing of health promotion activities.
2. The promotion of self-esteem and autonomy amongst client groups/recipients should be an underlying principle of all health promotion practice.
3. Health promotion should encourage people to value others whatever their gender, age, race, class, religion, culture, sexuality, ability or health status, and attempt to counter prejudice and discrimination wherever it occurs.

Social and Environmental Influences

4. Health promotion programmes should be relevant and sensitive to the nature of the intended client group, for example, the social, economic and cultural framework of the group.
5. Health promotion work should include recognition of and action focused on the social, economic and environmental determinants of health.
6. Health promotion work should aim to empower and enable people to exercise informed choice and influence structures and systems that have an impact on health.
7. Health promotion programmes which focus on specific issues should always be set in the wider political, social, economic, geographical, psychological and environmental context which has a bearing on health.
8. The sustainability of health promotion interventions needs to be considered within the context of the aims of any programme of activity. Health promotion interventions should aim to have a positive impact on both the immediate recipients and future generations of people.

Health Promotion Practice

A. An aim of health promotion practice is to bring about change in the social and economic environment to improve health and to reduce or eliminate inequalities in health at a local, national and international level.
B. Appropriate research and evaluation is an essential component of health promotion activity. Practitioners should endeavour to disseminate results and findings.
C. Practitioners have a responsibility for ensuring an accurate and appropriate information flow between the public, professionals, local and national agencies, and for taking the initiative and responding accordingly.
D. Practitioners will endeavour to provide services or information that they have at their disposal that would, in the light of current theory and/or evidence, maintain and promote health. They will endeavour to keep their knowledge of current developments in health promotion up to date.
E. Practitioners will have due regard to the confidentiality of information to which they have access, bearing in mind the requirements of the law.
F. Health promotion work should encourage all services and organizations to develop their health promotion role and to adopt the above principles of practice.
G. Health promotion activity is by its nature a collaborative endeavour. Practitioners should seek to actively collaborate with colleagues and others to promote health.
H. The methods and process of health promotion should be health promoting.

Ethical decisions in health promotion

You may find it helpful to use the questions an pages 48 – 49 to identify the issues relevant to each situation, and to decide what you would do.

Case A

A group of local people, led by a woman whose son died of a heroin overdose, have got together because they are concerned about drug misuse in the neighbourhood. They are afraid for the safety of their teenagers and younger children: drugs seem to be an established part of the teenage social scene, are easily available in the neighbourhood, and needles and syringes are found in local alleyways.

The group has decided that the best way to combat drugs is to go into local schools and scare the children off drugs with horror stories of bad 'trips' and addiction. They have recruited a former drug addict who is prepared to tell his story. They have asked the school nurse to help by getting them supplies of leaflets and supporting them in their approach to the schools.

The school nurse believes that the 'shock-horror' approach the group proposes has been shown by research into drug education to be ineffective. At best it will do no good, and at worst it could glamorize the drug scene and a make a hero out of the ex-addict. She believes that the local schools' approach is best: education on the facts of drug-taking and how to minimize harm from taking drugs, coupled with building up self-esteem, social skills and confidence for young people to deal with drug situations. The parents think this is far too soft, and believe that their idea for a hard-hitting approach will work for their children.

- **Identify the ethical issues in this situation.**
- **What do you think the school nurse should do, and why?**

Case B

An environmental health officer (EHO) wants to undertake some research into the impact of air pollution on asthma rates in a neighbourhood which straddles a main road. Town planning colleagues have told the EHO that they expect this road to become even busier soon because it will become the feeder road to a new bypass leading to a massive new out-of-town office development. The EHO has a well worked out research proposal and has the cooperation of local GPs which will enable him to see if there is any correlation between traffic flow, air pollution levels and asthma rates. If he can show a correlation, it will help to put health issues on the agenda of the Council's Planning Committee, so that the health impact of planning decisions will be taken into account in future.

He needs to secure a research grant to pay for the additional pollution measurements and traffic flow counts, and to collect and process the data from the GPs. If he does not start within the next month, he will miss the chance to collect vital baseline measurements before the expected increase in traffic when the bypass opens.

Despite applications to many sources, the only offer of research money he has received has come from a research trust which specializes in the impact of environmental pollution on respiratory disease. It is funded primarily by the tobacco industry. The trust assures the EHO that that they will not interfere with the research in any way, and the grant will be given with 'no strings attached'. The EHO is unhappy about accepting money from the tobacco industry, but this is now his only chance to get the research under way.

- **Identify the ethical issues in this situation.**
- **What do you think the EHO should do, and why?**

| Exercise 3.4 | Developing a code of practice |

Work in small groups of 3 or 4.

Consider the points in the *National Occupational Standards for Professional Activity in Health Promotion and Care – Values and Principles of Good Practice* and the *Society of Health Education and Health Promotion Specialists – Principles of Practice,* both reproduced above.

To what extent do you think you take account of these values and principles in your work?

Do you encounter any difficulties in putting these values and principles into practice?

Are there any values and principles you would like to amend?

Are there any values and principles you would like to add?

PRACTICE POINTS

- You need to recognize the range of approaches to health promotion which reflect different aims and values.

- Ethical issues and dilemmas are inherent in health promotion practice.

- You need to think through the process of how you will make ethical decisions.

- Professional codes of practice can help you to be clear about the underlying principles of your work and you should be familiar with the code of professional practice of any profession to which you belong.

- Good practice in health promotion means working to the specific values and principles of practice on which The National Occupational Standards in Health Promotion and Care are based. The Society of Health Education and Health Promotion Specialists *Principles of Practice* also provides helpful guidelines.

Recommended Reading

Two critical overviews of models of health promotion:
➤ Katz J & Peberdy A (1997) *Promoting Health – Knowledge and Practice.* Chapter 5, Theories and Models in Health Promotion. Basingstoke: Macmillan in association with the Open University Press.
➤ Naidoo J & Wills J (1994) *Health Promotion – Foundations for Practice.* Chapter 5, Models and Approaches to Health Promotion. London: Baillière Tindall.

On a client-centred approach to health promotion:
➤ Raeburn J & Rootman I (1998) *People Centred Health Promotion.* Chichester: Wiley.

On ethical issues in health promotion:

➤ Seedhouse D (1988) *Ethics – the heart of health care.* Chichester: Wiley.
➤ Naidoo J & Wills J (1994) *Health Promotion – Foundations for Practice.* Chapter 6, Ethical Issues in Health Promotion. London: Baillière Tindall.
➤ Katz J & Peberdy A (1997) *Promoting Health – Knowledge and Practice.* Chapter 6, Ethical Issues in Health Promotion. Basingstoke: Macmillan in association with the Open University Press.
➤ Duncan P (1995) Ethical Audit: should it concern health promoters? What should they do? *Journal of the Institute of Health Education* **33** (3), 72–75. (Provides a rationale for health promoters' concern with ethics and suggests a framework of 'ethical audit'.)

Notes and References

1   Some further reading on philosophy and ethics –
see *Recommended Reading* and:

Doxiadis S (ed.) (1987) *Ethical Dilemmas in Health Promotion*. Chichester: Wiley.

Doxiadis S (ed.) (1990) *Ethics in Health Education*. Chichester: Wiley.

Seedhouse D (1997) *Health Promotion – Philosophy, Prejudice and Practice*. Chichester: Wiley.

Downie R S, Fyfe C & Tannahill A (1990) *Health Promotion: models and values*, Part 2. Oxford: University Press.

Wall A (1989) *Ethics and the Health Service Manager*. London: King Edward's Hospital Fund.

Hunt G (ed.) (1994) *Ethical Issues in Nursing*. London: Routledge. (Deals with specific nursing issues but also general themes applicable to a wide range of health promoters, such as professional responsibility.)

Pike S & Forster D (eds) (1995) *Health promotion for all*. Chapter 5, Values and ethical issues. Edinburgh: Churchill Livingstone. (Discusses ethical issues in health promotion, particularly applied to nurses.)

2   Some articles and readings on models of health education/promotion since the 1980s are:

Burkitt A (1983) Health Education. In Clark J & Henderson J (eds) *Community Health*. Edinburgh: Churchill Livingstone.

Draper P (1983) Tackling the disease of ignorance. *Self Health* (1) 23–25.

Catford J & Nutbeam D (1984) Towards a Definition of Health Education and Health Promotion. *Health Education Journal* **43** (2 & 3), 38.

Tannahill A (1985) What is Health Promotion? *Health Education Journal* **44**(4), 167–168.

Downie R S, Fyfe C & Tannahill A (1990) *Health Promotion: models and values*, Part 1. Oxford: University Press.

French J (1990) Boundaries and horizons, the role of health education within health promotion. *Health Education Journal* **49**(1), 7–10.

French J & Milner S (1993) Should we accept the status quo? *Health Education Journal* **52**(2), 98–101.

Tones K & Tilford S (1994) *Health Education: effectiveness, efficiency and equity*. Chapter 1. London: Chapman and Hall.

Maben J & Macleod Clark J (1995) Health promotion: a concept analysis. *Journal of Advanced Nursing* **22**(6), 1158–1165. (On nurses' concepts of health promotion.)

3   For discussion about the 'lifestyle approach' and the impact of social factors on health, see: Graham H (1984) *Women, Health and the Family*. Chapter 12. Brighton: Wheatsheaf Books.

Graham H (1993) *Hardship and Health in Women's Lives*. Hemel Hempstead: Harvester Wheatsheaf.

Blaxter M (1990) *Health and Lifestyles*. London: Tavistock.

4   This exercise is based on an idea in the training manual for the Schools Health Education Project 5–13, published by the Health Education Council, London, and reproduced here by kind permission of the Council.

5   For a description of the 'empowerment' model of health education, see: Tones K & Tilford S (1994) *Health Education: effectiveness, efficiency and equity*. Chapter 1, pp. 22–32. London: Chapman and Hall.

Tones K (1997) Health education as empowerment. Chapter 4 in Sidell M, Jones L, Katz J & Peberdy A (1997) (eds) *Debates and Dilemmas in Promoting Health*. Basingstoke: Macmillan/Open University Press.

6   Katz J & Peberdy A (1997) *Promoting Health – Knowledge and Practice*. Chapter 5, Theories and Models in Health Promotion. Basingstoke: Macmillan/Open University Press.

7   One of the best known is Tannahill's model of three overlapping circles which together form health promotion. The three circles are comprised of prevention, health education and health protection:

Tannahill A (1985) What is Health Promotion? *Health Education Journal* **44**(4), 167–168.

Downie R S, Fyfe C & Tannahill A (1990) *Health Promotion: models and values*. Chapter 4, Health Promotion. Oxford: University Press.

8   Graham H (1993) *Hardship and Health in Women's Lives*. Hemel Hempstead: Harvester Wheatsheaf. Chapter 8, Making Ends Meet shows that many families are living on incomes which make it hard to survive, and looks at how low-income families spend their limited budget and at the strategies that mothers develop to keep their family in health and out of too much debt. Such strategies often include mothers going without food, heating and other basic necessities themselves so that their children can have them.

9 Some examples of successful health promotion initiatives in reaching 'hard-to-reach' groups are:

Cardale P (1992) Springing the Poverty Trap. *Nursing Times* **88** (29), July 15. (On bringing antenatal care to women who are homeless, in poverty or otherwise socially deprived.)

Gruer L (1993) Bringing a city wide service for exchanging needles and syringes. *British Medical Journal*, May 22, 1394–1397. (On developing services for drug misusers, for needle and syringe exchange and other health and social services.)

James J, Brown J, Douglas M, Cox J & Stocker S (1992) Improving the diet of under 5's in a deprived inner city practice. *Health Trends* **24** (4), 161–164.

Community Health Action, Issue 22, winter 91/92, has a number of articles on tackling the promotion of healthy eating in areas of poverty and deprivation.

10 In 1997, the government-backed Health Education Authority publicity promoted the notion of 'daily benchmarks' of 2 to 3 units of alcohol a day for women, and 3 to 4 units a day for men. This followed publication in December 1995 of: Department of Health (1995) *Sensible Drinking: The Report of an Inter-Departmental Working Group*. London: Department of Health. The new guidelines replaced ones which advocated a weekly sensible drinking limit of 14 units for women, 21 for men.

11 A good example of lay people working in partnership with professionals is the successful experience of using non-professional volunteer mothers working with disadvantaged first-time mothers to develop their parenting skills:

Johnson Z, Howell F & Molloy B (1993) Community mothers' programme: randomised controlled trial of non-professional intervention in parenting. *British Medical Journal* **36**, 1449–1452.

12 This question is addressed in: The Society of Health Education and Health Promotion Specialists (1996) *Income Generation – Moral Threat or Marvellous Opportunity?* Principles of Practice Standing Committee, Briefing Sheet No. 2.

13 The questions in this section (reproduced by kind permission of John Wiley & Sons) are based on the work of Seedhouse, which is recommended for further study:

Seedhouse D (1988) *Ethics – the heart of health care*. Chichester: Wiley.

14 For example, professional bodies such as the Community Practitioners' and Health Visitors' Association.

15 Care Sector Consortium (1997) *National Occupational Standards for Professional Activity in Health Promotion and Care – Introductory Guide*. London: Local Government Management Board.

16 These values and principles of good practice are from: Care Sector Consortium (1997) *National Occupational Standards for Professional Activity in Health Promotion and Care – Introductory Guide*. Sections 2.2 and 2.3. London: Local Government Management Board. (Crown copyright is reproduced with the permission of the Controller of Her Majesty's Stationery Office.)

17 This is reproduced with the kind permission of the Society of Health Education and Health Promotion Specialists. It is the *Principles of Practice* part of the *Principles of Practice and Code of Professional Conduct for Health Education and Promotion Specialists*, July 1997.

4 Who Promotes Health?

SUMMARY

In this chapter we identify the major agents and agencies of health promotion, and discuss their role. We cover international and national organizations, the Government, the Health Education Authority (and sister organizations in Scotland, Wales and Northern Ireland), the NHS, local authorities, local groups and many others. We include an exercise on identifying key local health promoters. We end the chapter with suggestions and an exercise about how you can improve your own health promotion role.

To some extent everyone is a health promoter, because everyone discusses health matters and gives advice and guidance to others from time to time. This usually happens informally, for example when parents are reminding children to clean their teeth, or when friends are discussing their experiences. Health promotion may also occur incidentally: for example, the availability of a wide variety of cheap fruit and vegetables in the summer means that it is easier for people to choose a healthy diet. So the greengrocer is unwittingly promoting health. These informal and unplanned sources of health promotion are very significant. Our aim here, however, is to identify the agents and agencies through which planned, deliberate programmes and policies are channelled.

Agents and Agencies of Health Promotion

Figure 4.1 indicates the most important agents and agencies of health promotion. Most agents have a variety of health promotion roles. For example, the environmental health departments in local authorities are involved in formal health education through educating caterers about food handling in kitchens, but they are also involved in environmental measures such as control of air pollution. And they have important duties related to the enforcement of laws such as food hygiene regulations and health and safety at work legislation.

An increasing number of agencies recognize that they have a role to play in promoting health, and are working together in collaborative partnerships. This widening ownership of health promotion is helping it to be more effective. As part of *The Health of the Nation*, the Department of Health produced guidance on how agencies can work together for better health.[1]

Fig 4.1   **Agents and agencies in health promotion.**

International organizations (World Health Organization, European Community)

Government (Department of Health, Department of Social Security, Ministry of Agriculture, Fisheries and Food, Department for Education and Employment, Central Office of Information, Department of the Environment, Transport and the Regions, etc.)

**National Health Service
— NHS Executive**

¥ Health Education Authority
¥ Health Education Board for Scotland
¥ Health Promotion Wales
¥ Health Promotion Agency for Northern Ireland

¥ Institute of Health and Care Development

¥ Regional Education and Development Groups

¥ NHS Trusts

¥ Health authorities and health boards

¥ Community health councils

¥ Health promotion specialists

¥ Health professionals
   doctors, dentists, nurses, health visitors,
   dietitians, chiropodists, etc.

**Local
government**

¥ Teachers, lecturers

¥ Planning officers

¥ Environmental
   health officers

¥ Health promotion/
   education officers

¥ Social services staff

¥ Housing officers

¥ Recreation and
   leisure officers

¥ Youth workers

**The Training
Agency**

¥ Training and
   Enterprise
   Councils

**Other national
organizations**

¥ National voluntary
   organizations and pressure
   groups, e.g. RoSPA, FOE

¥ Professional organizations

¥ Trade unions

¥ Churches and religious
   organizations

National organizations
and local branches,
e.g. NCT, MIND, Citizen s
Advice Bureaux
↓
local branches

Private preventive
medical services

National media, TV,
radio, newspapers, etc.

Local media

Police

Local community and
voluntary groups,
e.g. youth groups,
self-help groups

The informal network,
family, friends,
neighbours, etc.

Institutions
of higher
learning

Health and
Safety Executive

Workplace employers
(occupational health
services, personnel
officers, managers)

Manufacturers
and retailers

Industrial and
commercial
organizations

Natural health
practitioners

International Organizations

The European Community

The European Community is increasingly making an impact on health by, for example, setting standards for beach pollution and through directives regulating permitted food additives. The Maastricht Treaty introduced a new public health article 129, which focused on health protection and disease prevention. New areas for Community action in the late 1990s include health promotion, education and training. An annual report is also prepared on the health protection aspects of other Community policies.

The World Health Organization (WHO)

See Chapter 1, p. 14.

The role of the WHO in 'Health For All by the Year 2000' (HFA) is discussed in Chapter 1.[2] The WHO European programme is intended to achieve a shift away from a narrow medical view of health towards an understanding of the social influences on health. It emphasizes integration of health services with other related activities such as education, recreation, environmental improvements and social welfare. (This is often referred to as 'intersectoral action' or 'intersectoral collaboration' and, more recently, in *The Health of the Nation* documents as 'healthy alliances'.) The European Office of WHO (WHO EURO) is monitoring and reviewing member states' progress in reaching HFA year 2000 targets. Launched in June 1985, the WHO EURO 'Europe against Cancer' campaign has had considerable influence on cancer education, both in the UK and throughout Europe.[3]

The Government

Government departments, particularly the Department of Health, but also the Department of Social Security, the Home Office, the Department for Education and Employment, the Department of the Environment, the Department of Transport and the Ministry of Agriculture, Fisheries and Food, have an interest in, and responsibility for, health promotion, through the impact of legislation and economic and fiscal policies on health.

There is more about national strategies for health in Chapter 7 section on national health strategies

The publication of the Government's national strategies for health in the late 1980s and 1990s signalled a major change towards the pursuit of improved health, rather than focusing almost exclusively on the provision of treatment services and health care.

The Government has also taken a lead in tackling health problems in other areas, such as the problem of drug misuse. A three year strategy for tackling drugs in England, *Tackling Drugs Together*, was published in 1995.[4] The aims were to increase safety of communities from drug-related harm, to reduce the acceptability and availability of drugs to young people and to reduce the health risks and other damage related to drug misuse. It required health authorities to set up multiagency Drug Action Teams to produce a local plan, coordinate work, and create one or more Drug Reference Groups to bring together a wide range of people and agencies to work on issues at a more local level.

Other National and Local Organizations

The Training Agency. This is the country's national training authority.[5] It operates as an executive agency within the Department for Education and Employment, and reports to the Secretary of State. It is responsible for the development and delivery of government sponsored vocational education programmes.

Training and Enterprise Councils (TECs). These are independent companies, directed by local business leaders, with a budget transferred from the Training Agency. There are about 80 TECs in England and Wales with a remit to provide employment training for local businesses and individuals. It includes training for unemployed people so that they have the skills required for local jobs. Obviously the opportunity, and the competence, to work are important influences on health, and training may include opportunities for health education.

National Voluntary Organizations and Pressure Groups. There are many national organizations concerned with health promotion, some of which have regional and/or local branches. An example of an organization which has no local network is The Advisory Council on Alcohol and Drug Education (TACADE). Organizations which have local branches include the National Childbirth Trust (NCT), the National Association for Mental Health (MIND) and the Citizens Advice Bureaux. Most of these organizations produce educational material, and some run training courses for professionals and/or the public. Some organizations primarily act as pressure groups, for example Friends of the Earth.

Professional associations, such as the British Medical Association (BMA), the Royal College of Nursing (RCN), the Royal College of General Practitioners, and the Chartered Institute for Environmental Health, have been influential in policy making, in pressing for legislative changes and in the practice and training of their members in health promotion.

Trade Unions are active in promoting health and safety at work both through negotiating workplace conditions and through health and safety representatives. The Health and Safety Executive also oversees the implementation of health and safety at work legislation.

Commercial and Industrial Organizations. These have a role in safeguarding the public health. Examples include companies providing water, refuse removal companies, and the transport industries. In recent years, many facilities with a public health protection function have been privatized and this has produced new problems. For example, should water companies have the right to cut off supplies to consumers who do not pay their bills, when a possible consequence of this is the occurrence and spread of infectious diseases such as dysentery?

Manufacturers and Retailers. Manufacturers are increasingly taking the health and safety aspects of their products into account. These include manufacturers of children's wear and toys, food manufacturers, producers of 'green' household products, and pharmaceutical companies. Large supermarket chains have made an increasingly wide range of 'healthy' options available to the public, such as fat-reduced and low-sugar foods. These trends are due to increased consumer demands reflecting heightened awareness of health issues.

See Chapter 11.
The Mass Media. Health education is undertaken by national and local mass media, such as television, radio, newspapers and magazines.

Churches and Religious Organizations. Churches and religious organizations play an important part in developing values, attitudes and beliefs that affect health. Some provide training in skills, such as meditation, which can improve mental, emotional and spiritual health.

The National Health Service (NHS)

The Structure of the NHS

The structure and organization of the NHS can also influence health. Fundamental changes in the way the NHS is run were brought about with the 1990 National Health Service and Community Care Act. Overall policy and strategy for the NHS is now set by the NHS Executive, based at Quarry House in Leeds. The Executive also has regional offices.

One key feature of the NHS reforms was the division of the NHS into 'purchasing' and 'providing' functions. 'Purchasers' or 'commissioners' decide what health care is required for the population and purchase it, setting and monitoring contracts with local hospitals and community services. 'Providers' provide the services, working to the contracts they have won from the purchasers.

These 'internal market' reforms, set out in the 'Working for Patients' White Paper proposals (1989) transformed the structure and character of the NHS in the 1990s, by creating a competitive market within the NHS and between the NHS and other bodies such as the private and voluntary sectors.[6] The separation of hospital and community health services into NHS Trusts (independently managed units within the NHS) raised fears about the fragmentation of the NHS, and whether we shall continue to have a truly *national* health service. Concern about fragmentation was further fuelled by the GP fundholding scheme, whereby GPs are allocated funds to purchase care for their patients from the hospital of the GP's choice, instead of being sent to the hospitals of their health authority's choice.

The concept of health gain is discussed in Chapter 2.
On the other hand, health authorities could now place a new emphasis on purchasing for 'health gain'. Contracts for health services could focus on health outcomes, in terms of the improved health of the population served, and include health promotion as part of the contract.[7] In some ways, therefore, the NHS reforms were a positive force for driving national health improvement forwards, and in other ways the reforms created new barriers to the implementation of local strategies for health.

The change of government in 1997 brought a new approach, with an emphasis on removing the competitive 'market place' approach and moving towards working in a spirit of cooperation.[8] We wait to see what impact this will have.

National Health Promotion Agencies

The Health Education Authority[9] (previously the Health Education Council) was established as a special health authority within the NHS in 1987. Under its constitution, it is required to provide information and advice about health directly to members of the public and to support other organizations and people who provide health education to members of the public. It also has an input into wider public health policy through its advice to the Secretary of State for Health. The Authority published a strategy in 1993 which states that the HEA's strategic objective is to ensure that by the year 2000 the people of England are more knowledgeable, better motivated and increasingly able to acquire and maintain good health.[10] A new strategy is expected in 1997/98.

Like the rest of the NHS, the HEA works by winning contracts, from the Department of Health and other agencies.[11] Its work includes, for example, contracts for public health promotion programmes on promoting physical activity (*Active for Life*) and preventing skin cancer (*Sun Know How*).[12] It has also developed the 'Health at Work in the NHS' initiative, commissioned by the NHS Management Executive, which aims to ensure that, as an employer, the NHS promotes healthy workplaces and thereby contributes to the health and well-being of its employees.[13] The NHS employs five percent of the total working population, and in addition, NHS staff are an important influence on the health-related behaviour of the public, through demonstrating their own commitment to practices conducive to health ('practising what they preach').

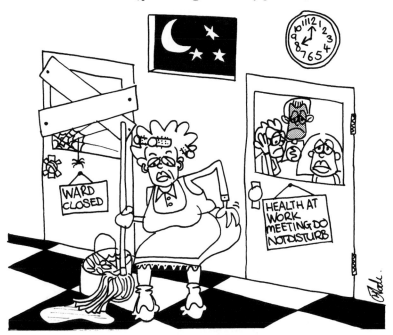

The NHS promotes healthy workplaces

The Health Education Board for Scotland (HEBS) is the national agency responsible for health education in Scotland.[14] It organizes programmes, projects, training, research and evaluation at national level, and supports health boards and local education authorities with their own health education.

The Health Promotion Agency for Northern Ireland and Health Promotion Wales are bodies performing similar functions for Northern Ireland and Wales.[15]

The Institute of Health and Care Development (IHCD) (the successor body for the operational functions of the NHS Training Division) is the national agency responsible for developing the human resources within the NHS and beyond. It works in partnership with other NHS, care and educational organizations, such as the Open University and the NHS Executive. It is a self-financing trading agency. (A development unit of the NHS Executive retains responsibility for overall policy and strategy.) Some products of the IHCD help to ensure that training in health promotion is covered in training schemes for NHS managers and health professions.[16]

Health Authorities and Boards

Following the NHS reforms in 1991, an increasing number of small Health Authorities (Health Boards in Scotland, Health and Social Services Boards in Northern Ireland) began to merge into larger ones. In 1996, all Health Authorities (HAs) merged with Family Health Services Authorities (FHSAs). FHSAs were previously the bodies responsible for primary health care services, and managed the contracts for local GPs, dentists, pharmacists and opticians; all these functions are now carried out by health authorities. A further change in 1996 was that Regional Health Authorities were abolished, and replaced with regional offices ('outposts') of the NHS Executive. In April 1996, the final position following these reorganizations was that there were one hundred HAs in England, divided into eight regions with between nine and sixteen HAs in each. Wales had five health authorities; Scotland had fifteen health boards and there were four health and social services boards in Northern Ireland. (We do not expect the Labour Government elected in 1997 to bring in further organizational change to this structure except that there may be mergers of smaller health authorities.)

As we outlined above, as a result of the 1990 NHS and Community Care Act, HAs now have the 'purchaser' role. They are responsible for purchasing the range of health services required to meet the needs of the population of the area served by the health authority. Services can be purchased from NHS Trusts (which are self-governing health services, usually hospitals and/or community services), private health care organizations, or voluntary organizations. Each HA has a Director of Public Health who is responsible for monitoring the health of the local community and determining health needs.

There has been concern that the extended roles of health authorities as commissioners of hospital and community services, and as managers of primary care services, has overshadowed the function of disease prevention and health promotion for their populations. A group of HA chief executives who believe in the central importance of health promotion and wish to stimulate debate and develop a shared understanding of best practice have joined together to form the Health Promotion Network.[17]

NHS Trusts

NHS Trusts are self-governing units of health services. Many run hospitals or groups of hospitals; others run community services; some run both hospital and community services; some run specific services such as ambulance services or services for people with learning difficulties. All these, of course, have a part to play in health promotion, particularly with opportunities for health education and preventive health work.

Local Specialist Health Promotion Services

Health Promotion Services (sometimes called 'specialist health promotion services') are an NHS service. They may be located in HAs, in NHS Trusts or organized as an 'agency' within HAs. In the early and mid 1990s, after the introduction of the NHS reforms, these services were subject to reorganization in order to fit into the new 'purchaser/provider' structure. Some are located within HAs, but most ended up in NHS trusts.[18] In addition to not fitting easily into the purchaser/provider divide, other factors such as short-term and decreasing funding,[19] and a perceived lack of a secure knowledge base, have compounded feelings of vulnerability about the future of health promotion specialists.[20] But wherever they are located, they are broadly responsible for the provision of expert advice, training, programmes and resources to support local health promotion. Health promotion specialists liaise with other health promotion agents and agencies both within and outside the NHS, to ensure that activities, wherever initiated, are coordinated and supported.[21]

Regional Education and Development Groups and Local Consortia

The NHS Executive has now devolved responsibility for the training of NHS staff to Regional Education and Development Groups and Local Consortia with a remit for purchasing education for NHS staff. The arrangements were formalized in April 1996 and views differ about whether they are either shaping up well or are a 'dog's breakfast.'[22] The intention is to make employers responsible for planning and commissioning education and training for their workforce. Consortia are made up of purchasers, providers (NHS and non-NHS) and GPs. The Consortia have training budgets and commission non-medical education and training. Each Consortium is represented on its area's Regional Education and Development Group, which also includes representatives of the NHS regional office.

Primary Health Care Teams

The WHO International Conference on Primary Health Care in Alma-Ata (1978) defined primary health care as:

> *essential health care ... made universally accessible to individuals and families in the community ... It forms an integral part both of the country's health system, of which it is the central function and main focus, and of the overall social and economic development of the community.*

Primary health care teams are the first point of people's contact with the National Health Service, bringing health care as close as possible to where people live and work. The role of health promotion in primary health care has been reviewed and government documents in the 1980s emphasized the importance of health education in primary health care settings.[23] The role of primary care in the NHS has been emphasized in the 1990s.[24] This has been underlined in the changes to GP contracts and with the identification of the role of primary health care teams in national strategies for health. Some GPs are now purchasers as well as providers (GP purchasers are referred to as 'fundholders') (see the previous section on the health service reforms) and the NHS Executive has evolved the concept of a 'primary care-led NHS'.[25] We expect that there will be some changes introduced by the Labour Government, including changes to fundholding and the development of the role of GPs in working with Health Authorities to commission health services.

Workbooks for primary care teams focusing on their role in prevention, especially of coronary heart disease and strokes, have proved useful.[26] The work of the HEA Primary Health Care Unit is contributing to focusing health improvement work on primary health care.[27]

In Britain, the work of primary health care is shared by a team. The exact membership of each primary health care team varies but it usually includes the following:

General practitioners. The GP is an independent contractor, and has a contract with a Health Authority, providing a comprehensive range of medical services for 24 hours a day, seven days a week, to those patients in the practice, and to those outside the practice in an emergency. GP contracts set targets for the GP in areas such as immunization and cervical cytology (smear tests for early detection of cervical cancer), and health promotion programmes. In the early 1990s, there were important changes in the contracts for GPs, and specific payments were introduced as incentives for undertaking health promotion work. In 1993 the GP contract was amended, in response to criticism of the arrangements for health promotion, and a system was introduced which allowed GPs to receive payments for health promotion services on specific topics linked to heart disease risk factors. In 1996, the system was changed again, so that GPs receive payment for health promotion programmes of their choice. These programmes have to be agreed by a local committee made up of GPs and health authority staff.

Practice managers. These are key people in enabling the smooth running of practices. They have overall responsibility for ensuring that patients are efficiently, confidentially and caringly received at the practice. They are responsible for appointing receptionists and for arranging in-service training for them. They have an important role in health promotion because they can control access to health information for patients. The role of the practice manager has become more complex as GP fundholding developed, and practice managers have a key role in managing the contracts and financial work involved.

Receptionists. The uniqueness of the receptionist's role and its inherent challenges have been recognized and courses are now available within colleges of further education. These emphasize the roles of the receptionist in health promotion and provide training in communication skills.

Practice nurses. These may hold clinics for people with chronic conditions such as diabetes and asthma, and provide encouragement, education and check-ups. Health promotion work such as screening clinics for heart disease, Well Woman and Well Man clinics, and helping patients to stop smoking, are also part of their health promotion role. An open learning package for practice nurses has been published by the English National Board for Nursing.[28]

The district nursing team. This includes the district nursing sister/charge nurse and a team of enrolled nurses and auxiliaries. They are responsible for assessing, implementing and evaluating the nursing needs of patients at home. They have an important role in the education of both patients and their carers.

Health visitors. Health visiting consists of planned activities aimed at the promotion of health and this is achieved through working one-to-one and in groups. Health visitors work with a large network of others concerned with health, sickness and social and educational services.

Community psychiatric nurses (CPN). With the implementation of the policy to transfer people with mental health problems out of hospitals and into the community, the community psychiatric nurse is often a key member of the Primary Health Care Team. CPNs are involved in all forms of care for the mentally ill and people with learning difficulties and in family counselling work.

Community midwives. Midwives provide services to all childbearing women during pregnancy and for between 10 and 28 days after the birth of a child. They work closely with the GP and the health visitor in parent education.

Some Primary Health Care Teams also include people with jobs specifically concerned with prevention and health promotion, such as health promotion nurses or primary care facilitators who specialize in helping practices to prevent heart disease.

Other Health Professions

Many other health professions, such as hospital nurses, dentists, hospital and retail pharmacists, opticians and the professions allied to medicine (such as chiropodists and dietitians) have a part to play in health promotion, especially in patient education.[29]

Community Health Councils

Community Health Council members can be an influence on health authority health promotion policies and plans. They may also carry out health education as part of their work with users of health services.

Health Services Outside the NHS

Alternative health practitioners. These include homoeopaths, chiropractors, osteopaths, acupuncturists and practitioners of herbal medicine. They can play a part in promoting health and relieving health problems, often using a more holistic approach than conventional medicine.[30] They are also known as complementary or natural health practitioners, and may be available on the NHS.[31]

Private agencies. Some of these are funded through insurance schemes and offer a range of health checks and preventive medical services.

Local Authorities

In the 1980s the 'new' public health was characterized by increasing involvement of Local Authority Departments in health issues, which often led to the restructuring of Local Authority Committees and Departments.[32] Many Local Authorities have health committees and full-time health officers responsible for promoting liaison and consultation between all departments of the Council, and with other bodies, on matters related to health. Health Officers are most frequently based in the Department of Environmental Health, but are sometimes part of a Health Unit directly accountable to the Chief Executive, or based in the Social Services Department.

A package produced by the Health Education Authority describes initiatives by Local Authorities.[33] The Health Education Authority also funded (in 1990) a three-year project to explore the health promotion potential within a local authority setting. The purpose of the project was to develop a national health promotion training and professional development strategy for local authority staff with a health promotion role; a training manual is available.[34] More recently, the HEA commissioned and published an audit of health promotion work in local authorities[35] and a guide on developing health strategy in local authorities.[36]

Environmental Health Officers. The measures necessary to deal with the physical factors in the environment which threaten health, in the widest sense, constitute what is known as 'environmental health'. The organization of environmental health services is mainly the function of Local Authority Environmental Health Departments, but may be combined with housing or recreation and leisure. National and local legislation gives power to these departments to take advisory and legal action on behalf of people who visit, live, or work in an area. The scope for health promotion by these departments is wide and constantly growing, along with new threats to the environment. Many departments appoint specialist officers to work on specific health issues, such as home safety or recycling.

The Local Education Authority. LEAs have responsibility for health education in schools and further education colleges through the work of teachers and lecturers.[37] LEAs may also have advisors with specific responsibility for health education, and other staff who provide advice, support and training in health education for teachers. With the introduction of Local Management of Schools (LMS), and LEA resource constraints in the 1990s, many of these posts have disappeared.

There have been considerable developments in school health education over the last twenty years: many major curriculum development projects have taken place, resulting in significant progress.[38] Other significant policies affecting health education include the National Curriculum introduced in 1989, the changing role of school governors and the shift of budget-holding responsibilities from local education authorities to schools themselves (LMS).

There is more about promoting health in schools in Chapter 16.

Social Services staff, including social workers, staff of residential homes and home helps, are often concerned with improving the health of clients. With the movement towards care in the community, the role of Social Services Departments in promoting the health of vulnerable groups such as elderly people, mentally ill people and people with learning difficulties is increasing.[39]

Many other local authority staff have a role in health promotion, such as recreation and leisure officers, housing officers and youth and community workers.

Other Local Organizations and Groups

There are numerous individuals and groups at local level who help to promote particular aspects of health. Some notable ones are as follows:

Institutions of Higher Education. Universities are responsible for the basic professional training of the professions with health promotion roles. They are also increasingly involved in post-basic and continuing education for health promoters, including running Health Education Certificate Courses.[40] The Open University has been very active, both in developing degree courses in health, especially useful to professionals without a first degree, and in producing community education material on health issues for the general public.[41]

Local Voluntary and Community Groups. A huge range of local voluntary and community groups exists, many of which undertake educational work on health matters. Patients associations, self-help groups, environmental action groups and youth groups are just a few examples.

Community based work in health promotion is discussed in Chapter 15.

Employers. Employers can be active in developing health-promoting policies and conditions in the workplace. Personnel officers and occupational health staff, in particular, are vital to the implementation of workplace policies and in promoting the well-being of staff.

There is more about promoting health in workplaces in Chapter 16.

Police and probation officers. The police protect the public from crime and violence, take action to prevent misuse of drugs and alcohol and help to ensure road safety. Prison officers and probation officers are involved in the health and well-being of prisoners and their families, and may also be involved in initiatives such as health-promoting prisons, health education about HIV/AIDS, and educational programmes on sensible drinking for drink/drive offenders.

The next exercise is designed to help you to identify the health promotion agents and agencies which are important for your work. There is much to gain by having good local knowledge of other people you can work with or refer people to.

The Informal Network

Finally, as we mentioned in the opening paragraph of this chapter, it is essential to remember that the whole informal network of family, friends and neighbours is of great significance in shaping people's health beliefs and behaviour and in providing healthy living conditions.

Improving Your Health Promotion Role

A number of factors affect the development of the health promotion role of professionals. The need for improved training is recognized. One of the difficulties

Exercise 4.1	What's on your patch? Finding out about your local agents and agencies in health promotion

Think of the geographical 'patch' where you work, and identify its boundaries as clearly as you can. For example, this could be the area served by a GP practice, the catchment area served by a hospital/health service or the geographical patch defined as your responsibility as an environmental health officer or community worker.

Identify as many health promotion agents and agencies on your patch as you can, using Figure 4.1 and the list above as a checklist.

It is likely that you will know some of them very well and others not at all. Identify any which it would be helpful to know more about and plan to find out about them.

If there are some that you know nothing about, such as the community groups which exist on your patch, identify people who do know about them (such as local health visitors, health promotion departments) and plan to find out more.

is how to fit more into the already overcrowded curriculum of basic professional training courses. It may help to identify the core competencies health promoters need (such as basic communication skills) and to ensure that these are taught as part of basic professional training.

Post-basic courses, such as Health Education Certificate courses, and post-graduate diplomas and masters degrees in Health Education and Health Promotion are increasingly available, often in a range of learning modes such as full-time, part-time, college-based or open learning. It is now possible for students to accumulate 'credits' which they can use to contribute towards higher qualifications. Training is being developed which meets occupational standards of competence in the workplace, with the emphasis moving towards assessment of competencies: employees demonstrate whether they are competent to carry out particular activities.

There is more about occupational standards in Chapter 2.

The Department for Education and Employment have established a framework for developing occupational standards, and under this initiative the Care Sector Consortium has developed occupational standards for health promotion work.

All these developments help to minimize the time students are 'off the job' for training, provide more flexible training opportunities, and help managers to assure the quality of the work performance of their staff. In the fast changing world of health and social care, ensuring that staff are competent to carry out new roles is an increasingly important focus of the work of managers.

A problem for students is that they use trained professionals as examples to follow ('role models'), but research has long since shown that trained professionals themselves may not have the necessary skills.[42] This is particularly true of health promotion skills in networking, joint working, facilitating, marketing and political skills, which have not traditionally been included in professional training.

Some professionals have too narrow a concept of health and what is meant by health promotion and by health education. Therefore they may only use individual behaviour change approaches and fail to take advantage of opportunities for using alternative or complementary approaches. Lack of knowledge about which approaches to health promotion are likely to be effective in different circumstances is also a problem. Furthermore, the health promotion and health education needs of the professionals themselves may not have been met. They may be exhorted to be a good example but they are often not given the help they need to make health choices and carry these through.

In addition, resource constraints may hinder the professions from achieving their potential in health promotion. There may be staff shortages and work overload, leading to less time available for long-term health promotion work.

The need for education and training of policy makers and managers has also been highlighted.[43] More resources need to be put into the design and evaluation of training programmes.[44]

On the positive side, there is ample evidence that people want more information and welcome health education from, for example, general practitioners.[45] Evidence concerning the effectiveness of professionals in promoting health is growing.[46] The Department of Health has reviewed the contribution of nurses, midwives and health visitors to national health strategy, and provided guidance on how to target their activities most effectively.[47] The professional associations have played an important part in updating concepts about the health promotion role of their members.[48]

The Health Education Authority and the NHS Training Directorate (now the IHCD) have jointly commissioned a project to produce learning and resource materials for health service managers which will assist with promoting and spreading good practices in the management of health promotion work related to the national health gain strategy.[49]

In summary, some strategies have proved very useful in improving the role of professionals in health promotion. But overall education and training for professionals remains an underdeveloped area, particularly the training of policy-makers and managers and training in the skills of networking, joint working, facilitation, marketing and influencing policy and practice.

The following exercise is designed to help you to identify factors which help and hinder you in carrying out health promotion work, and what you might to do to improve the situation.

Exercise 4.2	**What helps and hinders your health promotion work?**

This exercise is designed to help you to identify helping and hindering forces in your own situation.

In a stable system, the forces for producing changes are equally offset by forces opposed to change. It is essential to pinpoint all the possible helping and hindering forces, so that you can take steps to increase the power of helping forces, and decrease the power of the hindering forces. The disruption of the balance results in progress towards change.

For your own situation:
● make a list of *forces which help you* in your health promotion work;
● make a list of *forces which hinder you* in your health promotion work;
● identify *ways of increasing the helpful forces;*
● identify *ways of decreasing the hindering forces;*

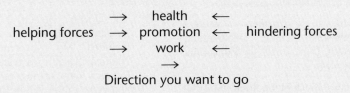

PRACTICE POINTS

- It is important to appreciate the whole range of agents and agencies with a health promotion role: informal and formal, local and national.

- Think about how you can best work together with other people and agencies.

- Ensure that you are clear about your own role in health promotion.

- Consider how you could improve your health promotion role, through education and training, or through identifying what helps and hinders your health promotion work and how the situation could be improved.

Recommended Reading

Health promotion by a range of different professionals in a variety of settings:

➤ Scriven A & Orme J (eds) (1996) *Health Promotion: professional perspectives*. Basingstoke: Macmillan/Open University. (Has chapters on health promotion in different settings: health service, local authority, education and youth organizations, voluntary sector and workplace.)

➤ Naidoo J & Wills J (1994) *Health Promotion: Foundations for Practice*. London: Baillière Tindall. (Chapter 13 discusses implementation in schools, workplaces and primary health care.)

➤ Tones K & Tilford S (1994) *Health education; effectiveness, efficiency and equity*. 2nd edn. London: Chapman & Hall. (Has chapters on health promotion in schools, health care settings, workplace and community.)

Two classic studies on informal sources of health education, and the role of women in family health:

➤ Blaxter M & Paterson E (1982) *Mothers and Daughters: A Three Generational Study of Health Attitudes and Behaviour*. London: Heinemann.

➤ Graham H (1984) *Women, Health and the Family*. London: Wheatsheaf Books.

Further reading on health promotion training needs:

➤ Simnett I & Lawrence T (1996) The role of health professions in health promotion: a review of current practice, training needs and training provisions. *Journal of the Institute of Health Education* **34**(3), 86–88.

Notes and References

1   Department of Health (1993) *Working Together for Better Health*. London: DoH.

2   WHO Regional Office for Europe (1985) *Targets for Health for All*. WHO, Scherfigsveg 8, DK-2100, Copenhagen, Denmark.

3   Department of Health (1993) 'Europe against Cancer', *Echo* (Health and Social Services in Europe and Overseas newsletter), July, p. 2.

4   White Paper *Tackling Drugs Together – a strategy for England 1995–1998*. Home Department, Department of Health, Department for Education, Cmd 2846. London: HMSO.

5   The Training Agency, Moorfoot, Sheffield, S1 4PQ. Tel: 01742 753275.

6   Secretaries of State for Health (1989) *Working for Patients*. London: HMSO.

7   Killoran A (1992) *Putting Health into Contracts*. London: Health Education Authority.

     Health Education Authority (1994) *Contracts for smoking prevention; current practice in the NHS*. London: HEA (Reviews progress in implementing policy on smoking prevention.)

8   The Queen's speech at the opening of the new Parliament following the general election in 1997 included 'My Government will improve the National Health Service .... They will bring forward new arrangements for decentralization and cooperation within the service and for ending the internal market.'

White Papers setting out the Government's intentions were published in December 1997: Secretary of State for Health (1997) *The New NHS: Modern, Dependable*. London: The Stationery Office.

A different White Paper was published for Scotland:

Department of Health/Scottish Office (1997) *Designed to Care: Renewing the National Health Service in Scotland*. London: The Stationery Office.

9   Health Education Authority, Trevelyan House, 30 Great Peter Street, London SW1P 2HW. Tel: 0171 222 5300. Fax: 0171 413 8900. http://www.hea.org.uk.

10 Health Education Authority (1993) *Strategic Plan 1993–1998*. London: HEA.

11 Health Education Authority (1995) *The New HEA: business prospectus for the HEA 1995/96*. London: HEA.

12 Health Education Authority (1996) *Keeping People Healthy – HEA Annual Report 1995/96*. London: HEA.

Health Education Authority (1997) *Working Together – HEA Annual Report 1996/97*. London: HEA.

13 Health Education Authority/NHS Management Executive (1992) *Health At Work in the NHS: Action Pack*. London: HEA.

14 Health Education Board for Scotland (HEBS). Woodburn House, Canaan Lane, Edinburgh EH10 4SG. Tel: 0131 536 5500. Fax: 0131 536 5501. http://www.hebs.scot.nhs.uk

HEBS publishes Annual Reports, a publications catalogue and strategic plan: Health Education Board for Scotland (1997) *Strategic Plan 1997–2002*. Edinburgh: HEBS.

15 Health Promotion Agency for Northern Ireland, 18 Ormeau Avenue, Belfast BT2 8HS. Tel: 01232 311611. The Agency publishes an Annual Report.

Health Promotion Wales, Ffynnon-las, Ty Glas Avenue, Llanishen, Cardiff, CF4 5DZ. Tel: 01222 752222.

Health Promotion Wales publishes an Annual Report and Catalogue of Publications.

16 For example, Health PICKUP is a modular training programme to develop the continuing management education needs of health care professionals. The modules include skills training in some of the core competencies required by health promoters: Meeting the Challenge of Change; Team Leadership for Quality Care; Communicating with Patients; Communicating with Organizations; and Using Research at Work.

The Institute of Health and Care Development, St Bartholomews Court, 18 Christmas Street, Bristol BS1 5BT. Tel: 0117 929 1029. Fax: 0117 925 0574.

17 Health Promotion Network (1996) Leader of the pack. *Health Service Journal* **12**, September, 28–29.

18 Milner S & French J (1997) *A Survey of Specialist Health Promotion Services in relation to purchasing and providing arrangements in England, Scotland, Wales and Northern Ireland carried out in November 1996*. North Cumbria Health Development Unit, Carlisle: Society of Health Education and Health Promotion Officers.

19 Milner S & French J (1997) A Survey of Specialist Health Promotion Services in relation to purchasing and providing arrangements in England, Scotland, Wales and Northern Ireland carried out in November 1996. North Cumbria Health Development Unit, Carlisle: Society of Health Education and Health Promotion Officers.

20 Nettleton, S and Burrows, R (1997) If health promotion is everybody's business what is the fate of the health promotion specialist? *Sociology of Health and Illness* **19**(1), 23–47.

21 For a review of the role of health education officers/health promotion specialists, see: Ewles, L (1993) Paddling Upstream for 50 Years: the role of health education officers. *Health Education Journal* **52/3**, 172–181.

22 Snell J (1997) Shaping Up. Special report on training. *Health Service Journal*, 6 March, pp. 3–8.

23 DHSS (1986) *Primary Health Care, an agenda for discussion*. London: HMSO.

DHSS (1987) *Promoting Better Health, The Government's Programme for Improving Primary Health Care*. White Paper (Cmd 249), London: HMSO.

24 For further reading on a primary care-led NHS, see:

Meads, G (ed.) (1996) *A Primary Care-led NHS: Putting it into practice*. London: Churchill Livingstone.

Office for Public Management (1997) *Achieving Health Gain through Health Promotion in a Primary Care-led NHS*. London: HEA.

The government has published a discussion document on the future of primary care: NHS Executive (1996) *Primary Care: The Future*. London: Department of Health.

25 NHS Executive (1995) *Developing NHS Purchasing and GP Fundholding: Towards a Primary Care-led NHS*. London: Department of Health.

The following three government white papers were issued in 1996, leading up to the NHS (Primary Care) Act 1997:
- *Primary Care – the future*
- *A Service with Ambitions* (looked at broad principles but included the concept of 'primary care-led NHS')
- *Choice and Opportunity*.

Following these publications, pilot initiatives were funded under 'Seizing the Opportunity' and 'Choice and Opportunity' schemes.

26 Tudor Hart J and Stilwell B (1988) *Prevention of Coronary Heart Disease and Strokes: a workbook for primary care teams*. London: Faber and Faber.

'Better Living, Better Life' is a resource for primary health care teams to help plan and implement health promotion programmes with patients. Produced by the Department of Health with the Royal College of General Practitioners, in consultation with many other agencies and individuals, it was circulated to every practice in England, Scotland and Wales in 1993. It is available as a full ring-bound version or a shorter book version, from the publishers:

Knowledge House Ltd, Redvers House, 13 Fairmile, Henley-on-Thames RG9 2JR. Tel: 01491 577151.

27 Primary Health Care Unit, Block 10, Churchill Hospital, Headington, Oxford OX3 7LJ. Tel: 01865 226061.

28 English National Board for Nursing (ENB) (1989) *HEALTH Promotion in Primary Health Care, an open learning package for practice nurses*. London: ENB with Learning Materials Design.

29 Books that focus on health promotion in clinical and hospital settings, using a practical topic-based approach, are:

Bright J (1997) *Health Promotion in Clinical Practice: Targeting the Health of the Nation*. London: Baillière Tindall.

McBride A (1995) *Health Promotion in Hospital: a practical handbook for nurses*. London: Scutari Press.

Books on health promotion specifically for nurses are:

Pike S & Forster D (eds) (1995) *Health promotion for all*. Edinburgh: Churchill Livingstone.

Dines A & Cribb A (eds) (1993) *Health Promotion: concepts and practice*. Oxford: Blackwell Science.

Three *Health of the Nation* publications which focus on the roles of specific health professionals are:

Department of Health (1993) *Targeting Practice: The Contribution of Nurses, Midwives and Health Visitors to the Health of the Nation*. London: DoH.

Institution of Environmental Health Officers (1993) *The Health of the Nation for Environmental Health*. London: The Institution of Environmental Health Officers.

Department of Health (1994) *Targeting Practice: The Contribution of State Registered Dietitians*. London: DoH.

On the role of pharmacists, see:

Health Education Authority & National Pharmaceutical Association (1994) *Health Promotion and the Community Pharmacist*. London: HEA.

30 Unattributed article (1992) Alternative Medicine on trial. *Which? Way to Health*. June, pp. 102–105.

31 Burch C (1993) Alternatives to the NHS. *Which? Way to Health*, August, pp. 125–127.

A series of three articles on complementary therapies covered regulations and standards, NHS funding and working relationships with the NHS:

Hodges C (1995) Complementary regulations. *Healthlines* **20**, March 1995, 11–13.

Nelson F (1995) Alternative forms of funding. *Healthlines* **21**, April 1995, 17–19.

Nelson F (1995) A marriage of convenience? *Healthlines* **23**, June 1995, 12–13.

32 See a case study by Peter Allen on Healthy Oxford 2000, in:

Simnett I (1995) *Managing Health Promotion: Developing health organisations and communities*, pp. 168–170. Chichester: Wiley.

33 Simnett I (1991) *Promoting Health – Local Authorities in Action*. London: Health Education Authority.

34 King M (1994) *Promoting Health: A health promotion training pack for local authorities*. Tameside Metropolitan Borough Council.

35 Moran G (1996) *Promoting Health and Local Government*. London: Health Education Authority and Local Government Management Board.

36 Health Education Authority and Local Government Management Board (1997) *Health on the agenda? A guide to health strategy development for local authorities*. London: HEA.

37 For further reading on health promotion in educational settings, see:

Nutbeam D, Haglund B, Farley P & Tillgren P (eds) (1990) *Youth Health Promotion: from theory to practice in school and community*. London: Forbes Publications.

Opportunities for Health and Education to Work Together: Linking the Health of the Nation targets to the National Curriculum. Available from:

Outset Publishing, Saffron House, 59 High Street, Battle, East Sussex TN33 0EN.

Cale L (1997) Health education in schools: in a state of good health? *International Journal of Health Education* **35**(2), 59–62. (Argues that school health education is not in good health, and must fight for its survival and growth in a rapidly changing educational climate.)

O'Donnell T & Gray G (1993) *The Health Promoting College*. London: Health Education Authority.

Simnett I (1996) How to become a health promoting college. *Healthlines*, July/August, 18–19.

38   National Curriculum Council (1990) *Curriculum Guidance 5*. Health Education National Curriculum Council, 15–17 New St, York YO1 2RA.

Lewis D (1993) Oh For Those Halcyon Days! – a review of the development of school health education over 50 years. *Health Education Journal* **52**(3), 161–171.

There is now a large and growing number of curriculum development materials, teachers' guides and classroom materials for health education in schools. These cover both broad health education programmes and work in specific subject areas such as alcohol, drugs, smoking, dental health, preventing heart disease and preventing child abuse. There are materials for primary, secondary and special schools, and colleges; and for use during initial teacher training, in-service training of teachers, and for use with school governors. For details, contact the Health Promotion Department in your local health authority, NHS Trust, or health board.

The Advisory Council on Alcohol and Drug Education (TACADE) produces material and runs in-service training. Address: 1 Hulme Place, The Crescent, Salford M5 4QA.

39   Department of Health (1989) *Caring for People: community care in the next decade and beyond*. White Paper (Cmd 849). London: HMSO.

40   Health Education Certificate courses for professionals are available on a day release or open learning mode, from universities and colleges of further and higher education in the UK.

The Open University also runs courses in health promotion. For further details contact The Open University, Walton Hall, Milton Keynes, MK7 6AA. Tel: 01908 653743.

41   For details of the Open University Community Education materials, contact:

Department of Community Education, The Open University, Walton Hall, Milton Keynes, MK7 6AA. Tel: 01908 653743.

42   Faulkner, A *et al.* (1985) *Communication in Nurse Education: Survey of schools of nursing. Research Project 1982–85*. London: Health Education Council.

More recent evidence suggests that the situation has not changed substantially. See: Mitchinson, S (1995) A review of the health promotion and health beliefs of traditional and Project 2000 student nurses. *Journal of Advanced Nursing* **21**, 356–363.

43   See, for example:

Fitzgerald L, Ashburner L and Ferlie E (1993) The Learning Curve. *Health Service Journal* **4**, 24.

Macleod Clark J, Wilson-Barnett J, Latter S and Maben J (1992) *Health Education and Health Promotion in Nursing – a study of practice in acute areas*. Executive summary and full report available from The Department of Nursing Studies, Kings College London, Cornwall House Annex, Waterloo Road, London SE1 8TX.

Cant S, Killoran A & Calnan M (1993) *Preventing Heart Disease – the role of the community nurse*. London: Health Education Authority.

44   Blinkhorn A S and Mackie I C (1995) Training to encourage health promotion – a case report. *Journal of the Institute of Health Education* **33**(3), 90–92.

45   See, for example:

Office for Public Management (1997) *Achieving Health Gain through Health Promotion in a Primary Care-Led NHS*, p. 42. London: Health Education Authority.

46   See, for example:

Killoran A (ed.) (1993) *Giving Up Smoking – does patient education work?* Summary report from the Health Education Authority. London: Health Education Authority.

47   Department of Health (1993) *Targeting Practice: The Contribution of Nurses, Midwives and Health Visitors to the Health of the Nation*. London: DoH

48   For example, the British Dietetic Association has trawled good practice related to the role of dietitians in The Health of the Nation:

Department of Health (1994) *Targeting Practice: The Contribution of State Registered Dietitians*. London: DoH.

The Institution of Environmental Health Officers has produced a document on the role of local authority environmental health services:

Institution of Environmental Health Officers (1993) *The Health of the Nation for Environmental Health*. London: Institution of Environmental Health Officers.

The Royal College of General Practitioners and the British Medical Association have produced an information pack for GPs:

Royal College of General Practitioners/British Medical Association (1996) *The Health of the Nation: What you can do about it*. An Information Pack from General Practitioners for General Practitioners. London: RCGP/BMA.

49   Health Education Authority (1996) *Health Improvement: A resource for managers in health and social care*. London: HEA.

2 PLANNING AND MANAGING FOR EFFECTIVE PRACTICE

PART SUMMARY

Part 2 aims to provide guidance on how you can:

- plan and evaluate your health promotion work using a basic framework;
- identify the views and needs of the clients/users/receivers of health promotion, and set priorities for your work;
- link your work to the efforts of colleagues and to local and national strategies;
- use an 'evidence-based' approach, through using published research, doing your own research when necessary, and auditing your work, thus ensuring that your efforts are effective and provide value for money;
- organize yourself and manage your work in order to be effective and efficient;
- develop skills to work more effectively with colleagues and people from other organizations.

In Chapter 5 we set out a seven-stage planning and evaluation cycle, which will help you to clarify what you are trying to achieve, what you are going to do, and how you will know whether you are succeeding.

In Chapter 6 we consider what a 'need' for health promotion means, and we describe the sources of information you require to identify the needs of a community, a group, or an individual person. We provide guidelines on how to assess needs and set priorities.

Chapter 7 provides guidance in greater depth on the knowledge and skills required to plan health promotion activities effectively. We include guidance on how you can contribute to strategic plans and complement what other people are doing.

In Chapter 8 we focus on how you can develop the skills to manage yourself and your work effectively, including managing information, writing reports, using time effectively, planning project work, managing change and working for quality.

Chapter 9 is about how to work with other people, including communicating with colleagues; coordination and teamwork; participating in meetings; and working in health alliances with other organizations.

5 The Basic Planning and Evaluation Process

SUMMARY

In this chapter we outline a seven-stage planning and evaluation cycle useful in the everyday work of health promoters:

1. identify needs and priorities;
2. set aims and objectives;
3. decide the best way of achieving aims;
4. identify resources;
5. plan evaluation methods;
6. set an action plan;
7. action!

We give examples of aims, objectives and action plans, and exercises on setting aims and objectives and using the planning framework to turn ideas into action.

This chapter is about planning and evaluation at the level of your own daily work in health promotion. It provides a basic framework which you can use to plan and evaluate your health promotion activities, whether you work with clients on a one-to-one or group basis, or undertake specific projects or programmes.

Planning is a process which ends up with a plan; at its very simplest, a plan should give you the answers to three questions:

- what am I trying to achieve?
- what am I going to do?
- how will I know whether I have been successful?

If you are really clear on these three issues you should be well on the way to effective and efficient health promotion work.

The first question 'what am I trying to achieve?' is concerned with identifying needs and priorities, then with being clear about your specific aims and objectives, which we discuss in more detail below.

The second question 'what am I going to do?' can be helpfully broken down into smaller steps:

- selecting the best way of achieving your aims from a variety of possible ways;
- identifying the resources you are going to use;
- setting a clear action plan of who does what and when.

The third question 'how will I know whether I have been successful?' means that you will need to include plans for evaluation in your overall plan. This highlights a very important point: that evaluation is an integral part of your overall plan, not tacked on as an afterthought. It is all too easy to plan a project, carry it out, and then think about evaluating it, often too late to capture the information you need.

Putting these together, we have a seven-stage flowchart (Figure 5.1).

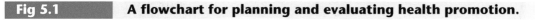

Fig 5.1   **A flowchart for planning and evaluating health promotion.**

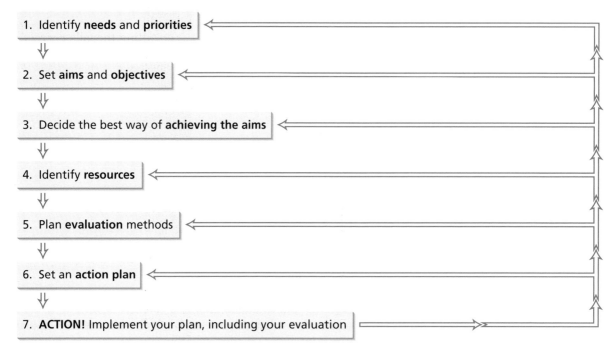

1. Identify **needs** and **priorities**

2. Set **aims** and **objectives**

3. Decide the best way of **achieving the aims**

4. Identify **resources**

5. Plan **evaluation** methods

6. Set an **action plan**

7. **ACTION!** Implement your plan, including your evaluation

There are three key points to note about using the flowchart. One is that the arrows on the flowchart lead you round in a circle. This is because, as you carry out your plan and evaluation, you will probably find things which make you re-think and change your original ideas. For example, things you might want to change could include: working on a client need you found you had overlooked; scaling down your objectives because they were too ambitious; or using different educational or publicity materials because you found that they were not as useful or effective as you had hoped.

The second point is that the main direction of the arrows is in an anti-clockwise direction, but, in reality, planning is not a tidy process. You may actually start at Stage 6 with a basic idea of something you would like to do. Then you think more about it, and this leads you to clarify exactly what your aims are (Stage 2). Next, you might think about what resources you are going to need (Stage 4) and realize that you do not have enough time or money to do what you had in mind. So you go back to Stage 2 and modify your aims. Then you think about the best way of achieving them (Stage 3) and work out an action plan (Stage 6). After that, you start to think seriously about how you will know whether you are successful (Stage 5) and you put your evaluation plans into your action plan (Stage 6 again). This does not imply that you are muddle-headed or 'doing it wrong'. On the contrary, you are continually reviewing and improving your plan, using the framework appropriately to help you keep on course.

The third point is that planning takes place at many levels. If you are embarking on a major project, you will need to take time to plan it in depth and detail. On the other hand, you may simply be planning a short one-to-one session with a client; in that case you will still need to plan, and to go through all the stages, but it may be a process which takes only a few minutes and does not even get written down.

For example, a chiropodist seeing a patient with a foot care problem may identify that the patient needs knowledge and skills in cutting toenails correctly. She decides that her aim is to give some basic information and training about this. She will know if she has been successful by getting feedback from the patient about how he managed next time she sees him. She identifies a leaflet that she can give him to reinforce what she says. She decides on an action plan of explanation, demonstration and then getting the patient to practise. She reviews the patient's toenail cutting skills next time she sees him, reinforcing or correcting as necessary. All this planning takes place inside the chiropodist's head, and is an integral part of her everyday professional practice.

We will now look at each stage of the planning and evaluation flowchart.

Stage 1. Identify Needs and Priorities

How do you find out what health promotion is needed? If you think you already know, what are you basing your judgement on? Who has identified the need: you, your clients or someone else? These questions begin to show that identifying need is a complex process, and we look at it in depth in the next chapter.

You may have a long list of health promotion needs you would like to respond to, but you cannot do everything, so another question is how you establish your priorities. Again, we discuss this in detail in the next chapter. All there is to say now is that you must have a clear view about which needs you are responding to, and what your priorities are.

Stage 2. Set Aims and Objectives

This is the point where you ask yourself 'what exactly am I trying to achieve?' and go on asking it until you have the answer very clearly defined.

People use a whole gamut of words to describe statements of 'what I am trying to achieve' – aims, objectives, targets, goals, mission, purpose, achievement, result, product, outcomes. Though there is no universal agreement about the precise meaning of these words, it can be helpful to think of them as forming a hierarchy (Fig. 5.2). At the top of the hierarchy are words that tell why your job exists, such as your job purpose or your mission. In the middle of the hierarchy are words that describe what you are trying to do in general terms, such as your goals or aims. At the bottom of the hierarchy are words that describe in specific detail what you are trying to do, such as targets or objectives.

Fig 5.2   **A heirarchy of aims.**

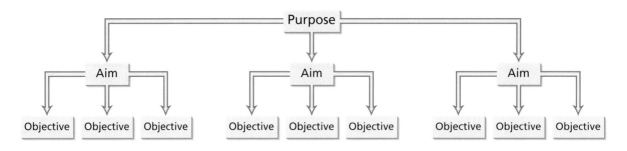

It is worth noting that objectives can be of different kinds. *Health* objectives are usually expressed as the outcome or end state to be achieved in terms of health status, such as reduced rates of illness or death. However, in health promotion work objectives are often expressed in terms of a step along the way towards an ultimate improvement in the health of individuals or populations. In health education work, *educational* objectives are framed in terms of the knowledge, attitudes or behaviour to be exhibited by the learner. Objectives can also be in terms of *other kinds of changes*, such as a change in health policy (e.g. introducing a no-smoking policy in a workplace), or health promotion practice (e.g. providing health information in minority ethnic languages or starting a coronary rehabilitation programme).

See the section below on setting educational objectives.

A further point is that the term 'targets' is increasingly used in health promotion. Targets usually specify how the achievement of an objective will be *measured*, in terms of quantity, quality, and time (the date by which the objective will be achieved). So, a *health target* can be defined as a measurable improvement in health status, by a given time, which achieves a health objective. This is the approach used in national strategies for health, such as *The Health of the Nation* and its successor strategy *Our Healthier Nation*.[1] The objectives are framed as *health* objectives, and the targets are framed as *health targets* (changes in rates of death or illness by a specific date) or *behaviour targets* (such as changes in population rates of smoking or drinking by a specific date).

There is more about national strategies and targets in Chapter 7 (section on National Health Strategies).

We now turn to how the individual health promoter sets aims, objectives and targets.

When planning health promotion initiatives, it is the levels of aims, objectives and targets that we need to focus on. (We choose to use the words aims, objectives and targets in our discussion here, but, as we said above, many other terms are used such as goals and outcomes.)

Your aims (or aim – there does not have to be more than one) are broad statements of what you are trying to achieve. Your objectives are much more specific, and setting these is a critical stage in the planning process.

Objectives are the desired end state (or result, or outcome) to be achieved within a specified time period. They are not tasks or activities. Objectives are:

■ **challenging.** The objective should provide you with a challenge. It should 'stretch' you.

Exercise 5.1	**Clarifying your purpose, aims and objectives**

Think about this example of a health promoter's purpose, aims and objectives: Mark is a health promoter working for a Local Authority. His *purpose* is to reduce inequalities in health in the population living and working in the borough. To do this, one of his *aims* is to improve levels of health knowledge of black and ethnic minority groups. One of his *objectives* is to improve access to health information through the use of videos. He sets a target of having a selection of ten health videos in six languages available in 25 shops within four months.

Now:

1. **Thinking of your own job, write down what you believe to be its mission or purpose.**
2. **Then give an example of one of the health promotion aims you are trying to achieve.**
3. **Finally, give an example of an objective you are trying to achieve, in fulfilment of the aim you selected.**

If you can't find a real-life example, make up an example of what you would like to do if you had the opportunity.

- **attainable.** On the other hand it should be both realistic and achievable within the constraints of your situation.
- **as measurable as possible.** You should try to identify your objectives in terms that are as measurable as possible, for example specifying quantity, quality and a time when they will be achieved (i.e. you are clear about your *targets*). For example (using the example in the exercise), an objective of 'to improve access to health information through the use of videos ...' has been improved by working out the appropriate number of videos and languages, and then specifying the target as 'to have ten videos in six languages ...'.
- **relevant.** It should be consistent with the aims of the organization and with the overall aims of your job.

It is often difficult to distinguish between aims and objectives and action plans. For example, a dietician who wants to improve the information she gives to patients may describe her aim as 'to produce an information leaflet' – but this is also her objective and her action plan! The answer is to think it through further, and ask 'Why produce a leaflet? What am I aiming to achieve by producing the leaflet?' It then becomes clearer that the aim is to improve patient compliance with dietary treatment, and one of the objectives is to improve patients' understanding of their dietary instructions. The action is to produce the leaflet. The importance of actually thinking through your aims and objectives in this way is that it helps you to be absolutely clear about *why* you are doing something, not just *what* you are doing. Failure to think through this stage means that health promoters waste time and energy ploughing ahead with 'a good idea' only to realize, too late, that what they are doing is not actually achieving what they want.

Exercise 5.2　Setting aims and objectives

Yewtree Scheme

The three practices at Yewtree Health Centre have agreed to establish physical activity assessment sessions, backed up by a display in the shared waiting area, with the aim of reducing the incidence of coronary heart disease in the practice populations.

The detailed objectives are:

1. To raise the users' awareness of the link between inadequate exercise and coronary heart disease, and the part which individuals can play in reducing their own vulnerability to the disease.
2. To assess, and advise about, individuals' physical fitness levels and help them to prepare an appropriate exercise action programme based on those results.
3. To monitor and evaluate, on a continuing basis, the effectiveness of the fitness testing, in respect of the resources involved and the reduction in vulnerability to heart disease.

Ask yourself the following questions:

1. **Do the objectives match the characteristics of objectives described above – are they challenging, attainable, as measurable as possible, and relevant?**
2. **How would you suggest changing the objectives?**

Setting Educational Objectives

If your health promotion activity is a health education programme, it is useful to plan in terms of *educational* objectives.

Educationalists traditionally often think of objectives (sometimes called 'learning outcomes') in terms of what the clients will gain. Furthermore, the objectives are considered to be of three kinds: what the educator would like the clients to *know, feel* and *do* as a result of the education. (In the language of the educationalist, these may be referred to as cognitive, affective and behavioural objectives.)

Objectives about 'knowing'. These are concerned with giving information, explaining it, ensuring that the client understands it, and thus increasing the client's knowledge. For example, explaining the pros and cons of vaccination to a baby's parents has the objective that they will *know* what the advantages and disadvantages of vaccinations are.

Objectives about 'feeling'. These objectives are concerned with attitudes, beliefs, values and opinions. These are complex psychological concepts, but the important feature to note now is that they are all concerned with *how people feel*. Objectives about 'feelings' are about clarifying, forming or changing attitudes, beliefs, values or opinions. In the example above, when a health educator is educating parents about vaccination, in addition to the 'knowledge' objective, there may be an objective about helping anxious parents to feel less worried about it.

Objectives about 'doing'. These objectives are concerned with a client's *skills* *and actions*. For example, teaching a routine of physical exercises, or teaching a diabetic how to give himself an injection, has the objective that clients acquire practical skills and are able to do specific tasks.

In health education, educational objectives are rarely concerned exclusively with knowing, feeling or doing – a mixture is usually required. For example, when advising a mother about feeding her toddler, a health educator probably has several objectives in mind, which she may be planning to achieve within three home visits:

- the objective of ensuring that the mother *knows* which foods are nourishing for her child and which are best given in restricted amounts;
- the objective of changing the mothers erroneous *belief* that sugar is essential to give her child energy, and *relieving her anxiety* that her healthy child's 'food fads' may cause serious ill-health;
- the objective that the mother learns what to *do* at meal times when her child has a tantrum over eating his food.

Case studies 5.1 and 5.2 — Aims and objectives for health promotion projects

Case study 5.1

Jim is an environmental health officer. His project is to tackle the problem of smoky atmospheres in pubs. This fits in with the overall purpose of his job, which is to work for a health-enhancing environment. Jim works out that his **aim** is to work with local publicans to set up smoke-free areas in pubs. He researches the subject in detail, looking at the results achieved from similar projects and working out how much time and money it is likely to take. He then decides that it is reasonable to set his **objective** as:

- within six months, to have raised awareness of the feasibility and advantages of a smoke-free area with 10 publicans, and worked with at least five to set up smoke-free areas.

Case study 5.2

Sue is a nurse specializing in coronary care. Her project is to run patient education programmes so that discharged patients know how to look after themselves. This fits in with the overall purpose of her job, which is to care for patients while they are in hospital, and maximize their chances of a healthy life afterwards.

Sue decides that her **aim** is that patients will have participated in a cardiac rehabilitation programme for post-heart-attack patients. Her **objectives** are:

- that every patient, before he leaves hospital, will know what he is advised to do about diet, exercise, smoking and stress control;
- that every patient will be confident and competent to put this advice into practice;
- that every patient, and his carers and relatives, will have had an opportunity to discuss questions and anxieties with a qualified member of the staff.

Sue's programme is a continuous course of group sessions each week, with each session focusing on a specific issue. So each individual session also has a set of objectives. Objectives for the session on 'Eating well when you go home', for example, include:

- patients will understand the basic principles of a healthy diet: low fat, low salt, low sugar and high fibre:
- patients will know which foods they can eat in unlimited amounts, which they should restrict and which they should avoid;
- patients will know what their ideal weight should be;
- patients who are overweight will have devised a personal weight-loss plan.

To summarize the key points about setting aims and objectives:

- the focus is on *what you are trying to achieve*;
- be as specific as possible – avoid vague, woolly notions of what you want to achieve;
- express your objectives in ways which can be measured if possible – how much? how many? when?
- do not get bogged down in terminology – it does not matter whether you talk about goals, aims, objectives, targets or outcomes – the key principle is to *be very clear about what you are trying to achieve*.

Stage 3. Decide the Best Way of Achieving the Aims

Occasionally, there might be only one possible way of accomplishing your aims and objectives. Usually, however, there will be a range of options. In Case Study 5.1, Jim has a number of options about how he achieves his objective of raising awareness with publicans of the feasibility and advantages of smoke-free areas in pubs. He could write to the breweries, he could drop leaflets in the pubs, he could lobby consumer groups to take up the cause, he could find out if there are any local meetings of publicans and ask to speak at them, he could conduct a campaign in the local media, he could write to the trade journals which publicans read, or he could try to meet each publican face-to-face. Or he could do two or more of these together.

You are therefore faced with the problem of how to identify the best option. There is no one 'best buy' for health promotion as a whole. Some factors to consider include:

- which methods are the most appropriate and effective for your aims and objectives? (This is explored in more detail below.)
- which methods will be acceptable to the consumers?
- which methods will be easiest?
- which methods are cheapest?
- which methods are the most acceptable to the people involved?
- which methods do you find comfortable to use? (Bear in mind that you may feel uncomfortable with some methods at first, but that this can be overcome with experience to build your confidence.)

There is more about *evidence for success, cost effectiveness* and *value for money* in Chapter 7, and Part 3 of this book covers the use of these methods and how to develop the necessary competencies.

Looking at the first of these questions, which methods are most appropriate and effective for your aims? there is an accumulated body of evidence which helps to identify effective methods for particular aims.[2] Table 5.1 identifies the range of aims, grouped into categories, and the appropriate and effective methods for achieving them. This provides a general guideline, to which there may be exceptions.

You may have decided on more than one of these categories of aims. For example, the inputs which contribute towards changing the behaviour of individuals can be complemented by societal changes, so that together they are more effective than either intervention alone. (This is known as 'synergy'.) So, for example, to reduce the over-consumption of alcohol by young people, you could:

- provide health education about alcohol as part of school personal and social education programmes;
- provide educational rehabilitation programmes for young drink–drive offenders;
- work with young people to promote the social acceptability of drinking non-alcoholic drinks;
- lobby for an increase in alcohol taxation.

The example in Figure 5.3 shows the range of aims and methods which might be used to promote healthy eating. We do not suggest that all of these would be used by a health promoter at any one time – they are given here to illustrate the range of possibilities.

Stage 4. Identify Resources

What resources are you going to use? You need to clarify what resources are already available (which may be more than you think at first), what you are going to need, and what additional resources you are going to have to acquire, and whether you will need money. A number of different kinds of resources can be identified:

You. Your experience, knowledge, skills, time, enthusiasm and energy are a vital resource.

People who can help you. It helps to identify all the people with something to offer. This may include colleagues and other people with relevant expertise who can advise and help you to make your plans, clerical and secretarial staff who can help with administration, technicians and artists who can help with exhibitions, displays and teaching/publicity materials.

Your client or client group. Another key resource. Clients may have knowledge, skills, enthusiasm, energy and time, which can be used and built upon. In a group, clients can share their knowledge and previous experience and in this way help each other to learn and change. An ex-client can be a very valuable resource too. For example, someone who has successfully lost weight, an ex-smoker or a person who has undergone a particular experience can be great help to clients who are grappling with similar problems and experiences.

People who influence your client or client group. These may include clients' relatives, friends, volunteers, patients associations and self-help groups. It may also be possible to harness the help of significant people in the community who are regarded as opinion-leaders or trendsetters; this group might include political figures, religious leaders or pop stars.

Existing policies and plans. For example, if you are planning to do work on 'safer sex' to help prevent the spread of sexually transmitted diseases and HIV, and reduce unwanted pregnancies, find out if there is already a policy on promoting sexual health in your health district. If there is, you can use it to back up the work you plan to do. Also find out whether your work fits into national strategies for health.

Table 5.1	Aims and Methods in Health Promotion	
Aim		**Appropriate method**
Health awareness goal Raising awareness, or consciousness, of health issues		Talks Group work Mass media Displays and exhibitions Campaigns
Improving knowledge Providing information		One-to-one teaching Displays and exhibitions Written materials Mass media Campaigns Group teaching
Self-empowering Improving self-awareness, self-esteem, decision-making		Group work Practising decision-making Values clarification Social skills training Simulation, gaming and role play Assertiveness training Counselling
Changing attitudes and behaviour Changing the lifestyles of individuals		Group work Skills training Self-help groups One-to-one instruction Group or individual therapy Written material Advice
Societal/environmental change Changing the physical or social environment		Positive action for under-served groups Lobbying Pressure groups Community development Community-based work Advocacy schemes Environmental measures Planning and policy-making Organizational change Enforcement of laws and regulations

Existing facilities and services. Find out what facilities already exist and whether these are fully utilized; for example, sports centres offering facilities for exercise and local classes or groups on cooking for healthy eating.

Material resources. These might include leaflets, posters, display/publicity materials, or, if you are planning health promotion involving group work, you need resources such as rooms, space, seats, audiovisual equipment and teaching/learning materials.

Fig 5.3   **Aims and methods for the promotion of healthy eating.**

AIM: Health awareness

Possible **methods:**
• articles in local newspapers
• exhibition on healthy eating and weight control, including
  weighing machine, height/weight charts, information on
  physical activity and healthy eating cookery demonstrations
• posters on nutritional themes in health service premises
• programmes on local radio

AIM: Social change

Possible **methods:**
• working with parents and teachers to encourage
  the sale of nutritious foods in school tuck shops
• working with NHS caterers to devise lower fat,
  higher fibre hospital food for patients and staff
• lobbying food manufacturers to include
  clearer information on food labels

AIM: Knowledge

Possible **methods:**
• nutrition teaching as part of home economics
  and health education in schools
• advice and help for patients from
  health professionals in clinical settings
• talks on aspects of nutrition to community groups

**PROMOTION OF
HEALTHY EATING**

AIM: Behaviour change

Possible **methods:**
• groups for healthy eating and weight control
• individual support for patients on special diets
• groups and cooking clubs to develop skills
  and confidence in preparing healthier meals
  for families
• recipes and ideas for nutritious packed
  lunches for schoolchildren

AIM: Self-awareness,
       attitude change
       decision-making

Possible **methods:**
• informal group work with antenatal clients and
  pre-retirement groups
• work with individual clients on whether to lose
  weight, cut down on salt, or increase fibre

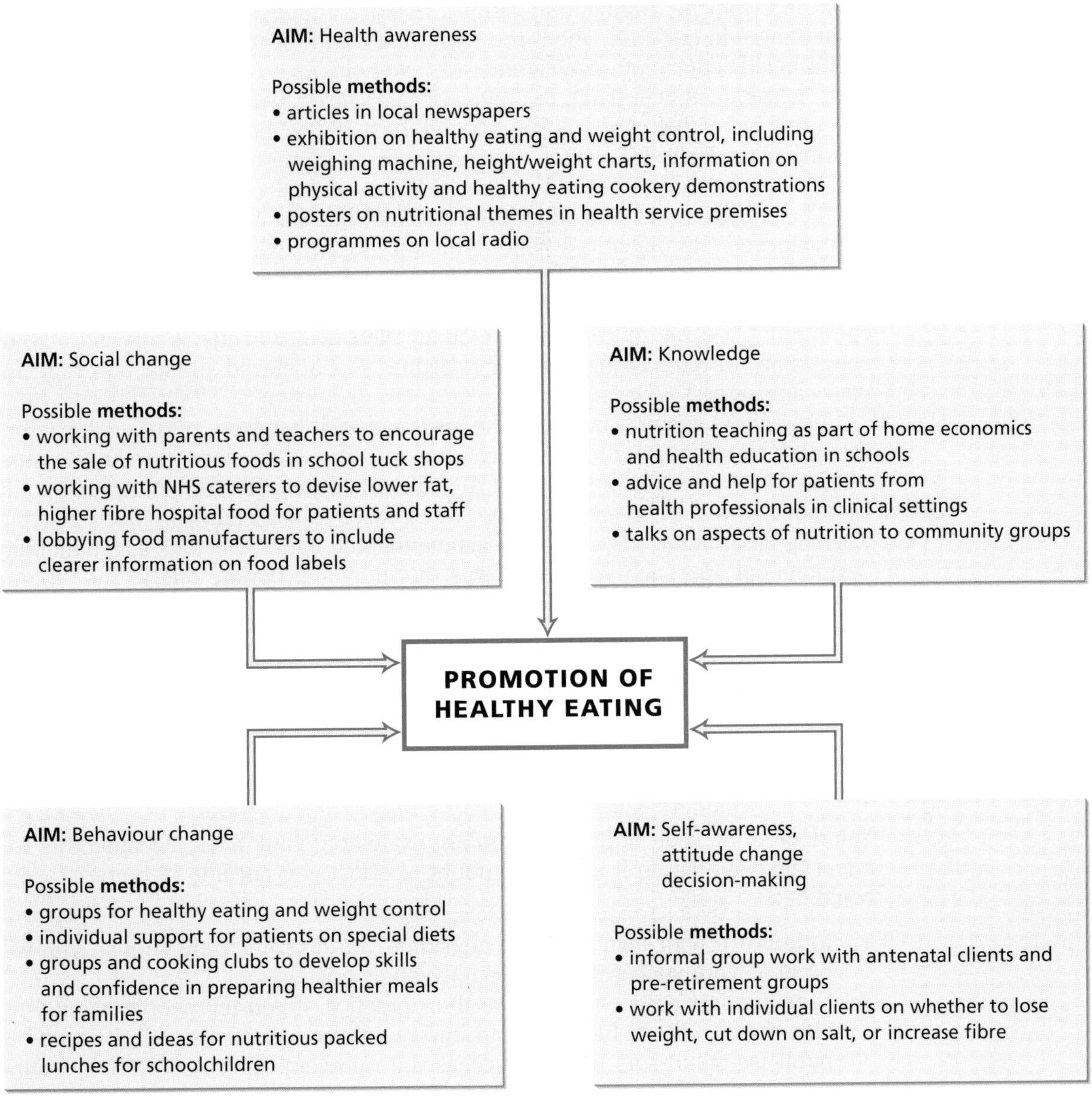

Stage 5. Plan Evaluation Methods

How will you know whether your health promotion is successful? And how will you measure success? There are no easy answers to these crucial questions about evaluation. On a large scale, sophisticated research is required. This should not deter health promoters; modest methods of evaluating the everyday practice of health promotion can, and should, be used routinely.

Defining Terms

What is meant by 'evaluation'? Simply, making a judgement about the value of something – in our case, about the value of a health promotion activity (whether it is a health education programme, for example, or a community project or an awareness-raising campaign to change local policy). Evaluation is the process of assessing what has been achieved and how it has been achieved. It means looking critically at the activity or programme, working out what was good about it, what was bad about it, and how it could be improved.

The judgement can be about the *outcome* (*what* has been achieved): whether you achieved the objectives which you set. So, for example, it could be about whether people understood the recommended limits for alcohol consumption as a result of your 'sensible drinking' education, whether people in a particular community became more articulate about their health needs as a result of your community development work, or whether you achieved media coverage for your campaign.

Judgement can also be about the *process* (*how* it has been achieved): whether the most appropriate methods were used, whether they were used in the most effective way, and whether they gave value for money. So, for example, it could be about considering whether the video-based discussion you used in your teaching programme was the best teaching method to use, whether the community development approach you chose was the most appropriate one in the circum-stances, or whether you would have achieved more public awareness with less money if you had opted for a media 'stunt' with possible free news coverage rather than an expensive advertising and leaflet campaign.

Some other key terms often used in discussions about evaluation are defined in the notes at the end of this chapter.[3]

Why Evaluate?

You need to be clear about why you are evaluating your work, because this will affect the way you do it and the amount of effort you put into it. Some reasons could be:

1. to improve your own practice: next time you do something similar, you will build on your successes and learn from any mistakes;
2. to help other people to improve their practice: if you tell people about your experiences, it can help them to improve their practice as well. It is vital to publicise failures as well as successes, to prevent other people re-inventing square wheels;
3. to justify the use of the resources that went into the work, and to provide evidence to support the case for doing this work in the future;
4. to give you the satisfaction of knowing how useful or effective your work has been; in other words, for your own job satisfaction;
5. to identify any unplanned or unexpected outcomes that could be important; for example, a publicity campaign to deter young people from taking drugs could have the opposite effect by unwittingly 'glamorizing' drug-taking and making it appear to be a more commonplace activity than it really is.

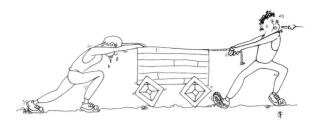

Publicise failures as well as successes, to prevent other people re-inventing square wheels

Who For?

Who will be using your evaluation data? The answer to this affects what questions you ask, how much depth and detail you go into and how you present the information.

If you are solely assessing how well a health education session went, for your own benefit so you can change it appropriately next time you run a similar session, you will simply make a judgement on how you think it went based on your observation and the learners' reactions, and make a few notes. But if you are writing a report for your manager, or for a body which you want to fund the work, you need to think through what questions those people will expect to be answered, and how much detail they will want.

For example, a group of health visitors evaluating a pilot scheme for a telephone advisory service at evenings and weekends need an evaluation report after six months for their manager who is funding the service. What will the manager need to know? At the very least, she will probably need a clear indication of the use made of the service (how many people used it? what were the characteristics of the users, e.g. were they first-time parents? how much was it used? what sort of issues did people ring about?), what the clients gained from it, and how much it cost. It would be helpful for the health visitors to ask their manager what evaluation data will be required at the planning stage of the project, so that the appropriate data can be collected from the start.

Assessing the Outcome

Looking first at *outcome* measures, you need to go back to the objectives you set, and plan how you are going to get the answer to the question 'have I achieved these objectives?' Objectives are about changes you aim to make: changes in people's knowledge or behaviour, for example, or changes in policies or ways of working. Large long-term health promotion projects may also have objectives about changes in health status. The following list indicates the kinds of changes which may be reflected in your objectives, and what methods you might use to assess or measure those changes.

Changes in Health Awareness Can be Assessed by:

- measuring the interest shown by consumers, e.g. how many people took up offers of leaflets, how many people enquired about preventive services;
- monitoring changes in demand for health-related services;
- analysis of media coverage;
- questionnaires, interviews, discussion, observation with individuals or groups.

Changes in Knowledge or Attitude Can be Assessed by:

- observing changes in what clients say and do: does this show a change in awareness and attitude?
- interviews and discussion involving question-and-answer between health promoter and clients;
- discussion and observation on how clients apply knowledge to real-life situations and how they solve problems;
- observing how clients demonstrate their knowledge of newly-acquired skills;
- written tests, or questionnaires which require clients to answer questions about what they know. The results can be compared with those taken before the health promotion activity or from a comparable group that has not received the health promotion.

Behaviour Change Can be Assessed by:

- observing what clients do;
- recording behaviour. This could be regular records such as numbers attending a health promotion clinic or bringing their children to be vaccinated. It could be a periodical inventory, such as a follow-up questionnaire or interview to check on smoking habits six and twelve months after attending a stop-smoking group. Records of client behaviour can be compared with those of comparable groups in other areas, or with national average figures.

Policy Changes Can be Assessed by:

- policy statements and implementation, such as increased introduction of 'environmentally-friendly' products in everyday use, or healthy eating choices in workplaces and schools;
- legislative changes, such as increased restriction on tobacco advertising;
- changes in the availability of health promoting products, facilities and services, such as low-cost recreational facilities or more smoking cessation advice;
- changes in procedures or organization, such as more time being given to patient education.

Changes to the Physical Environment Can Be Assessed by:

- measuring changes such as levels of pollutants in the air, traffic or pedestrian flows or the amount of open green space available to the public within a defined area.

Changes in Health Status Can be Assessed by:

- keeping records of simple health indicators such as weight, blood pressure, pulse rates on standard exercise or cholesterol levels;
- health surveys to identify larger-scale changes in health behaviour or self-reported health status;
- analysis of trends in routine health statistics such as infant mortality rates or hospital admission rates.

Help with these is given in Chapter 7 and in Part 3 of this book. It will be seen from this list that common methods are observation, asking questions, holding discussions and giving questionnaires.

Assessing the Process

Having looked at assessing the outcome, we now turn to assessing the process. This means looking at what went on during the process of implementation, and making judgements about it: was it done as cheaply and quickly as possible? Was the quality as good as you wished? Were the appropriate methods and materials used? You may, for instance, achieve your objectives, but in a time-consuming, costly or inefficient way, so it is important to evaluate the process as well as identifying whether you have achieved your desired outcome.

How are you going to assess the process? We suggest three key aspects: measuring the input, self-evaluation by asking yourself questions and getting feedback from other people.

Measuring the input. This is essential if you are going to make judgements about whether the outcome was worthwhile. You need to record everything that went into your health promotion activity, in terms of time, money and materials. Then you can make an informed judgement about whether the outcome was worth the cost.

Self-evaluation. Ask yourself 'What did I do well?' 'What would I like to change?' and 'How could I improve that next time?' All kinds of health promotion can be subjected to this kind of process evaluation, whether it is one-to-one health education with a client, facilitating a self-help group, undertaking community work, developing and implementing policies or lobbying for organizational changes.

An important point to note about self-evaluation is the value of emphasizing the positive. It is all too easy to criticize oneself in a negative, destructive way, which is unhelpful because it erodes confidence. Always look for the positive, identify the things you feel pleased with, and look for constructive ways forward about things which could be improved.

Feedback from other people. Giving and receiving feedback is an essential skill for every health promoter. Getting feedback from a trusted colleague on your work performance is a valuable form of peer evaluation. Asking for, and getting, feedback from your manager should be part of the regular monitoring of See section in Chapter 10 Asking Questions and Getting Feedback. your performance.

Obtaining feedback from the clients or users themselves should also be part of assessing the process of every intervention. The important thing is to encourage an atmosphere of openness and honesty, where problems can be confronted without people feeling blamed or judged as bad people. It can be done in many ways; simply observing clients and users accurately is an important tool. Do they look anxious or relaxed? Do they look interested and alert or bored and detached? You can also ask for feedback in various ways – through a suggestions box, through a sensitive and accessible complaints procedure, through noting any spontaneous verbal feedback you receive or through asking questions.

Stage 6. Set An Action Plan

Now that you know:

- what you are trying to achieve and have identified the best way to go about it,
- how to evaluate it,
- what resources you need,

you can get down to planning in detail exactly what you are going to do. This means writing a detailed statement of who will do what, with what resources and by when.

It is helpful, especially if you are tackling a large project, to break down your plan into smaller, manageable elements ('bite-sized pieces'). One way of breaking it down is by thinking in terms of key events. Draw up a schedule which shows the key events that are planned to happen at particular points in time. Key events plans specify deadlines that must be met by the people involved and can be useful in planning health promotion campaigns, for example.

Another way of breaking down a large project is by milestone planning. This is different from key events planning: instead of listing events, it lists a series of dates at fixed intervals (the 'milestones') and shows what must have happened by each of them.

Stage 7. Action!

This is the stage in which you actually *do* your health promotion, remembering to evaluate the process as you go along.

To summarize planning:

> *I once did meet six serving men (or women)*
> *They served me well and true*
> *Their names were what and why and when*
> *And how and where and who!*

| Example 5.1 | **Action plans** |

A **key events plan** drawn up by a health visitor who plans to set up a health stall in a local supermarket could look like this:

1. *Discuss with my manager* at October meeting.
2. *Identify support from colleagues* by November.
3. *Approach supermarket manager* (before Christmas rush); agree space and times.
4. *Convene planning group* of colleagues and health promotion officer in January to sort out who will do what and when, and evaluation plans, and identify the resources required.
5. *Set up first stall* in March.

A brief **Milestone plan** for the early stages of setting up a community health project could be like this, in a framework of three-monthly 'milestones':

January–March 1990	Steering group agrees job description for community health worker. Job advertised.
By end of June 1990	Interviews; appointment made. Community worker takes up post.
By end of September 1990	Community worker induction programme completed.
By end of December 1990	First progress report to Steering Group.

| Exercise 5.3 | **Ideas into action: planning a health promotion project** |

Work alone or in a small group

Think of an area of health promotion where there is an identified need, and it is within the remit of your job to meet that need. It could be an established area of work such as antenatal education, patient education, teaching food hygiene, or an area of new work you would like to tackle. (If you are not currently in a job which involves health promotion, think of a health-related project you would like to tackle in your personal life, or a project for any voluntary/community group you are associated with, or just imagine what you would like to do if you had the opportunity.)

Work through the following stages of the planning cycle. Start by writing each of the following headings at the top of a separate large sheet of paper, and then work through them:

1. **Aims and objectives**
   - Ask yourself 'What am I trying to achieve?' Identify your broad aim, or aims, then be more specific and identify your objectives.
2. **The best way of achieving my aims**
   - Think of all the ways in which you could achieve your aims and identify the best way.
3. **Resources**
   - Identify the resources you already have available and any extra ones you will need.
4. **Evaluation**
   - Ask yourself 'How will I know if I am succeeding?' Identify how you will evaluate both the process and outcome of your work.
5. **Action plan**
   - Identify who will do what, with what resources, and by when.

Be aware that when you are thinking about one section, it may have implications for the others, so you may find yourself going back to modify and refine what you have already written.

PRACTICE POINTS

- Health promotion work benefits from being planned and evaluated in a systematic way.

- The following 7-stage planning cycle can help you to do this:

  1. Identify needs and priorities: find out what your clients need, and work out your priorities.
  2. Set aims and objectives: be clear about exactly what you are trying to achieve, and by when.
  3. Decide the best way of achieving aims: think about which methods are: likely to be effective; will be acceptable to your clients; will give value for money; you have the competence to use.
  4. Identify resources: people (their time, knowledge and skills), things (existing policies and plans, facilities, educational materials) and money.
  5. Plan evaluation methods: work out why you need to evaluate and who for, and what you will do.
  6. Set an action plan: who will do what, with what resources and by when.
  7. Action: this is the stage where you actually do your health promotion, remembering to evaluate as you go along.

Recommended Reading

On Planning

An outline and discussion of several models of programme planning:
➤ Naidoo J & Wills J (1994) *Health Promotion: Foundations for Practice*. Chapter 12: Planning Health Promotion Interventions. London: Baillière Tindall.

A short straightforward guide to judging success in health promotion and to planning in settings of schools, workplaces, communities and the use of mass media:
➤ Whitehead M & Tones K (1991) *Avoiding the Pitfalls*. London: Health Education Authority.

On evaluation of Health Promotion Activities:

A useful discussion and guide to evaluating health promotion:
➤ Katz J & Peberdy A (1997) *Promoting Health: Knowledge and Practice*. Chapter 16, Evaluation in health promotion: why do it? and Chapter 17 Evaluation design. Basingstoke: Macmillan/Open University Press.

An in-depth look at questions of defining success, issues in evaluation research, indicators of success and measures of performance, which reviews effectiveness in different settings of schools, health care, workplace and communities, and the use of mass media:
➤ Tones K & Tilford S (1994) *Health Promotion: Effectiveness, Efficiency and Equity*, 2nd edn. London: Chapman and Hall.

On Planning and Evaluation of Health Alliances

A useful framework for planning and evaluating health promotion work by alliances of agencies working together:
➤ Funnell R, Oldfield K & Speller V (1995) *Towards Healthier Alliances: a tool for planning evaluating and developing healthy alliances*. London: Health Education Authority.

Notes and References

Since the mid-1990s, a number of organizations and academic centres have published reviews of effectiveness which summarize evidence from research in specific topics or approaches. For details of these, and other research reports on the effectiveness of health promotion, see Chapter 7 (section on Evidence-Based Health Promotion).

1   Secretary of State for Health (1992) *The Health of the Nation: A Strategy for Health in England*. London: HMSO.

Secretary of State for Health (1998) *Our Healthier Nation: a contract for health*. A consultation paper. London: The Stationery Office.

2   Early reviews of studies which showed the effectiveness of different health promotion interventions were:

Gatherer A, Parfit J, Porter E & Vessey M (1979) *Is Health Education Effective?* London: Health Education Council.

Bell J & Billington D (eds) (1985) *Annotated Bibliography of Health Education Research Completed in Britain from 1948–1978 and 1979–1983*. Edinburgh: Scottish Health Education Group.

A more recent overview and discussion is in

Tones K & Tilford S (1994) *Health Promotion: Effectiveness, Efficiency and Equity*, 2nd edn. London: Chapman and Hall.

3   Some terms often used when discussing evaluation are:

Evaluation: the process of assessing what has been achieved and how it has been achieved.

Effectiveness: what has been achieved, that is, the outcome.

Efficiency: how the outcome has been achieved, that is, how good is the process (in terms of, for example, value for money or the use of time).

Input: everything that goes into a programme or activity, including money, time, staff and materials.

Outcome: the end-product of the programme or activity, expressed in whatever terms are appropriate. For example, the outcome might be expressed in terms of changes in people's attitudes or knowledge, changes in health policy, changes in the uptake of services or changes in the rate of illness.

Process: what happens between input and outcome.

Impact: this is sometimes used to describe short-term outcomes. For example, the impact of a programme to encourage women to attend for a breast cancer screening test (mammogram) might be assessed in terms of how many women attended; the long-term outcome would be a change in the rate of women who died of breast cancer.

Monitoring: the process of regularly reviewing achievements and progress towards goals.

Qualitative: the term used to describe methods of assessment which express the outcome in words rather than numbers, and describe how good/bad the outcome was according to specified criteria. Assessment is usually based on observations or accounts of people's experiences.

Quantitative: The term used to describe methods of assessment which are expressed in terms of numbers.

For example, the evaluation of a breast screening programme may include qualitative data collected in focus group discussions with patients, and could include users' descriptions of their experience ('it was painful'; 'it was quick and well-organized'; 'it was embarrassing'), and quantitative data such as x number of women attended over y period of time, which is $z\%$ uptake by the women sent invitations, with an average through-put time of m minutes per patient and n percentage called back for further assessment. Often both qualitative and quantitative data are used to evaluate health promotion programmes.

6 Identifying Health Promotion Needs and Priorities

SUMMARY

We start with an analysis of the concept of need. We follow with a section discussing four factors for you to consider when identifying health promotion needs (the scope, reactive/proactive choices, putting the user at the centre and adopting a marketing philosophy), and an exercise on the 'user-friendliness' of services. In the next section, on finding and using health information, we identify varieties and sources of information and include exercises on gathering and applying information. There follows a framework for assessing health promotion needs, with a case study and an exercise. In the final section we focus on setting priorities, and include exercises on analysing the reasons for health promotion priorities and on setting priorities.

Identifying the people who are intended to benefit from health promotion activities (sometimes called **target groups**) is a complex process which takes place at many levels, from global and national to the level of local communities, groups, families and individuals. These people may be referred to as **users**, by which we mean those who use health promotion services, such as smoking cessation groups, maternity services, and pest control services. In some cases people **receive** help rather than **use** it, for example receiving advice, information or health education. Alternatively, people may be called **consumers**, **customers**, **clients** or, of course, **patients** if they are receiving preventive medical services. Sometimes potential users are as important to identify as current users, because a service may not be accessible or attractive to some groups of users. Positive action may be necessary for some people to get the same out of existing services as everybody else.

Going one stage further and identifying people's needs, and prioritizing them, is also a complex and difficult process. There is a bottomless pit of needs, and only finite resources available to meet them, so difficult choices have to be made.

At global, national and regional level, the assessment of health promotion needs, and the formulation of policies and plans to meet those needs, are part of the work of the World Health Organization (WHO), government departments, the Health Education Authority in England (and its equivalents in Scotland, Wales and Northern Ireland), and NHS Executive Regional Offices among others.

At a more local level in the NHS, it is the responsibility of the health authority or health board, who are charged with purchasing health care for their population. The Director of Public Health has a key role. At local authority level health policy is usually the responsibility of a health committee, with its membership drawn from local councillors and attended by senior officers from a range of departments. Increasingly, health authorities, local authorities and other agencies are undertaking joint information-gathering related to health promotion needs, and developing joint plans. Identifying needs at these larger-scale levels is outside the scope of this book. Our concern in this chapter is with the level of work undertaken by health promoters working with individual clients, families, groups and communities.

See the section on *Local health policy* in Chapter 16

Before looking further at how we can meet the needs of the users and receivers of health promotion, it is worth considering first what may be meant by a need.

Concepts of Need

It is useful to think of four kinds of need.[1]

1. Normative Need – Defined by the Expert

Normative need is need defined by an expert or professional according to her own standards; falling short of those standards means that there is a need. For example, a dietitian may identify a certain level of nutritional knowledge as the desirable standard for her client and she defines a need for nutrition education if her client's knowledge does not reach that standard. This normative need is based on the value judgements of professional experts, which may lead to problems. One is that expert opinion may vary over what is the acceptable standard, and the other is that the values and standards of the experts may be different from those of their clients.

Some normative needs are prescribed by law, such as food hygiene regulations.

2. Felt Need – Wants

Felt need is the need which people feel; in other words, it is what they want. For example, a pregnant woman may feel the need for information about childbirth. Felt needs may be limited or inflated by people's awareness and knowledge about what could be available, so, for example, people will not feel the need for knowing their blood cholesterol level or the sex of their unborn child if they have never heard that such a thing is possible.

3. Expressed Need – Demands

Expressed need is what people say they need; in other words, it is felt need which has been turned into an expressed request or demand. Commercial weight control groups and exercise classes are examples of expressed need; they are provided in response to demand.

Not all felt need is turned into expressed need or demand. Lack of opportunity, motivation or assertiveness could all prevent the expression of a felt need. Lack of demand should not be equated with lack of felt need.

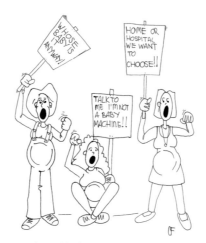

Expressed need is felt need turned into demand.

Expressed needs may conflict with a professional's normative needs. For example, a patient may express a need for a considerable amount of information on his medical condition, and this may be far more than a nurse is able or willing to give. The converse may also happen, with the nurse wishing to tell the patient far more than he wants to know.

4. Comparative Need

Comparative need for health promotion is defined by comparison between similar groups of clients, some of whom are in receipt of health promotion and some who are not. Those who are not are then defined as being in need. For example, if Company A has health policies about smoking at work and provides 'healthy' food choices in the staff dining room and Company B does not, it could be said that there is a comparative need for health promotion in Company B. This assumes that the health promotion in Company A is desirable and ideal, which of course it may not be.

To summarize:

Need, like beauty, is in the eye of the beholder.[2]

Need, Demand and Supply

The 1990s have seen a dramatic increase in public debate over need, demand and supply of health services and indeed other public sector services such as education. We are now aware that levels of service can vary across the country, and between GPs and hospitals even in the same neighbourhood. The 'need' for services may be similar or different, but it is clear that the supply is unevenly distributed. Some services may be funded in some parts of the country, but not in others. It is also clear that demand often outstrips supply, which means that people do not always get the health care they want, or indeed that health professionals believe they need. Health Authorities and other public bodies, faced with demands they cannot meet because they have a finite pot of money to spend, have to prioritize. Sometimes this is called 'rationing': limiting the supply of health care and only providing it according to specified criteria. This issue of uneven provision of services also applies in prevention and health promotion, with different levels of provision in different health authorities and boards. However, there are no reliable comparative figures because there is no clear definition of what constitutes health promotion and therefore 'counts'.

Identifying Health Promotion Needs

How does a worker in health promotion set about identifying the needs of people? We suggest four key areas it is useful to think about first: the boundaries of your job, the balance of your work between being reactive and proactive, to what extent you are putting your clients first, and the usefulness of adopting a marketing philosophy. We address each of these in turn.

The Scope

How to do this is discussed in Part 3 on Developing Competence in Health Promotion.

For some workers the task of identifying needs has already been done to some extent. For example, dental hygienists working in a dental surgery with individual patients already have the clearly identified task of educating patients in oral hygiene. But they may want to think carefully about how they can make their service as person-centred and user-friendly as possible. And they will certainly have to identify and respond to the individual needs of each patient.

Other workers, however, have more choice and scope in the range of health promotion activities they can undertake. Health visitors and community workers may have considerable scope, but the degree of autonomy they have will vary according to the policy of their managers and the resources available. All health promoters will need some competency in being responsive to the health promotion needs of their clients, and will need to be clear about the boundaries of their work: which health promotion activities are within their remit to undertake, and which are not, however desirable they may be. For example, a family planning nurse may be asked to undertake educational work with young people in schools, but is this within the boundaries of her job?

Reactive or Proactive?

It is useful to make an initial distinction between being reactive and proactive when identifying needs. Being reactive means responding (i.e. reacting) to the needs and demands which other people make. Pressure from vested interest groups and the media may introduce bias into how needs are perceived, and produce pressure to react. Being proactive means taking the initiative and deciding oneself on the area of work to be done. It may include saying 'no' to the demands of other people if these do not fit existing policies and priorities.

Being reactive or proactive can be related to the approaches to health promotion which were discussed in Chapter 3. Using a client-directed approach means being reactive to consumer's expressed needs, whereas using a medical or behaviour change approach probably means being proactive. This is particularly true of preventive medical interventions such as immunization campaigns. In practice, there is usually a balance to be struck between being reactive and proactive.

Putting Users' Needs First

Whose needs should come first – the users' or the providers'? There may be conflict between the two; for example, users may want a family planning service open on Saturdays but providers are unable to provide this because of difficulties of getting staff to work at weekends. However, we identify several trends which have emphasized putting the views and needs of users at the centre of the provision of health promotion:[3]

- the emphasis on the user as a unique person;
- the trend towards professionals working in partnership with lay people;
- the emphasis on improving the availability of, and access to, services which promote health, for example, leisure and recreational services, preventive health services;
- the trend towards a client-centred approach to health education with self-empowerment of the client the key aim;
- the trend towards more user participation in the planning and evaluation of health promotion activities.

Two other trends which play a part are the growth of the wider consumer movement since the 1960s, and the influence on service provision of market models in the late 1980s and 1990s. An interest in the techniques of commercial enterprise is now widespread amongst public sector managers. Health service managers are recommended to use market research, among other methods, to find out about the experience and perceptions of patients and the community.[4]

One of the most important ways of making activities more responsive to users and receivers is to give them more control over what happens to them. There are an increasing number of local authority and health authority initiatives aiming to give users more choice.[5]

Adopting a Marketing Approach[6]

We referred to the growth of the consumer movement in health services and market models above; 'marketing' is a term frequently used in relation to health promotion.

Marketing is often associated solely with commercial businesses and making profits, and with the activities of sales and advertising. How, then, does it relate to health promotion, and, more specifically, to the question of identifying needs?

Usually, health promoters work in the public or voluntary sector, and are not generally required to make profits, and so they are different from commercial enterprises. But the health promoter could be more effective and efficient through adopting a marketing approach.[7] The fact that health is obviously a 'good thing', which therefore does not need a 'hard sell', and that health promotion services often emphasize person-to-person involvement, has tended to convince health promoters that they are in touch with their clients/users and that marketing may have nothing more to offer. However, there is increasing recognition that this is not so.

Although the phrase 'the customer is always right' originated in the service industries, there are many cases where this is patently not practised. For example, people are placing an increasing value on their time, and resent it if they are kept waiting because the professional's time appears to be more valuable than their own.

What would 'adopting a marketing approach' mean in the context of health promotion? In general usage, marketing is the management skill of identifying opportunities for satisfying customers' requirements and, by doing so, maximizing profits. In the context of health promotion, we suggest the following definition of marketing:

> *Marketing is the management skill of identifying opportunities for satisfying consumers/clients' requirements and, by doing so, maximizing the protection and/or improvement of their health.*[8]

So the output is health, not profits. Fundamentally, marketing is an attitude of mind. It is about identifying consumer needs and satisfying them in the most efficient way, so that the maximum output is achieved in terms of people's health. Through adopting this approach, health promotion activities can benefit from greater effectiveness and efficiency, and from improved consumer satisfaction. In certain circumstances this may involve using specific marketing techniques, such as market research. It also means being much more responsive to the consumers' needs and wants, tailoring services to these rather than to the providers' ideas of what they think people should have. A marketing approach means making services 'user-friendly'. The following exercise provides a checklist to assess how user-friendly your health promotion services are:

Exercise 6.1   **How user-friendly are your services?**[9]

Think of a health-related service you provide as part of your job, or if you can't, one which you use as a client (such as your family planning clinic, GP or dentist.)

Below is a list of ten factors which may affect how users view the service. Rate the service on each factor using a scale from 1 (very poor) to 5 (excellent). The maximum score is 50. How does the service measure up?

1. **Availability of service** – do the times suit the user?
2. **Accessibility** – easy access by public transport? Easy car parking?
3. **Quality of service** – what are the standards, reliability, results?
4. **Speed of service** – do appointments keep to schedule?
5. **Friendly service** – a warm, welcoming atmosphere, continuity of relationship?
6. **Good environment** – safe, warm, clean, comfortable?
7. **Information about the service** – is it widely available, inviting, accurate, easy to understand?
8. **Reputation of the service** – do local people rate the service highly?
9. **Attitudes** – is there an understanding and acknowledgement of the user's circumstances and feelings?
10. **Responsiveness of the service** – is the service relevant to local people, does it reach all potential groups of users, are suggestions encouraged and complaints handled sensitively?

We now return to the central questions: how can needs for health promotion be identified, and once identified, what criteria can the health promoter use to decide whether, and how, to respond?

Finding and Using Information

The starting point for defining health promotion needs is information of various kinds from a range of sources. If information is being gathered on a local area for the first time, it would be helpful to share the work, and the findings, with colleagues. For example, health visitors may have done a neighbourhood profile as part of their training; the local Health Authority Health Promotion Department may have gathered information; the local Health Authority Public Health Department will certainly have collected health data on the local population. Gathering and updating all these different kinds of information is an ongoing project for every health promoter and sharing the burden makes sense. Working with colleagues needs to go hand in hand with developing good links with local people, in order to gear health promotion more effectively towards active participation of users and receivers.

We will now look at the major kinds of information and how they may help to identify health promotion needs.

Epidemiological Data

Epidemiology is the study of the distribution and determinants of disease in communities. Epidemiological data indicate how many people are affected by a health problem, how many people die from a particular health problem, and who are most at risk (for example, men or women? which age groups? which ethnic group? which social class? which occupation? which geographical area? fat or thin people? smokers or non-smokers? sedentary or active people?).

Detailed discussion of the sources and limitations of epidemiological data is outside the scope of this book, and further reading is suggested in note[10] and *Recommended Reading* at the end of this chapter. The important point to make here is that epidemiological data provide essential information on the health of the population, the causes and risk factors related to ill-health, and consequently, the potential for prevention and health promotion.

Mortality and morbidity data are collected nationally, and some data are also available on a regional and local basis. (Mortality data are concerned with causes of death; morbidity data are concerned with types of illness and disability.) Mortality data are derived from death certificates; morbidity data are derived from a wide range of sources, including general practice records, hospital records, sickness absence certificates, child health records, returns of notifiable diseases, disability registers and many others. In addition, surveys such as the government's General Household Survey, and surveys carried out for research purposes provide a considerable amount of health information.

Your local Health Authority or Health Board should be able to provide a copy of the Annual Public Health Report for the local population including mortality and morbidity data (such as admission rates for particular conditions). This is for the population as a whole and possibly also broken down to the level of the population of smaller areas such as electoral wards. It might be helpful to compare data for the whole population and electoral ward data (for a neighbourhood) on, for example:

- The major causes of death.
- The key causes of childhood admission to hospital.
- The main conditions for which adults are admitted to hospital.

Exercise 6.2   **Gathering Local Public Health Information**

Look at a copy of your local Annual Public Health Report. You should be able to get one from your Health Authority or Health Board. Or you should be able to see one in your local Health Promotion Department library, or your local public library.

Annual Public Health Reports vary in style and content, but they will all tell you about the health of your local population. Browse through yours, and note what information it contains. For example, does it tell you:

- What are the major causes of death?
- What are the main reasons why people are admitted to hospital?
- What are the major risk factors for ill-health; for example, is there information on how many people smoke in your local population?
- How many people have had communicable diseases (i.e. diseases that can be caught from other people) such as measles and sexually transmitted diseases?
- Which are the neighbourhoods with the poorest health?
- What steps are being taken to prevent ill-health and promote good health?

Does it tell you anything else which will help you in health promotion work?

Lifestyle Data

There is an increasing amount of information available about people's health-related behaviour and lifestyle, such as physical activity, sexual behaviour, smoking and drinking. This is available on a national basis from survey data.[11] You may also find that your own Health Authority or Health Board has done a lifestyle survey of your local population, and published the findings in a report.

Socioeconomic Data

The planning or information departments of local councils should be able to help with information about housing, employment, social class and social/leisure/recreation/shopping facilities. Many produce summaries of census data. It might be helpful to compare district/borough/city and electoral ward data on, for example:

- unemployment;
- household amenities;
- income;
- ethnicity.

It is advisable to ask for figures which are as full and recent as possible. Much data is obtained from the census which only takes place every ten years, and data from the 1991 census will not be updated until information from the 2001 census becomes available.

By setting illness alongside socioeconomic data, you may be able to see particular patterns of inequalities in health in your area. The Annual Public Health Report of your Health Authority or Health Board or reports from your local authority may look at this issue in detail. For example, they may have tables and maps which show areas of particular social deprivation and high health need in your locality.

Professional Views

The views of fellow health promoters reflect experience and perceptions accumulated over the years which it would be foolish to ignore. What do other workers in your area, such as teachers, youth workers, social workers, GPs, health visitors, district nurses, environmental health officers, police officers, community workers and religious leaders, consider to be the major health concerns?

Public Views

There is more about research methods for finding out people's views in Chapter 7 (section on *Doing Your Own Small Scale Research*).

There are several methods of obtaining the views of the public at large. These range from informal discussions/interviews to large scale surveys using questionnaires or in-depth interview techniques.

A number of attempts have been made to classify the various ways of involving users in the planning of services.[12] Identifying priority groups and thinking clearly about them will influence the choice of methods used to contact and involve them.

It is best to start with the characteristics of the groups and then design the best approach. For instance, how large are the relevant groups? Do they have particular age, class or ethnic structures? What makes it a 'group' (geography, membership, current use of services and facilities)? Are the members of the group mobile? Do they have easy access to transport facilities? What times of day are they likely to be available for meetings? Be absolutely clear about what sort of relationship you are proposing to have with local groups and individuals.

This is discussed in detail in Chapter 15, Working with Communities.

For example if the plan is simply to establish consultation mechanisms, there may be hostility if local people have played a stronger role in other circumstances.

The groups involved may include the Community Health Council (established by the 1973 NHS Act to represent the user's voice in the NHS), local voluntary organizations and community groups such as self-help groups, black and minority ethnic groups, pensioners' clubs, tenants associations, and a variety of local advisory groups or planning subcommittees, in addition to groups of key clients such as mothers. Gathering views informally is a useful dipstick but there are of course problems about the accuracy and representativeness of subjective information. However, these subjective data can usefully feed into the wider framework.

One of the most powerful ways of finding out what it is really like for users is to experience a service first-hand.[13] This can result in individual workers radically changing their working practices. However, it may not always be possible to translate this into general changes in the way services are delivered.

There is more about research methods for finding out people's views in Chapter 7 (section on *Doing Your Own Small Scale Research*).

You may want to consider undertaking some first-hand research but first think about how much time and money it will take. Will the results justify the costs? If you still think it is worth doing, who could do it? If it is very small scale you could perhaps undertake it yourself, maybe in collaboration with some colleagues.

Exercise 6.3	Using Services Which Promote Good Health or Prevent Ill-health: user views

Find out about some services available locally, designed for the public, staff and/or health students (whichever is relevant to you), which aim to promote health or prevent ill-health. (The public library, Personnel Department of your employer, NHS Trust or College may be able to provide information about what services are available). These could include fitness testing, swimming facilities, exercise classes, screening tests or the Resources and Information service of your local Health Promotion Department.

See also the section on Working for Quality in Chapter 8 for information on quality in health promotion services.

Select one of these, appropriate and acceptable to you, and visit it. Make notes about what happens. Look back at the previous section in this chapter, on Adopting a Marketing Approach, if you need to remind yourself about how to make a service responsive to its users.

- **Is the service easy to find?**
- **Is transport easily available/is there easy access for parking your car?**
- **Are the opening times convenient to you?**
- **If there is a charge for the service, is it affordable and good value for money?**
- **How are you welcomed at reception? Are you given all the information you need? Do you feel at ease? Are the staff friendly?**
- **What do you think about the environment – is it safe, clean and comfortable?**
- **What do you think about the quality of the service you received? Do you have any ideas about how it could be improved? Will you use this service again?**
- **What have you learnt as a service user which you can now apply to health promotion practice?**

Local Media

The opinions and data collected will provide you with a picture at a particular point in time. Monitoring local radio, TV and papers will give a view of any major changes in the community. All this adds to the profile of local information which is building up, providing a basis for planning health promotion.

Assessing Health Promotion Needs

The assessment of health promotion needs can be approached systematically by asking a series of key questions. The answers will help you to decide whether to respond to a particular need, and if so, how.

1. What Sort of Need is it?

Is this a normative, felt, expressed or comparative need?

In a parent education class, for example, what kind of need is being met: the normative needs decided by the health professional, the felt or expressed needs of the parents or comparative needs decided after looking at what was available elsewhere?

2. Who Decided that there is a Need?

Whose decision is it: the health promoter's, the client's or both?

Sometimes the answer to this question is not immediately obvious, because the need has emerged after discussion between the health promoter and client. People do not always know what they need or want, because their awareness and knowledge of the possibilities is limited. The health promoter may help by raising awareness and knowledge of health issues; in this way she may create a demand (an expressed need) for health promotion. For example, the public's demand for non-smoking in restaurants only came after health promoters had raised awareness of the hazards of passive smoking, which gave people the confidence to express their feelings about how unpleasant it is eating in a smoky atmosphere. The ideal situation is a joint decision by clients and health promoters.

3. What are the Grounds for Deciding that there is a Need?

Is there any evidence of need in the form of objective data, such as facts and figures? If *local* data are not available, has the information been collected in other localities and is it reasonable to assume that the same conditions will apply? Be aware of the pitfall that gathering data can be a delaying tactic to avoid doing something about an obvious problem. For example, surveys have shown that elderly people without cars find it difficult to get to hospitals when there is poor public transport. It is reasonable to assume that this applies in most localities with poor public transport. So, only collect information if the answer to a question is really not known. Have the views of the clients been sought? Do they see this as a need?

4. What are the Aims and the Appropriate Response to the Need?

Health promotion cannot solve all problems or meet all health needs. First, you need to be clear what the need is, then what your aims are for meeting that need, then the appropriate way to meet it.

For example, there may be an identified need to increase the uptake of immunization. The aim is to achieve an 80% uptake rate. You then need to decide the appropriate way to achieve it. It would be all too easy in this case to say that 'there is a need for a health education campaign to get parents to have their children immunized' because messages about attending immunization clinics may be seen to be the answer. But this may make no difference because the appropriate response is to educate the health professionals who are found to be withholding immunization wrongly when a child has only a mild cold, and to move the time and place of the clinics so that working mothers without cars are able to bring their children.

See the section on setting aims and objectives in Chapter 5 for a more detailed discussion of setting aims and objectives and identifying appropriate responses.

In the following case study, we assess an identified need for health promotion, applying the four assessment questions.

Case study 6.1	**Assessing Health Promotion Needs**

A community clinic[14]

The health visitors and primary care manager in a clinic wanted to make it into a focus for the local community. They felt that the clinic was an under-used local asset, and that the health visitors were failing to meet local needs and should extend their client group beyond mothers and babies to include more elderly and middle-aged people, and schoolchildren. They also wanted to extend their role to become health advisers and counsellors.

The health visitors believed that offering an improved service would give them more satisfying jobs. They put considerable time and energy into planning how to achieve these goals. Yet much of the project never got off the ground and in the end the service remained virtually unchanged.

Although some reasons for this, such as staff changes, were outside the project's control, lack of clear ideas about how best to achieve the changes they wanted weakened the project from the start.

1. What sort of need is it?

Those involved in the project were anxious not to reinvent the wheel and made a number of contacts with other health visitors who had developed similar schemes.

This is a normative need based on a professional view. It is also a comparative need based on what other clinics provide.

2. Who decided that there is a need?

The professionals (the health visitors).

The views of existing and potential client groups were not sought. A letter was sent to existing users of the service informing them of the proposed changes. No attempt was made to find out the needs and views of the additional client groups the health visitors wished to serve, although a plan was made to administer a questionnaire (see Question 3 for the outcome of this).

The other members of the primary health care team were not involved, and the receptionists were unsure about what was being proposed. Local community groups and other local health promoters had not been involved in drawing up the plans.

3. What are the grounds for deciding there is a need?

The grounds were the comparative under-use of the clinic, as perceived by the health visitors and primary care manager.

The proposed changes were not tied into the major priorities and objectives for the Community Directorate, and the manager of the Directorate was not involved in discussions. As a result a proposal to gather information from users about their need for services which the clinic could provide was the subject of cuts.

4. What are the aims and the appropriate response to the need?

The aims were not clear, and therefore the appropriate response to achieve the aims were not clearly thought through either.

One aim seemed to be to make the clinic accessible and attractive to a wider range of groups in the community. Who these potential users were, and what their specific needs were, remained unknown.

Another aim seemed to be for the health visitors to spend more time in face-to-face contacts with clients, acting as advisers and counsellors. Drop in sessions were put on and advertised on a poster at the clinic. These sessions were found to be under-used and almost only existing users – mothers and babies – were attending them. This is not surprising when there was so little marketing of the new service. Attempts at proper counselling sessions were often frustrated by the receptionists continuing to put 'phone calls through.

Exercise 6.4	Assessing a health promotion need

Use the following questions (discussed above in detail) to assess a health promotion need which you have identified in your own work, or one which you are likely to meet.

1.   What sort of need is it?
2.   Who decided that there is a need?
3.   What are the grounds for deciding that there is a need?
4.   What are the aims and appropriate response to the need?

Setting Health Promotion Priorities

You may have a huge workload of health promotion needs which you feel should be met, but there are always constraints on time, resources and energy. Spreading efforts a mile wide and an inch deep is probably useless and concentrating effort on priority areas is more effective and rewarding.

Before attempting to set priorities it is helpful to analyse current 'real life' practice and recognize the wide range of criteria which will affect such decisions. (See Exercise 6.5.)

The need to prioritize is vital, but one difficult issue to consider is how to approach work with people whose health experience is poorest. It is automatic to consider that these people should be top priority, but it is important to stop and think whether focusing all health promotion effort on those most at risk will, in the end, be of greatest benefit.

It is possible to consider two broad approaches to tackling a health issue, such as reducing the incidence of coronary heart disease, called the 'high-risk' and the 'whole population' approaches.[15]

The 'high risk' approach identifies people particularly at risk such as smokers, people who are obese and those with high blood pressure, and work with these people to change lifestyle factors and treat their raised blood pressure. But there may be poor return for effort, as these groups could include 'hard core' heavy smokers with poor diets who have no intention of changing, or people so overwhelmed with other issues in their lives that tackling smoking and eating habits is impossible.

The 'whole population' approach works at a community rather than individual level, with, for example, strategies to improve access to cheap healthy food, increase skills and confidence in producing healthy meals for families, and community development approaches to build up social support. At the same time, supporting changes at a wider population level, such as clamping down on under-age sales of cigarettes, and lobbying for better provision of income support, could result in better health gain across whole populations.

Generally, both approaches need to be taken (not necessarily by the same health promoters), and complement each other.

There can be no watertight method for setting priorities because priorities ultimately depend upon the value-judgements of the workers involved but it may be helpful to work through the checklist in Exercise 6.6.

| Exercise 6.5 | Analysing the 'real-life' reasons for health promotion priorities |

Identify a health promotion activity which has a high priority in your work. This could be work which you undertake with a number of clients (e.g. antenatal education) or just one (e.g. a particular patient); it could be part of your usual work or a special event such as a campaign. (It will be especially helpful for the purposes of this exercise if you can identify an area of work which has recently become a priority.)

Now work through the following tasks.

1. Identify who it was who decided that this work should take priority (e.g. you? your seniors? your clients? all three?)
2. List **all the possible reasons** why this work has priority – include the reasons that you are sure about as well as any that are speculation.
   Your reasons could include any of the following and probably many more:
   - I feel that it's important.
   - It is established policy of senior officers.
   - We've always done it and saw no reason to change.
   - There was pressure from the public.
   - It was in response to a crisis.
   - We had to be seen to be doing something.
   - There is new evidence of need.
   - There is evidence that the work has been effective in a similar area.
   - Someone has a personal enthusiasm for it (a bee in her bonnet).
   - It was the current national/local theme (e.g. World AIDS Day).
   - We had a new staff member with special expertise which we wanted to use.
   - We had to economize and be more efficient.
   - It was politically expedient.
3. Identify what you think the most important reasons are. Do you think that they are sound reasons for setting priorities?

| Exercise 6.6 | Setting Priorities for Health Promotion |

1. Health promotion issues, approaches and activities

Do you define your priorities in terms of:
- issues which have an influence on health (e.g. poverty, unemployment, racism, ageism, inequalities)?
- health promotion approaches (e.g. medical, behaviour change, educational, client-centred, societal/environmental change)?
- health promotion activities (preventive health services, community-based work, organizational development, economic and regulatory activities, environmental measures, health education programmes, healthy public policies)?
- health problems (e.g. heart disease, food poisoning, cancer, HIV/AIDS, overweight, mental health problems)?

Why?

2. Consumer groups

Who are the people your health promotion is aimed at:
- policy-makers and planners?
- individual clients or service users?
- families?
- selected groups?
- the whole community? If so, how do you define your 'community'?

Why?

3. Age groups

Do you define your priority consumer groups further in terms of age: children, young people, parents, older people, etc.?

Why?

4. 'At-risk' groups?

Do you define your priority consumer groups further in terms of high-risk categories, such as smokers, people with high blood pressure, unemployed people or those living on low incomes?

If so, why? Have you examined the evidence leading to the identification of these 'at-risk' groups?

If your group includes people with highest health needs, for example people living in areas of social deprivation with many health and social needs, do you know whether there is evidence that work focusing on specific issues will be successful? Would you get more health gain for your effort if you focused on whole populations rather than those most in need?

5. Effectiveness

See Chapter 7 for information on how to collect evidence.

Have you any evidence that health promotion in your priority areas is likely to be effective?

Have you any evidence that it will provide good value for money?

How could such evidence be collected?

6. Feasibility

Is it feasible for you to spend time with your priority groups?

Do you have access to these groups?

Do you have credibility with these groups?

Do you have the skills and resources to work with these groups?

7. Working with other people

Do you know what work is already being done with your priority groups, by other health promoters, community groups and voluntary organizations?

Are you sure that your work will complement any other work which is going on – and not be seen as duplication or interference?

Does your work fit in with existing local strategies and plans for health promotion?

8. Ethics

Are there ethical aspects to your work which you need to consider?
Is your work ethically acceptable to you?
Will it be acceptable to your consumer groups?
Will it be congruent with their values?
How may the desired outcome affect their lives?

9. Add anything else which you feel it is important to consider.

Now identify your top *priority* and add any other high *priorities*

PRACTICE POINTS

- You will have some scope for making choices about the range of health promotion activities which you undertake. These choices must be based on a careful assessment of health promotion needs. The starting point for doing this is through gathering various kinds of information.

- The views of users and receivers of services are paramount, therefore developing skills in gathering information directly from them is especially important.

- You can assess health promotion needs systematically through asking four key questions: what kind of need is it? who decided that there was a need? what is the evidence for deciding that there is a need? what is the appropriate response to the need?

- Like all health promoters, you have a duty to regularly re-assess priorities, through analysing whether your activities are targeted effectively, are feasible, complement the work of other practitioners and are acceptable to local people.

- Priorities depend ultimately on the value judgements of those involved. Best practice involves in-depth discussion on these matters with other health promotion workers and local people.

Recommended Reading

An in-Depth Look at the Concept of Need

➤ Doyal L & Gough I (1991) *A Theory of Human Need*. London: Macmillan.

On Marketing

➤ Morden A R (1994) *Elements of Marketing*, 3rd edn. London: DP Publications. (Comprehensive introduction to the theory and practice of marketing.)

➤ Irons K (1997) *The Marketing of Services: a total approach to achieving competitive advantage*. Maidenhead: McGraw-Hill. (Written for service-providing organizations.)

Basics of Epidemiology

➤ Barker D V P & Rose G (1997) *Epidemiology in Medical Practice*, 5th edn. London: Churchill Livingstone.

Studying and Measuring Health of Populations

➤ Bowling A (1997) *Measuring Health*, 2nd edn. Buckinghan: Open University Press.
➤ McConway K (ed.) (1994) *Studying Health and Disease*. Health and Disease series, Book 2. Buckingham: Open University Press.
➤ Naidoo J & Wills J (1994) *Health Promotion: Foundations for Practice*. Chapter 3: Measuring Health. London: Baillière Tindall.
➤ Katz J & Peberdy A (1997) *Promoting Health: Knowledge and Practice*. Chapter 12: What counts as evidence in health information?; Chapter 13: Studying Populations; Chapter 14: Analysing Numerical data. Basingstoke: Macmillan Open University Press.

Notes and References

1   This is a classic analysis of the concept of 'need', based on:

Bradshaw J (1972) The concept of social need. *New Society*, 30 March.

2   Cooper M (1975) *Rationing Health Care*, p. 20. London: Croom Helm.

3   Winn E & Quick A (1989) *User friendly services – guidelines for managers of community health services*. London: King's Fund Centre.

4   Department of Health and Social Security (1983) *Management Inquiry Report* (The Griffiths Report), p 9. London: DHSS.

5   Simnett I (1991) *Promoting Health – Local Authorities in Action*. London: Health Education Authority.

6   Morden A R (1993) *Elements of Marketing*, 3rd edn. London: DP Publications.

Irons K (1997) *The Marketing of Services: a total approach to achieving competitive advantage*. Maidenhead: McGraw-Hill. (Written specifically for service-providing organizations.)

7   For example, see:

Eadie D & Smith C (1995) The role of applied research in public health advertising: some comparisons with commercial advertising. *Health Education Journal* **54** 367–380 (On the relevance to public health advertising of methods and techniques from commercial advertising.)

Arnold-McColloch R & McKie L (1995) The potential application of social marketing techniques in health promotion. *Journal of the Institute of Health Education* **32**(4), 120–124. (Draws out the advantages of employing social marketing techniques in health information campaigns.)

8   This is adapted from a definition of marketing in:

Willsmer R L (1976) *The Basic Arts of Marketing*, p.7. London: Business Books.

9   This exercise is based on one in:

English National Board (1989) *Health Promotion in Primary Health Care – an open learning package for practice nurses*. Introduction, p. 8. London: English National Board with Learning Materials Design. (Reproduced by kind permission of the English National Board.)

10   Useful overviews of the health status of the population in Britain are:

Jacobson B, Smith A & Whitehead M (1991) *The Nation's Health: a strategy for the 1990s*, revised edn. London: King Edwards Hospital Fund for London.

Department of Health (1997) *Health Survey for England 1995*. Joint Health Surveys Unit, on behalf of the Department of Health. Published in full and summary versions by HMSO, London. (National survey of adults and children, covering topics including asthma, hay fever, eczema, lung function, accidents, disability, blood pressure, self-assessment of general health, obesity, alcohol and smoking.)

11   Some useful sources of lifestyle data are:

The Health Education Authority publish *Health Updates* which contain data on the health behaviour of populations in relation to specific topics. These include Coronary Heart Disease (1993), Sexual Health (1997), Physical Activity (1995), Smoking (1996), Alcohol (1997), Workplace Health (1997)

Health Promotion Wales produce Technical Reports on health surveys, such as: *Health-related behaviours in Wales 1985–1993: Findings from the Health In Wales survey*. Technical Report 8.

Health Education Authority and Office for National Statistics (1997) *Health in England 1996 – what people know, what people think, what people do*. London: HEA. (Looks at health knowledge, attitudes and behaviour of adults aged 16–64 in England.)

Health Education Authority (1995) *Health and Lifestyles: Black and minority ethnic groups in*

England. London: HEH. (Report of a study to assess health-related behaviour, attitudes and information needs of black and minority ethnic groups using questionnaires and interviews.)

Aggleton P (1996) *Health promotion and young people*. London: Health Education Authority. (Examines patterns of illness and death in young people, their risk-taking and health-protecting behaviours, and the effectiveness of different health promotion interventions.)

12   Maxwell R & Weaver N (eds) (1984) *Public Participation in Health*. London: King Edward's Hospital Fund for London. (Identifies a spectrum, ranging from consumer protection, through open managerial decision-making, full management participation by public representatives, to heightened individual and communal responsibility and power.)

13   Personal experiences of the health service from a user's point of view are recounted in occasional articles in the *Health Service Journal*, for example:

Coker N (1997) Smoke and Dust. *Health Service Journal*, **107**, 17 July p. 29.

McQueen R (1997) Hip, hip hooray! *Health Service Journal*, **107**, 16 January, p.27.

Friend B (1997) Sickness benefit. *Health Service Journal*, **107**, 7 August, pp. 24–27.

14   This case study is based on a more detailed one in:

Winn E & Quick A (1989) *User Friendly Services – guidelines for managers of community health services*, pp. 22–24. London: King's Fund Centre.

15   Whent H (1997) High risk v. whole population strategies. *Healthlines*, Issue 43, June, pp. 14–16. (Helpful discussion of pros and cons of high risk vs. whole population approach.)

Fowler G (1996) The population and individual strategies. Chapter 21, pp 301–308, in

Lawrence M, Neil A, Mant D & Fowler G (eds) *Prevention of cardio-vascular disease: an evidence based approach*. Oxford General Practice Series 33. Oxford: University Press. (Clear account of the two approaches.)

7 Skills of Effective Planning

SUMMARY

In this chapter we look at particular aspects of knowledge and skill which help you to plan successful health promotion. These are: linking your work into broader health promotion plans and strategies; basing your work on evidence of success; getting value for money; using published research; doing your own small scale research; audit.

Health Promotion Strategic Planning

By 'strategy', we mean a broad plan of action which specifies what is to be achieved and how to achieve it. This provides a framework for more detailed planning. Strategic planning is at a broad-brush level, and for health promoters there will usually be plans at a local Health Authority or local government level. These plans will themselves be informed by strategy at a higher level, such as national strategy.

So for individual health promoters, whether you work in the NHS, a local authority or another agency, your work can be seen as making a contribution to a larger plan. For example, the nurse in a GP practice who helps a patient to stop smoking is making her contribution to her Health Authority's strategy to reduce smoking, which in turn is contributing to the overall target to reduce smoking set in national strategies for health.

The value of strategies at district and national level is in focusing efforts on agreed priorities, and providing a framework for setting objectives and monitoring progress towards their achievement.

International Health Promotion Strategies

In health promotion, we have international planning led by WHO, which set European targets for health in 1985[1]. These have now been rather overtaken by a new focus on national targets.

See also Chapter 1.

National Health Strategies

The first national strategies in the UK

There has been considerable progress in strategic planning at national level in the late 1980s and 1990s. In the UK, Wales was first in 1989 with a strategy from the Welsh Office NHS Directorate, *Strategic Intent and Direction for the NHS in Wales*, and a series of planning documents for health in Wales published in 1990 by the Health Promotion Authority for Wales (now Health Promotion Wales).[2]

In England, the Department of Health issued a consultation document *The Health of the Nation* in 1991, followed by the *Health of the Nation* national strategy for health in England in 1992.[3] This identified five priorities (called Key Areas) for action: coronary heart disease and stroke; cancers – lung, skin, breast and cervical; mental illness; HIV/AIDS and sexual health; and accidents. It set objectives in each Key Area, with a total of 27 targets. (We have put an example in Table 7.1). The importance of the targets was that they set out quantified and measurable achievements to aim for, and provided yardsticks against which progress could be monitored. Targets were set in terms of mortality (death rates), morbidity (illness rates), or changes in health behaviour (such as the percentage of the population who smoke).

Table 7.1	**Health of the Nation: Example of Objective and Targets**	
Key Area	**Objective**	**Targets**
Coronary heart disease and stroke	To reduce the level of ill-health and death caused by coronary heart disease and stroke, and the risk factors associated with them.	Example: To reduce death rates for CHD in people under 65 by at least 40% by the year 2000 (from 58 per 100,000 population in 1990 to no more than 35 per 100,000). Other targets cover CHD in older people, strokes, smoking, blood pressure, obesity, diet and alcohol.

Many more *Health of the Nation* documents were issued following the initial launch in 1992, including Key Area Handbooks which gave examples of good practice and suggestions for action in the five Key Areas.[4]

In 1996, a consultation document was issued which proposed a sixth key area: the environment. Proposed targets focused on outdoor air quality, air quality in the home, radon (a naturally-occurring radioactive gas which can accumulate in buildings), noise pollution and lead in drinking water.[5]

In Scotland, *Scotland's health – a challenge to us all* was published in 1992[6] and in Northern Ireland, *The Regional Strategy for Health and Personal Social Services 1992–1997* was produced in 1991.[7]

So, for the first time, we had national strategies for health (as opposed to strategies for health *services*), with a clear emphasis on planning for improving, maintaining and restoring *health*, rather than planning for health care and treatment services. Health promotion had a key part to play in these strategies, although effective treatment and care continued, of course, to play a part. Improving health had become a prime mission of the NHS. The aim of health authorities had been reoriented, to some extent, towards improvement in the health of the population for which they were responsible.

The four national documents differed in their breadth and emphasis. England's *The Health of the Nation* had been welcomed because it put health promotion on the agenda, but it had also been criticized for largely failing to acknowledge the socioeconomic determinants of health. It mentioned inequalities as 'variations' in health status, and looked to the lifestyle change model of health promotion as the way forward. It emphasized the value of multiagency working, which it termed 'healthy alliances'.[8]

The Welsh strategy took a broader view, and included 'emotional health and relationships', 'physical disability and discomfort' and 'healthy environments' in its priorities for action. Its strategy documents identified the 'health skills' required to safeguard health and lead socially fulfilling lives: knowledge, attitudes, self-confidence, coping and relationships, parenting, safety and first-aid, self-help and mutual support.

Scotland's strategy emphasized the importance of environmental factors, and the Northern Ireland strategy included discussion of the impact of 'material deprivation' on health. All four, however, emphasized lifestyle factors as crucial; smoking, drinking, exercise, and sexual behaviour featured prominently.

How successful were these national strategies? A report in 1996 from the National Audit Office on progress towards *The Health of the Nation* targets concluded that, while the initiative was making an impact, progress was uneven and slow.[9] It concluded that although good progress was being made to cut the number of deaths from heart disease, strokes, and certain cancers, rising levels of obesity, alcohol drinking by women and smoking by children threatened to undermine health gains significantly.

In the areas where targets were being reached, and trends in death, illness and health behaviour were going in the right direction, it is impossible to say how far this good news was due to efforts to implement the strategy.[10] For example, there was a decrease in the rate of accidental deaths (many due to road accidents) in children. But why? It could have been because of improved education about accident prevention or a safer environment (such as more traffic calming schemes). Or it could have been because more injured children were saved from dying with better or quicker treatment, or maybe even because more parents were afraid to risk letting their children out to play, walk to school or cycle on the roads, so that their exposure to life-threatening risks was reduced.

1997 – New Directions in National Strategies

There were significant developments following the change of government in 1997. The Labour government reviewed England's strategy, *The Health of the Nation*, and proposed a revised strategy published in early 1998 as a Green Paper for consultation entitled, *Our Healthier Nation*.[11] Scotland's strategy went through a similar process, with a consultation paper, *Working Together for a Healthier Scotland*. Key features of these proposed strategies are set out in Box 7.1.

In Wales, new guidance was issued on the development of local strategies for health. 15 health gain targets were set with target dates of 2002 or 2010[12]. The targets covered cancers, heart disease, strokes, accidents, suicides, low birth weight babies, back pain, arthritis, mental health, smoking, consumption of fruit and vegetables, alcohol consumption, and dental caries.

| Box 7.1. | **New Directions in Public Health** |

Our Healthier Nation, issued for consultation in early 1998, set out proposals which embodied a new emphasis on health gain, tackling the root causes of ill-health, and reducing inequalities in health ('the health gap').

It set out *two key aims*:
- to improve the health of the population as a whole by increasing the length of people's lives and the number of years people spend free from illness
- to improve the health of the worst off in society and to narrow the health gap.

It proposed a national contract for health, with *four priority areas*:
- heart disease and stroke
- accidents
- cancer
- mental health.

One national *target* was proposed for each of these priorities, to be reached by year 2010.

A draft *national contract* for each priority was set out, with ideas for what could be done at three levels (government and national; local; and at the level of individual people), addressing four areas for action (social and economic; environmental; lifestyle; and services).

In addition to working on the four national priorities, the paper proposed that health authorities should identify *local priorities and targets*, in collaboration with a range of partners such as local authorities and voluntary and community groups. These local priorities should tackle pressing local problems and aim to reduce local health inequalities.

Three *settings* for action were proposed:
- healthy schools – focusing on children
- healthy workplaces – focusing on adults
- healthy neighbourhoods – focusing on older people.

Proposals for Scotland, set out in *Working Together for a Healthier Scotland*, were broadly similar, except that five priorities were proposed, three of which were the same as England's. These five were:
- heart disease and stroke
- cancer
- teenage pregnancy
- dental and oral health
- accidents.

In Northern Ireland, a new strategy for 1997–2002 was published: *Health and Wellbeing: into the next millennium*.[13] This set the overall direction for both health and personal social services, identified priorities and key areas for action: family and child health and welfare; physical and sensory disability; learning disability; mental health; circulatory diseases; cancers; and other non-communicable diseases of diabetes, respiratory diseases and back pain. Specific aims and (in some cases) quantitative targets were set.

Local Health Strategies

Most statutory agencies at a local level (Health Authorities or Health Boards, local authorities) produce their own local strategies which fit in with national strategies. In England, for example, many Health Authorities set their own local targets for the Key Areas specified in *The Health of the Nation*. They also monitor their achievement of the targets. The task of setting local strategies was given new impetus in 1997/98 with the publication of the white papers outlining the Labour government's plans for the NHS in England, Scotland and Wales.[14] A key feature of these white papers was that health authorities or boards, in collaboration with local authorities and other partners, were required to develop *health improvement programmes* (HIPs) for their populations. HIPs are local plans covering prevention and health promotion as well as treatment and care, and should incorporate work on the national health strategies.

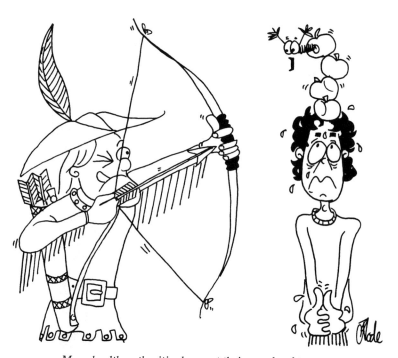

Many health authorities have set their own local targets.

What is the relevance of national and local strategy to the everyday work of a health promoter? In a nutshell, the key point is to identify how your own health promotion work **contributes** to a broader strategy, and how it **complements** work that other people are doing. This can increase your job satisfaction as you see that you are not alone but are part of a broader movement, increase the chance of successful funding and managerial support, and decrease the chance of unhelpful duplication of effort.

Figure 7.1 illustrates the many people in a range of agencies who may be contributing to the aim of increasing physical activity in the population, complementing each other's efforts.

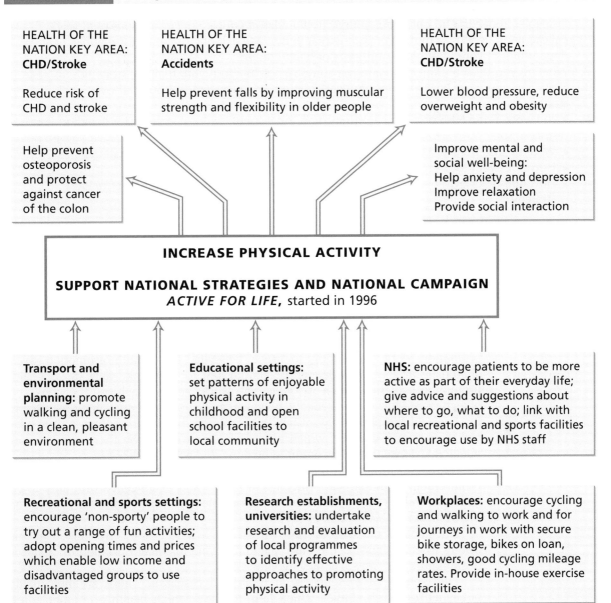

Fig 7.1 **Contributing to a National Strategy: Health of the Nation. Local complementary contributions to promoting physical activity.**

HEALTH OF THE NATION KEY AREA: **CHD/Stroke**

Reduce risk of CHD and stroke

HEALTH OF THE NATION KEY AREA: **Accidents**

Help prevent falls by improving muscular strength and flexibility in older people

HEALTH OF THE NATION KEY AREA: **CHD/Stroke**

Lower blood pressure, reduce overweight and obesity

Help prevent osteoporosis and protect against cancer of the colon

Improve mental and social well-being: Help anxiety and depression Improve relaxation Provide social interaction

INCREASE PHYSICAL ACTIVITY

SUPPORT NATIONAL STRATEGIES AND NATIONAL CAMPAIGN *ACTIVE FOR LIFE*, started in 1996

Transport and environmental planning: promote walking and cycling in a clean, pleasant environment

Educational settings: set patterns of enjoyable physical activity in childhood and open school facilities to local community

NHS: encourage patients to be more active as part of their everyday life; give advice and suggestions about where to go, what to do; link with local recreational and sports facilities to encourage use by NHS staff

Recreational and sports settings: encourage 'non-sporty' people to try out a range of fun activities; adopt opening times and prices which enable low income and disadvantaged groups to use facilities

Research establishments, universities: undertake research and evaluation of local programmes to identify effective approaches to promoting physical activity

Workplaces: encourage cycling and walking to work and for journeys in work with secure bike storage, bikes on loan, showers, good cycling mileage rates. Provide in-house exercise facilities

Evidence-Based Health Promotion

The term **evidence-based** has now come into common use, especially in the phrase 'evidence-based medicine'.[15] It means that we should aim to do only those medical activities which we have evidence will work successfully. So, for example, someone believing that decisions about health care interventions should be

Exercise 7.1   **Finding out about national and local health promotion strategies**

1. Have a look at the national strategy for health in your country (see section on National Health Strategies above to find out about yours). Try libraries at educational institutions or at work, colleagues in health promotion or planning at your place of work, or contact the public health department of your local health authority or health board.
2. What do you think are the good and not-so-good points about your national strategy?
3. How does your own health promotion work contribute to the aims set out in the national strategy?
4. If you work in the NHS or a local authority, find out if there is a local strategy for health in your district. If so:
    *   What do you think are the good and not-so-good points about your local strategy?
    *   How does your local strategy relate to your national strategy?
    *   How does your own health promotion work contribute to the aims set out in the local strategy?

based on evidence would argue that we should not undertake operations which research has shown do not benefit patients. This is the reason why, for example, it now uncommon to take out a child's tonsils, whereas years ago it was very common practice. Research over time has shown that it doesn't do the good doctors had hoped it would. The same arguments can be applied to health promotion work. According to those believing that health promotion work should be driven by evidence, we should aim to undertake only those health promotion activities which we *know* will work, and will achieve the aims and objectives we have set. Arguably, however, as David Seedhouse demonstrates in his book on the philosophy of health promotion, health promotion is driven by *both values and evidence*, which are often intertwined.[16] So there are two key questions: do we think this ought to be done *and* will it work?

So, health promotion must be based on sound scientific research. This is a requirement of the ethical principles of justice and beneficence (the duty to do good), as well as the political demand to be able to justify policies and practice on the basis of reliable evidence.

But another question is: how do we know what works? We looked at this briefly when discussing the basic planning cycle for health promotion: Stage 3, deciding the best way of achieving your aims.

See Chapter 5 (section on Stage 3 of the planning cycle).

We discuss how you can find and appraise research later in this chapter.

One source of evidence is in published research. There are now many published research studies which help to show which health promotion interventions work best.[17]

Often it is not one single activity which produces results, but a combination of activities, of which you may be involved in just one. In the case study of physical activity (Fig. 7.1.), we indicate a range of action which is likely to contribute to an increase in physical activity levels. Another example is child accident prevention work, where research indicates that we need a combination of educating people about safety and accident prevention, coupled with legislation and changes in the environment which make accidental injuries less likely.[18] For example, to reduce road accidents, we need a combination of road safety education for drivers and pedestrians, well-designed and maintained roads which include features such as traffic-calming schemes to slow motorists down, speed cameras to detect and deter speeding motorists, and legislation to enforce drink-driving laws. To reduce home accidents, we need education of parents and child carers on reducing risks around the home; provision of affordable or free loans of home safety equipment such as fireguards and smoke alarms; and legislation on safety standards for buildings and manufacturing items for the home such as flame-retardant furniture. Research shows that for many health promotion issues, a combination of complementary activities is the most effective.[19]

A major problem with the evidence-based approach is that there is not always evidence to hand. The particular piece of work you plan to undertake may not have been done before, and indeed the particular set of circumstances in which you are working will be unique. So the best that can be done is to be aware of what the published research in *related* areas of work tells you, and to reflect on how what was learned might apply to your circumstances.

It also helps to think carefully about what constitutes evidence. Evidence is not necessarily confined to formal research. The views of local people are evidence. Your own experience is evidence; your job as a health promoter is to use your judgement to decide whether the evidence available applies to your clients and circumstances, and if so how. For example, GPs quote a number of factors which they believe provide evidence that health promotion is effective, including: 'I'm convinced because I have seen changes in the health of my patients over the last eight or nine years – patients don't keep coming back, they are more aware of their physical health, have better control of their sugar levels, blood pressure, diabetes and so on'.[20]

In addition, you can plan carefully and evaluate or audit what you do. In this way, you will be building up your own body of knowledge about what is effective.

We discuss audit later in this chapter.

Finally, it is also important to bear in mind that your decision about whether to do a particular piece of health promotion work is ultimately a moral and ethical one. You could decide that it is your responsibility to intervene, even though you have little or no information about what might work.

The next section discusses how you can find, and use, published research.

Using Published Research[21]

Health promoters not only need to be well informed about relevant research, but to *use* their knowledge of research findings to improve their practice. Familiarity with research findings can also give you ammunition to use in making a case for more, or different and better, health promotion. Scanning journals and digests (which highlight recent articles of interest to health promoters) should be part of your everyday working life.[22]

How to do a Literature Search

However, you may sometimes wish to find out about research on a particular topic, perhaps because you are proposing to introduce new health promotion work and want to know what has been shown to work best. For example, imagine you are a nurse working in cancer care and you are considering introducing a counselling service for women who are undergoing mastectomy (surgery to remove a breast, usually because of breast cancer). You want to know if research shows what the needs and concerns of these women are and how best to meet them. Where do you start?

First you need to clarify exactly what your research question is. It pays to take time to discuss this with colleagues. For the mastectomy counselling service, you could also discuss it with someone who has recently had a mastectomy. What did she find helpful, and what was unhelpful?

Once you are clear about what it is that you want to find out, list no more than six key words which feature in your question. The cancer care nurse might include the words mastectomy, needs, and counselling in her list. Then write words that mean the same thing (these are referred to as 'synonyms'), or are close in meaning, by each key word. For example, you might put breast cancer as an alternative to mastectomy, and advice as an alternative to counselling. These key words and their synonyms/alternatives will be helpful when you go to the library. Here you will find 'abstracting journals' – these are publications that summarize published material in a particular subject area.[23] There are also research digests available on CD-ROM[24]. In addition, many journal articles include a list of key words after the title, and this will help you to know whether the article is of interest to you. When you have found a few references, you can start by reading the most recent one. This will in turn provide you with more references. Once you are underway, the next problem is to avoid being swamped by information. Here again, your key words are useful in stopping you from being side-tracked and in keeping your research question in mind.

It is important to keep records of what you read. Doing this may seem a chore, but it will save you time in the long run. There are computer programmes designed to help you store and retrieve references, but if you are using a paper system you can write up a separate index card for each article or book. For a book, you need to record:

- Author's (or editor's) surname and initials
- Year published
- Title and subtitle
- Edition if not the first
- Chapter, or numbers of pages, if you are only going to refer to part of the book
- Place of publication
- Publisher

For articles in journals you need to record:

- Author's surname and initials
- Year of publication
- Title and subtitles of article
- Journal title
- Volume and part numbers
- The inclusive page numbers of the article
- Date of publication

If you are gathering research evidence which will be used to inform a health promotion decision or action, then the first thing you need to know when reading an article is whether it is a report of actual research, or just a knowledgeable account of facts and opinions. The first thing that may help you to know about this is the *abstract*. This is a summary of why a study was done and what are the main findings. Abstracts usually take the form of a paragraph at the start of an article. Research reports also usually follow the following format:

- **Introduction** – background to the study
- **Literature review** – summary of previous and related research
- **Method** – a description of how the study was carried out
- **Results** – the findings of the study
- **Discussio**n – a discussion of the findings
- **Conclusions** – the implications of the findings
- **References** – all the studies and books referred to in the article

Having identified an article as a report of research which was actually carried out, you now need to read it critically, bearing a few crucial questions in mind:

When was the research carried out? Although the article is recent, it could be reporting on research which was carried out some years previously and has now been superseded by more up-to-date research.

Why was the research done? Do you see the need for this research? Will it contribute new knowledge on the subject? Will this knowledge be useful in practice?

How was the research carried out? Did it use methods and tools which were likely to provide answers to the questions posed by the researchers? What type of research was carried out? For example, if the researchers wanted to find out what works in changing the behaviour of sedentary people with angina to cause them to take more exercise, then **experimental research** would be required. (This is research which establishes a relationship between cause and effect, often through studying subgroups of people, where the *experimental* subgroup experience the intervention under consideration, and the *control* subgroup do not.) Another type of research is **action research**. This is used to find out exactly how to implement changes, or solve problems, in a specific situation, through watching and documenting in a systematic manner, how the changes are introduced.

Does the researcher draw reasonable conclusions from the results? This can be the most difficult question to answer, especially if you are blinded by statistics. If you are not sure that you understand, get help! This is of crucial importance if you are thinking of implementing the findings.

How could or should this research affect health promotion practice or policy? Even if the research was not carried out in your specialty or particular area of work, it could have implications for them. For example, findings about how best to communicate with patients who are very anxious after a heart attack, could be used to help to improve communication with patients who have cancer.

Through asking these, and other, questions you should be able to come to a judgement about whether a piece of research is sound. It should have:

- been carried out by competent researchers;
- used sound research design;
- contained sound baseline data;

For further discussion of research see the next section on 'Doing your own small scale research'.

■ used any research instrument (such as a questionnaire) which has been piloted (which means tried and tested first to iron out any problems) and validated (which means that it has been tested to show that it really does measure what it was supposed to measure).

So, you do not need to *do* research yourself – you can improve your effectiveness through examining research findings and considering whether and how they apply to your work. However, in certain situations you may wish to carry out a modest piece of research yourself. We discuss this in the next section.

Doing Your Own Small-Scale Research

There may be times when you might want to undertake some research yourself. For example, you may be studying for a qualification in a particular aspect of health or health promotion, and the course may include a research project. Or you and a group of colleagues may have uncovered an unmet health promotion need, and your health authority has agreed to fund a study to look in more detail at the need and how it could best be met.

We have included suggestions for further study on research skills in 'Notes and References' throughout this section, and in the 'Recommended Reading' at the end of the chapter.

By research, we mean a planned, systematic gathering of information for the purpose of increasing the total body of knowledge. Research involves gathering information which is not readily available. If you are inexperienced, it will be important for you to get some help from an experienced researcher, right from the start. The following information should also help, but it should not be used as a guide to doing research on its own.

The research process involves carrying out some specific tasks, which are set out in Box 7.2.

Box 7.2.	Research tasks

1. Define the purpose of the research.
2. Review the literature.
3. Plan the study and the method(s) of investigation.
4. Test the method by carrying out a pilot study.
5. Collect the information.
6. Analyse the information.
7. Draw conclusions based on the findings of the analysis.
8. Compile the research report.

Although the tasks will tend to be carried out in the sequence set out in the box, this is not necessarily so. For example, you may write parts of the research report as you go through each task, so that all the relevant information is set down as you go along. And you may have a much clearer idea about the purpose of the research *after* you have read the literature on other investigations in your area of interest.

The most important task in this list is the first one – the kind of question you want to answer will form the basis of the whole project. For example, suppose that you want to know what is the best way to encourage a particular group of patients with angina to take more physical activity. This question is concerned with ways of motivating a specific group of patients. The experts in this field are psychologists, so it is to the body of psychological research literature that you will turn for soundly-based principles. However, you may instead be concerned to know which of a number of alternative effective ways to motivate patients to take more physical exercise are best value for money. If so, you will want to look at cost-effectiveness studies and make use of the work of health economists. It is vital that you are clear about the practical reasons why you are engaging in this research. If you are very sure about why you are doing it, who will use the findings and for what purposes, then you are likely to come up with some useful answers. If you get distracted by interesting but irrelevant information, your research could be confused and therefore flawed.

Time spent on task 3, planning, always proves to be a good investment. If you are going to apply for funding, your planning must include investigating sources of funding and the particular interests of different potential funders. Most tasks take longer than you think they will, and you will need to allow plenty of time for consulting people; for example, to arrange interviews with people. Ethical issues and the need to apply for permission from ethical committees must also not be forgotten.[25] They will want to see the research proposal and may require additional information about issues such as confidentiality.[26]

You will also need to consider ways of collecting the information you need. Any information collected needs to be valid and reliable. By **validity** we simply mean actually measuring what you purport to measure. For example, if you are attempting to measure the success of health education in persuading a group of people to take more physical exercise, a valid measure would be to directly observe whether or not they spend more time doing physical activities. Asking them to complete a written questionnaire may not give valid responses because research shows that people may respond to questions and questionnaires as they think the experts want them to. By **reliability**, we mean that if the research is repeated, it gives the same results.

Basic Tools of Research

There are a number of basic tools used in health promotion research. Some of these are now briefly discussed.

Questionnaires[27]

These are useful when you want to collect information from relatively large numbers of people. They should be kept as simple as possible, but this does not mean that they are easy to design. A great deal of care is needed in the formulation of questions to ensure that valid conclusions can be drawn from them. Questionnaires are most useful for collecting information that is quantifiable, such as factual knowledge. Advantages of questionnaires include: they can be answered anonymously, and respondents may therefore be more truthful; they can be given to a whole group of people at the same time, so using respondents' and researcher's time effectively.

They should always first be piloted (tried out) on a small sample of people from the group for whom the questionnaire is intended. You will then be able to identify any questions which have been misinterpreted, and can redesign them.

The response rate to questionnaires can be low, and you may need to think about the implications of this (for example, will the results really reflect the views of the target population?). Also, some people hate filling in forms and even if they fill one in may do so casually, without giving it careful thought.

You need to consider right from the start how the information collected will be analysed. Decisions about whether a computer will be needed to analyse the information may affect the design of the questionnaire. Consultation with a statistician and/or an experienced researcher may be helpful at this point.[28]

You have to put a lot of effort into the design of quantitative questionnaires by clarifying closed questions with defined ways of responding (such as tick boxes), so that they will give accurate results. On the other hand, qualitative questionnaires (those with open questions which can be responded to in a variety of ways) are easier to design, but it can be very complicated to analyse the responses. There is no 'right' way to solve these problems: it is a matter of trading off the advantages of one approach against the disadvantages.

Personal interviews[29]

With face-to-face interviews you can develop rapport and encourage people to talk more openly. You may find out things which you did not think to ask about, but which are very relevant. The main advantage of personal interviews is that there is more scope for initiative by the interviewee. For example, the interviewee can seek clarification, and may be able to express views and opinions more easily verbally than in writing. The disadvantage is that unless you are very skilled, you may bias the response, that is, you may get the responses which you want to get or expect to get. For example, asking 'you do feel better, don't you?' biases the answer towards 'yes', whereas 'do you feel better?' removes this bias.

The basic skills of asking questions are discussed in Chapter 10.

Interviews can be one-to-one or with groups. They can be organized through using pre-prepared questions (this is often described as a **structured interview**) or allowed to flow more freely. At one extreme, you could design an interview schedule which looks like a questionnaire. At the other extreme, you might simply have three or four broad headings which you wish to discuss (a **semi-structured interview**). Special techniques, such as focus groups, have also been developed.[30] (Focus groups concentrate on a particular issue through 'focusing' on pre-determined questions.)

Discussion of interview techniques is beyond the scope of this book, but see the suggestions for further reading at the end of the chapter.

Participant and Non-Participant Observation

Observation can include observing behaviour, such as how well a person performs an exercise routine, and physiological observations, such as monitoring weight. **Participant observation** happens when the researcher is also actively involved in what is being observed, such as actively contributing to discussions in a meeting. **Non-participant observation** means that the researcher takes no part in what is being observed. Advantages of participant observation are that the researcher may be more aware of what is going on, including less tangible things such as the mood of a group of people. However, the researcher may have difficulty in making objective observations and also may find it difficult to record what is happening, so that information could be lost. The non-participant researcher may find it easier to make objective observations, and may be able to plan and record observations more easily. On the other hand, having an observer who does not participate can seem threatening. People may thus fail to open up or not behave as they normally do. This could have a big effect on what is observed, and invalidate the research.

Sampling

If it is too expensive or time consuming to collect information from the whole population or group you are interested in, then you need to select individuals so that you avoid getting a biased response. The techniques of random sampling or quota sampling can be used to ensure that the sample is representative of the whole population.

Random sampling. This involves identifying people at random from a list of the whole group. For example, imagine you are a practice nurse. Using the practice age–sex register, you could decide at random on a number between 1 and ten, say 5, and send out questionnaires to the 5th, 15th, 25th, 35th and so on persons on the list.

Quota sampling. This uses your knowledge of a particular group to help set criteria about who to include in the sample. Criteria you might use include age, sex and ethnicity. Once the group has been divided into segments, using your criteria, you can use a proportion from each segment for your sample. This ensures that people with certain characteristics are not over- or under-represented.

Convenience sampling. This means that researchers question the people they can get hold of at the time. This is biased, but accepting that it is very difficult to avoid bias altogether, it is important to decide whether the particular bias which has been introduced is acceptable. It will also be important to discuss this aspect of the research in the report, in order to avoid misleading readers.

The Research Report

The final stage of your research will be to make available the findings to all those with an interest through a written report. Readers may be interested in assessing the validity of the findings for themselves; in repeating the research in similar circumstances and avoiding any pitfalls; or in applying the research findings in the context of purchasing or providing health promotion work. So the report should be written with the objective of helping readers to use it in these ways.

See also the section on Report Writing in Chapter 8, and the section on Written Communication in Chapter 10.

You may need to consider producing more than one version of the report for different groups of readers; for example, a two-page summary for community groups, and a full report for your health authority.

The contents of research reports may include the information set out in Box 7.3. Not every point will be applicable to a particular report, which should be written with the needs of the readers in mind.

Finally, a warning: in a field like health promotion, interpretation of research data is a complex matter, often because of underlying differences of opinion on what is health and what constitutes success. It is therefore all too easy for the

| Box 7.3. | **Checklist of Research Report content. Source: adapted from Partridge and Barnitt (1987)[31]** |

- A statement about the purpose of the research, the background circumstances and the questions to be answered.
- The reasons for carrying out the research.
- A review of the literature to assess the current state of knowledge.
- The information which the research was designed to collect.
- A description of the population sample studied, the sampling methods and response rates.
- A description of the methods used for collecting the information and the reasons for selecting these methods.
- A discussion of the ethical implications.
- Descriptions of the methods used for analysing the information and the reasons for selecting these methods.
- A description of the pilot study and any changes which were made as a result.
- The findings and all statistical data (where appropriate) on which the conclusions were based.
- A discussion of the findings, stating clearly the limitations of the study and providing recommendations for further research.
- An account of the difficulties encountered, how they were dealt with and whether they affected the results.
- A reference list providing information about all source material.

sceptical to dismiss research findings. So it is extremely important that any health promotion research is of good quality. Poor research is worse than no research because it wastes resources and misleads.

Value For Money

When planning, you need to think about not just what resources you need, but also the wider question of whether you are getting value for money. Health economics is a discipline which provides a way of thinking about value for money and making efficient use of scarce resources. It is not about doing things more cheaply, but about choosing priorities and making the best choices with the resources available. To help with this the economist focuses on costs and outcomes. 'Costs' involve much more than money: they may include people, equipment, buildings and intangible costs, such as distress. 'Outcomes' include length of life and also things that are difficult to measure, such as relief of stress.

Opportunity cost. This is an important concept. If resources are scarce, doing one thing means giving up the potential benefits of doing another thing. So, for example, money devoted to drugs mass media campaigns cannot be used on drug education in schools. All health promotion activities involve the use of resources which are expected to produce benefits, but at the same time incur opportunity costs (benefits which will be forgone). It is often a matter, in practice, of getting the right *balance* between alternative activities, for example, in health education about drugs, between national advertising and local educational activities.

Cost–benefit analysis. This is the process of comparing benefits with costs. Failing the cost–benefit test does not mean that an activity is not worth investing in, but it does mean that the cost of pursuing these benefits, in terms of other benefits which will have to be forgone, cannot be justified. Formal cost–benefit analysis is a complex process, not least because it is difficult to decide how different benefits should be measured and valued. Nevertheless, it can be useful to apply the basic concepts of analysing the costs and the benefits, when you are allocating resources.

Cost-effectiveness analysis. This means comparing the costs and outcomes of alternative activities to achieve the same goal.[32] It can be used when it is possible to measure the outcomes of alternative activities in the same unit of measurement, such as measuring blood pressure. For example, supposing that research had shown that exercise, drugs and diet (or a combination of these) were effective in lowering high blood pressure; these interventions could then be costed to see which ones were the most cost-effective. This approach is used in considering alternative health interventions; for example, the Department of Health has reviewed the options available to reduce coronary heart disease and stroke in terms of effectiveness and cost-effectiveness.[33]

For examples of using a cost effectiveness approach and other concepts from health economics in health promotion research, see Note[34].

Audit and Evaluation

What is 'Audit'?

See Chapter 5.

Audit is the systematic examination of the operations of a service, followed by the implementation of recommendations to improve quality. Basically, an audit will scrutinize how the service carries out each stage of the planning/evaluation cycle which we described in Chapter 5. Strengths and weaknesses will be revealed, and ways of overcoming weaknesses will be identified. Audit can either involve an internal review by the people responsible for delivering a service, or scrutiny by an independent external auditor. For example, all NHS Trusts now have clinical auditors who audit the clinical activities of the Trust.[35] At national level, the Audit Commission is responsible for auditing NHS activities.[36] The audit cycle normally starts with the specification of standards or criteria, followed by the collection of data, the assessment of performance, the identification of the need for change and implementing the improvements (see Fig. 7.2).

It is in the nature of cycles that you can, in practice, start anywhere. So you might start with collecting data on performance, assess performance, and one of the recommendations could be the need to specify standards. The difficulty with auditing health promotion practice is that it is often embedded in other work. For example, audit of health promotion in clinical settings may involve scrutinizing issues about relationships, communication and staff training and supervision, all of which are vital to the quality of health promotion work, but non-clinical. In addition, the most serious problems are often between professions and departments and agencies, in the areas of communication and coordination, while audit is usually conducted on a uniprofessional basis (for example medical audit).

For further reading on quality standards, see Chapter 8 (section on 'Working for Quality').

However, there are a number of good reasons why it may be wise to make a start on auditing health promotion on a uniprofessional basis.[37] Many services

Fig 7.2   **An audit cycle.**

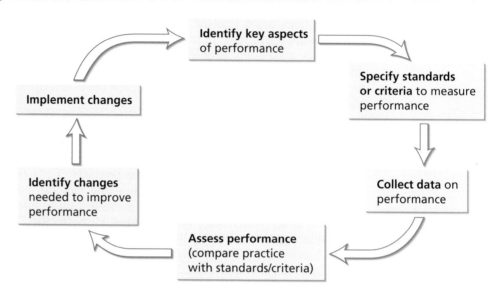

are structured by profession. Audit may be unfamiliar and may seem threatening to health promoters. Most existing experience of audit, and proof of its value, is within each profession (for example, within nursing audit and medical audit). This experience can help. Problems which involve other professions, departments or agencies can be noted and later tackled through establishing interprofessional or interagency health promotion quality groups.

Many of the tools described in the section above on 'Doing your own research', can also be used in audit. So, for example, you could study the satisfaction of patients with information and education provided to them while in-patients, through a telephone survey after discharge. When telephoning them, you would need to reassure patients that participation in the survey was voluntary, and that their comments would be completely confidential. The sort of things you might like to ask them are set out in the Box 7.4.

Box 7.4.   **Patient satisfaction with health education and information: telephone survey schedule**

- When you were in hospital, what information were you given about your illness?
- Do you now feel you have sufficient information about what was wrong with you?
- Were you able to discuss your anxieties with anyone while you were in hospital?
- Who did you prefer to discuss things with? *Prompt: Was it a nurse, a doctor, another professional or a domestic helper?*
- Did you have sufficient privacy to feel able to open up? *Prompt: Did you have access to a comfortable, private room for private conversations?*

- What instructions were you given about your health? *Probe: instructions about medication or how to look after yourself and avoid risks in future. How were these provided: through verbal instructions, in writing, through pictures or diagrams? Did you fully understand the instructions? If not, why do you think you had difficulties?*
- Did you have enough information to look after yourself after you left hospital? *Prompt: Do you need any more information to look after yourself now?*
- What other information would you have liked?
- How would you like information to be provided? *Prompt: in a leaflet, through one-to-one discussion, or through group sessions?*
- Have your relatives (or your spouse, or the person you live with) been provided with information? *Prompt: Do you think they have had sufficient information?*
- Do you feel confident about looking after your own health now? *Prompt: If not, what further help and support would you like?*

Audit, Research and Evaluation

Evaluation is discussed in detail in Chapter 5.

Audit, research and evaluation are complementary activities. Research is concerned with generating new knowledge and new approaches, which can be applied beyond the specific context where the study was done. Evaluation involves making a judgement about one specific intervention or project, which is the focus of its concern. Audit seeks to improve the performance of a continuing service, such as an environmental health service or a midwifery service, through reviewing its practice. All three are crucial to the pursuit of evidence-based health promotion.

You should not need to do a detailed evaluation of everything you do, because you will be basing what you do on techniques and materials which have already been evaluated by others and form part of the published evidence. What you *should* do is to audit your health promotion practices regularly to check whether what you have planned and the techniques you have chosen are working properly. One problem inhibiting health promoters from doing this is a lack of audit skills.[38] If you need further training in how to carry out an audit of your health promotion practice, it would be worth finding out about local opportunities for training in clinical audit – the basic concepts can be applied to

See the section on Working for Quality in Chapter 8.

health promotion. Another area to pursue could be training related to measuring and improving quality or quality assurance. Quality cycles and audit cycles are very closely related and the purpose of audit is to improve quality. You could also discuss, with your manager, local arrangements for performance appraisal (mechanisms for checking on and improving the performance of staff), professional development plans, and supervision, since these too are all related to audit.

For further reading on audit, see the suggestions at the end of the chapter.

From the viewpoint of the individual client or patient, we need to audit their total experience of a service, including non-clinical or non-technical aspects, and these include health education and health promotion practice.

■ It is important to identify how your health promotion work contributes to local and national strategies. Your effectiveness depends not only on what you do, but on how well your work complements, and avoids conflict with, that of other health promoters.

■ All health promoters have a duty to regularly appraise relevant research, and to base their work on evidence of effectiveness, when such evidence exists.

■ Evidence is not confined to formal research: the views of your clients are evidence; your own experience is evidence.

■ Doing research involves specialized skills, and it should not be attempted unless you have developed the appropriate competencies which the particular type of research requires.

■ When planning, you need to think about whether you are getting value for money, through using the ways of thinking developed in health economics.

■ Any service should regularly take stock of how it operates and identify how things can be improved.

Recommended Reading

National Strategies for Health

Find the most up-to-date version of the national strategy for health in your country. You should be able to find out what it is and possibly borrow a copy from:

- your local NHS health promotion department
- national health education/promotion libraries (Health Education Authority, Health Education Board for Scotland, Health Promotion Wales, Health Promotion Agency for Northern Ireland see Chapter 4 Notes 9, 14, 15 for addresses)
- your local health authority or board
- libraries in colleges and universities running health courses.

In early 1998, the most recent versions were:

For England
➤ Secretary of State for Health (1998) *Our Healthier Nation: a contract for health. A Consultation Paper.* London: The Stationery Office.

For Scotland
➤ Department of Health Scottish Office (1998) *Working Together for a Healthier Scotland: a consultation paper.* London: The Stationery Office.

For Wales
➤ Welsh Office (1989) *Strategic Intent and Direction for the NHS in Wales.* Welsh Office NHS

Directorate: The Welsh Health Planning Forum. This was updated in a letter from the Welsh Office to health authorities, NHS trusts, local authorities and others, 11 June 1998, headed *New Strategic Plans.* Letter ref. DGM (97) 50. A new strategy on public health was expected in 1998.

For Northern Ireland
➤ Department of Health and Social Services (1997) *Health and Wellbeing: into the next millennium.* Belfast: DHSS. Full and summary version available from: Department of Health and Social Services, Belfast. Tel 01232 524732

On Evidence-Based Health Care and Health Promotion

➤ Muir Gray J A (1996) *Evidence-based Health Care.* London: Churchill Livingstone. (Includes basic issues such as the nature of research and study design along with ways of accessing relevant research, critical appraisal of research, and methods of implementing research findings. It is written so that it is accessible to non-clinicians and clinicians alike, and is recommended for any professional working in, or training for, the health service.)
➤ Katz J & Peberdy A (1997) *Promoting Health: Knowledge and Practice.* Chapter 12, What counts

as evidence in health promotion? Basingstoke: Macmillan/Open University Press.

➤ Sidell M, Jones L, Katz J & Peberdy A (1997) (eds) *Debates and Dilemmas in Promoting Health.* Basingstoke: Macmillan/Open University Press. (Section 2: *Questioning the evidence base of health promotion* looks in depth at what counts as evidence in health promotion and includes chapters about epidemiological, economic and social work approaches to collecting and assessing evidence.)

See also *Notes and References 17* (below) for a list of effectiveness studies and reviews.

On Finding and Using Published Research

➤ Ogier M (1998) *Reading Research: or how to make research more approachable,* 2nd edn. London: Baillière Tindall/Royal College of Nursing.

On Doing your Own Research:

➤ Bell J (1993) *Doing Your Research Project: A guide for first-time researchers in education and social science,* 2nd edn. Buckingham: Open University Press. (Guidance on how to do small-scale research projects.)

➤ Maslin-Prothero S (ed.) (1997) *Baillière's Study Skills for Nurses.* London: Baillière Tindall. (Includes study skills; reading skills; using libraries and information technology; how to do literature searches; and writing skills (including writing reflectively for academic publications.)

➤ McConway K (ed.) (1994) *Studying Health and Disease,* revised edn. Open University Health & Disease series, Book 2. Buckingham: Open University Press. (Broad introduction to main methods of research and investigation used in the area of health and disease.)

➤ Katz J & Peberdy A (1997) *Promoting Health: Knowledge and Practice,* Chapter 13, Studying populations; Chapter 14, Analysing numerical data; Chapter 18, Enquiring and reporting. Basingstoke: Macmillan/Open University Press.

Useful Series on Research in the *Health Education Journal*

➤ Secker J, Wimbush E, Watson J & Milburn K (1995) Qualitative methods in health promotion research: some criteria for quality. *Health Education Journal* **54**, 74–87. (Review of qualitative research methods in health promotion.)

➤ Fraser E, Bryce C, Crosswaite C, McCann K & Platt S (1995) Evaluating health promotion: doing it by numbers. *Health Education Journal* **54**, 214–225. (Review of the quantitative approach to evaluation in health promotion.)

➤ Milburn K, Fraser E, Seeker J & Pavis S (1995) Combining methods in health promotion research: some considerations about appropriate use. *Health Education Journal* **54**, 347–356. (A critical assessment of the use of combined qualitative and quantitative methods in health promotion research.)

➤ Richardson J T E (ed.) (1996) *Handbook of Qualitative Research Methods for Psychology and the Social Sciences.* Leicester: British Psychological Society. (On qualitative research methods.)

On Value for Money and Health Economics in Health Promotion

➤ Tolley K (1994) *Health promotion: how to measure cost-effectiveness.* London: Health Education Authority. (A framework for evaluating the cost-effectiveness of health promotion.)

On Audit of Health Promotion Practice

➤ Simnett I (1995) *Managing Health Promotion: Developing healthy organisations and communities.* Chapter 5. Chichester: Wiley.

➤ Simnett I (1996) Auditing quality in health promotion work. *British Journal of Health Care Management* **2** (4), 205–207.

➤ Malby R (ed.) (1995) *Clinical Audit for Nurses and Therapists.* London: Scutari. (Detailed information on audit methods and skills.)

➤ Ovretveit J (1992) *Health Service Quality: An introduction to quality methods for health services,* pp. 62–75. Oxford: Blackwell Science. (This book also contains a useful quality audit checklist, which could be adapted for auditing health promotion. Appendix 2, pp. 166–168.)

Notes and References

1   WHO Regional Office for Europe (1985) *Targets for Health for All*. Copenhagen, Denmark: WHO.

2   Welsh Office (1989) *Strategic Intent and Direction for the NHS in Wales*. Welsh Office NHS Directorate: The Welsh Health Planning Forum.

The Health for All in Wales strategy was developed and produced by the Health Promotion Authority for Wales following widespread consultation during 1987 and 1988. The strategy was published as a series of planning documents:

Strategies for Action (Part A)

Health Promotion Challenges for the 1990s (Part B)

Strategic Directions for the Health Promotion Authority (Part C)

3   Secretary of State for Health (1992) *The Health of the Nation: A Strategy for Health in England*. London: HMSO.

Also published at the same time were a summary version, and a very short 'popular' version intended for the general public and available in English and ten ethnic minority languages.

4   Significant publications for health promoters included:

Department of Health (1993) *Key Area Handbooks* on:

CHD and Stroke

Cancers

Mental Illness (2nd edition published in 1994)

HIV/AIDS and Sexual Health

Accidents

Working Together for Better Health (1993), a handbook of guidance on forming and operating alliances for health.

Ethnicity and Health; a guide for the NHS (1993), about applying the Health of the Nation strategy to ethnic groups.

Variations in Health – what can the Department of Health and the NHS do? (1995), on health inequalities by social class, sex, region and ethnicity.

Targeting Practice: the contribution of nurses, midwives and health visitors to the Health of the Nation (1993).

Targeting Practice: the contribution of State Registered Dietitians (1994).

Health of the Nation Briefing Pack (1997), 2nd edn (series of loose leaf fact sheets on objectives, targets and progress towards meeting the targets.)

Also available on the Department of Health Web site (http://www.open.gov.uk/doh/dhhome.htm)

Target was a quarterly *Health of the Nation* newsletter, which became the newsletter for *Our Healthier Nation* (Health of the Nation's successor strategy) in July 1997.

Information on *Health of the Nation* publications is available from the Department of Health, Health Strategy Unit, Room LG04/05, Wellington House, 133–155 Waterloo Road, London SE1 8UG. Tel. 0171 972 4466.

5   Department of Health & Department of the Environment (1996) *Health of the Nation Consultation Document: The Environment and Health*. London: Department of Health.

6   Scottish Office (1992) *Scotland's health: a challenge to us all*. Edinburgh: HMSO.

7   Department of Health and Social Services (1991) *A Regional Strategy for the Northern Ireland Health & Personal Social Services 1992–1997*. Belfast: HMSO.

8   Department of Health (1993) *Working Together*. London: HMSO.

For further comment on the reality of working in 'healthy alliances', see:

Ewles L (1993) Hope Against Hype. *Health Service Journal* 103 (5367): 26 August.

Ewles L (1998) Working In Alliances: an inside story. Chapter 20 in Scriven A (ed.) *Health Alliances in Health Promotion: Theory and Practice*. Basingstoke: Macmillan

9   National Audit Office (1996) *Health of the Nation: a progress report*. London: HMSO.

For a summary of the National Audit Office report on *The Health of the Nation*, see:

News focus 'Variations on a theme.' *Health Service Journal*, 22 August 1996, pp. 12–13.

10   For a review of *Health of the Nation*, its choice of targets, how well it has performed, and whether some of the successes have anything to do with the strategy, see: Appleby J (1997) Feelgood Factors. *Health Service Journal*, 3 July 1997, pp. 24–27.

11   Secretary of State for Health (1998) *Our Healthier Nation: a contract for health*. A consultation paper. London: The Stationery Office.

Department of Health Scottish Office (1998) *Working Together for a Healthier Scotland: a consultation paper*. London: The Stationery Office.

12   Letter from the Welsh Office to health authorities, NHS trusts, local authorities and others, 11 June 1998, headed *New Strategic Plans*. Letter ref. DGM (97) 50.

13   Department of Health and Social Services (1997) *Health and Wellbeing: into the next millennium*. Belfast: DHSS.

14   Secretary of State for Health (1997) *The New NHS: Modern, Dependable*. London: The Stationery Office.

Department of Health Scottish Office (1997) *Designed to Care: Renewing the National Health Service in Scotland*. London: The Stationery Office.

Secretary of State for Wales (1998) *NHS Wales: Putting Patients First*. London: The Stationery Office.

15   Holloway P J & Worthington H (1997) What does 'evidence-based medicine' mean? *International Journal of Health Education* **35**(2), pp. 40–43. (Explains how decisions may be made using evidence by applying the principles of scientific method.)

16   Seedhouse D (1997) *Health Promotion: Philosophy, Prejudice and Practice*. Chapter 4. Chichester: Wiley. (Seedhouse argues that health promoters have a responsibility to arrive at their opinions through reflecting on both values and evidence and should be continually prepared to question, and if necessary to revise, their judgements.)

17   Since the mid-1990s, a number of organizations and academic centres started to publish reviews of effectiveness which summarized evidence from research in specific topics or approaches. Notably, these include:

- A series published by the Health Education Authority, starting in 1996:

  Health promotion in older people for the prevention of heart disease and strokes (1996)

  Health promotion in childhood and young adolescence for the prevention of unintentional injuries (1996)

  The effectiveness of video for health promotion (1996)

  Health promotion with young people for the prevention of substance misuse (1997)

  Health promotion with young people for the prevention of alcohol misuse (1997)

  Effectiveness of mental health promotion interventions – a review (1997)

  Forthcoming titles include:
  Oral health
  Healthy eating

- A series of *Effective Health Care Bulletins* produced by a consortium of the Nuffield Institute for

Health, University of Leeds and the NHS Centre for Reviews and Dissemination, University of York, with funding from the Department of Health, and published in association with Churchill Livingstone. The range of issues covered is wider than health promotion, but relevant titles include:

Brief Interventions and Alcohol Use (1993)

Preventing Falls and Subsequent Injury in Older People (1996)

Preventing Unintentional Injuries in Children and Young Adolescents (1996)

Preventing and Reducing the Adverse Effects of Unintended Teenage Pregnancies (1997)

The Prevention and Treatment of Obesity (1997)

Mental health promotion in high risk groups (1997)

Available from: Subscriptions Department, Pearson Professional, PO Box 77, Fourth Avenue, Harlow CM19 5BQ

- A series of reviews from the Health Promotion Research Programme, University of Bristol, Canynge Hall, Whiteladies Road, Bristol BS8 2PR. Titles are as follows:

No 1 *Health Visitor Prevention of Child Home Accidents* (1996)

No 2 *Promotion of Breastfeeding Maintenance* (1996)

No 3 *Smoke-Free Pubs* (1996)

No 4 *Life Education Centres* (1996)

No 5 *Effects of Drug Education on School Leavers* (1997)

No 6 *Primary Care to reduce Falls in Older People* (1997)

- A series of Dutch guides (in English) to effectiveness in health education and health promotion covers a wide range of issues, including sexual health, patient education, mental health, drug abuse, school health, oral health, tobacco control, accidents, exercise and cancer. Available from: Dutch Centre for Health Promotion and Health Education, PO Box 5104, 3502 JC Utrecht, The Netherlands.

There is also an increasing number of reviews published ad hoc by a variety of bodies. For example, useful ones include:

Harvey I (1995) *Prevention of Skin Cancer: a review of available strategies* Health Care Evaluation Unit, Department of Social Medicine, University of Bristol

Hogg C (1996) *Preventing Children's Accidents: a guide for health authorities and boards* Child Accident Prevention Trust, 18–20 Farringdon Lane, London EC1R 3AU

Aggleton P (1996) *Health promotion and young people*. London: Health Education Authority. (Examines patterns of illness and death in young people, their risk-taking and health-protecting behaviours, and the effectiveness of different health promotion interventions.)

Lawrence M, Neil A, Mant D & Fowler G (eds) (1996) *Prevention of cardiovascular disease: an evidence based approach*. (Oxford General Practice Series 33). Oxford: OUP. (Reviews risk factors for CHD and evidence for the clinical effectiveness of reducing them; evidence for the effectiveness of implementation; practical recommendations for CHD prevention in GP clinical practice.)

Aggleton P (1997) *Success in HIV Prevention*. Horsham: AVERT. (Discusses the most effective ways of working with young people, gay men and drug users on HIV prevention.)

Sprod J, Anderson R & Treasue E (1996) *Effective Oral Health Promotion*. Technical report 20. Cardiff: Health Promotion Wales.

It is increasingly difficult to keep up with the growing volume of research evidence for effectiveness which is accumulating through published reports of evaluated interventions. They are published in health promotion journals and many other journals focused on health and social care, medicine, community work, community nursing, environmental health and others. One helpful way to keep in touch is through the lists of *Journal Articles of Interest to Health Educators* and *Current Awareness Bulletin* published by the Health Education Authority, Trevelyan House, 30 Great Peter Street, London SW1P 2HW.

For a discussion of effectiveness reviews, see:

Research and Evaluation Division, Health Education Board for Scotland (1996) Guest editorial: how effective are effectiveness reviews? *Health Education Journal* 55, 359–362.

For further thoughts on the question of evidence in health promotion see:

Macdonald G, Tones K & Veen C (1996) Evidence for success in health promotion: suggestions for improvement. *Health Education Research* **11** (3), 367–376.

18   Health Education Authority (1996) *Health Promotion Effectiveness Reviews: Health Promotion in Childhood and Young Adolescence for the Prevention of Unintentional Injuries*. London: HEA.

NHS Centre for Review and Dissemination University of Leeds (1996) *Preventing Unintentional Injuries in Children and Young Adolescents*.

Hogg C (1996) *Preventing Children's Accidents: a guide for health authorities and boards*. London: Child Accident Prevention Trust.

19   Other examples are teenage smoking prevention work:

Staed M, Hastings G & Tudor-Smith C (1996) Preventing adolescent smoking: a review of options. *Health Education Journal* **55**(1), 31–54.

Preventing teenage pregnancy:

NHS Centre for Reviews and Dissemination, University of York (1997) *Preventing and Reducing the Adverse Effects of Unintended Teenage Pregnancies*.

20   Office for Public Management (1997) *Achieving Health Gain through Health Promotion in a Primary Care-Led NHS*. London: Health Education Authority. p. 42.

21   This section is partly based on:

Ogier, M. (1996) *Reading Research: or how to make research more approachable*. London: Baillière Tindall/Royal College of Nursing.

22   One helpful way to keep in touch is through the lists of *Journal Articles of Interest to Health Educators* and *Current Awareness Bulletin* published by the Health Education Authority, Trevelyan House, 30 Great Peter Street, London SW1P 2HW.

23   For example the DHSS publishes a 'Nursing Research Abstract' four times a year, which includes both published research and work in progress and is available in nurse libraries.

24   These are available via computer links. Access and advice is usually available from librarians in colleges and universities, and from specialist libraries such as the Health Promotion Information Centre at the Health Education Authority.

25   For further reading on ethical issues in research, see:

Ayer S (1994) Submitting a Research Proposal for Ethical Approval. *Professional Nurse*, September, pp. 805–806.

Behi R and Nolan M (1995) Ethical Issues in Research. *British Journal of Nursing* **4**(12), 712–716.

26   For more on writing a research proposal, see:

Parahoo K and Reid N (1998) Research Skills No. 3: Writing a Research Proposal. *Nursing Times* **84**(41), 49–52.

27   For guidance on designing questionnaires, see:

Stone D H (1993) Designing a questionnaire. *British Medical Journal* **307**, 1264–1266.

28   For basic concepts of statistics and their application in the design of research, see:

Bowers D (1996) *Statistics from Scratch: An introduction for health care professionals.* Chichester: Wiley.

29   For more on interviewing: Britten N (1995) Qualitative interviews in medical research. *British Medical Journal* **311**, 22 July, 251–253.

30   For guidance on conducting focus groups, see:

Ambler D (1993) Improving quality requires consumer input: using focus groups. *Journal of Nursing Care Quality* **7**(2), 34–41.

Morgan D (1993) *Successful Focus Groups: Advancing the State of the Art.* London: Sage Publications.

31   Partridge C J and Barnitt R E (1987) *Research Guidelines: A Handbook for Therapists.* London: Heinemann.

32   For more on aspects of health economics see:

On health economics and priority setting in health care:

Mooney G (1994) *Key Issues in Health Economics.* Hemel Hempstead: Harvester Wheatsheaf.

On cost effectiveness and prevention:

Tengs T O (1996) Enormous variation in the cost-effectiveness of prevention: implications for public policy. *Current Issues in Public Health* **2** (1), 13–17.

On performance indicators, targets and value for money as applied to health promotion:

Buck D, Godfrey C & Morgan A (1996) *Performance Indicators and Health Promotion Targets.* University of York, York YO1 5DD: Centre for Health Economics.

33   Department of Health (1995) *Assessing the Options: CHD/Stroke – Target Effectiveness and Cost Effectiveness of Interventions to Reduce CHD and Stroke Mortality.* London: Department of Health.

34   Examples of studies on the cost-effectiveness of health promotion include:

Buck D (1997) The cost-effectiveness of smoking cessation interventions: what do we know? *International Journal of Health Education* **35**(2), 44–52.

O'Neill C, Cupples M and McKnight A (1996) Cost effectiveness of personal health education in primary care for people with angina in the greater Belfast area of Northern Ireland. *Journal of Epidemiology and Community Health* **50** (5), 538–540.

Hughes D & McGuire A (1996) The cost-effectiveness of family planning service provision. *Journal of Public Health Medicine* **18** (2), 189–196.

Langham S, Thorogood M, Normand C and Muir J (1996) Costs and effectiveness of health checks conducted by nurses in primary care: the Oxcheck study. *British Medical Journal*, May 18, 1265–1268.

Wonderling D, McDermott C, Buxton M & Kinmouth A (1996) Costs and the cost effectiveness of cardiovascular screening and intervention: the British Family Heart Study. *British Medical Journal*, May 16, 1269–1273.

Wonderling D, Langham S, Buxton M & Normand C (1996) What can be concluded from the Oxcheck and British family heart studies: commentary on cost effectiveness analyses. *British Medical Journal*, May 18, 1274–1278.

Reid D (1996) How effective is health education via mass communications? *Health Education Journal* **55** (3): 332–344.

35   For an example of clinical audit of health promotion, see:

Learmonth A, Jackson M & English C (1997) Calling in the Auditors. *Healthlines*, March, pp. 8–9.

36   See, for example:

Audit Commission (1995) *Dear to Our Hearts? Commissioning Services for the Treatment and Prevention of Coronary Heart Disease.* London: HMSO.

37   These reasons are adapted from those set out in:

Ovretveit J (1992) *Health Service Quality: An introduction to quality methods for health services,* p. 65. Oxford: Blackwell Science.

38   Fox J (1997) Clinical audit and the practice nurse. *Practice Nursing* **8**(6), 18–20.

8 Skills of Personal Effectiveness

SUMMARY

This chapter is about developing skills to manage your health promotion work effectively. We cover managing information; writing reports; using time effectively; managing project work; managing change; and finally, working for quality. We include cases studies and practical exercises.

Management Skills in Health Promotion

See also chapters 5, 6, 7.

Working well in health promotion means not only having a clear view of your aims and plans, but also having management skills to implement your plans.

It is not easy to define what management is, but in general terms we can say it is about being effective and efficient in your work. **Effectiveness** is the extent to which the results you set out to achieve are actually achieved. **Efficiency** is about how you achieve those results compared with other ways of achieving them.

We have already discussed some important aspects of management, such as setting aims and objectives, setting priorities, planning and evaluating work. A comprehensive introduction to management is beyond the scope of this book, but interested readers are provided with some suggestions for further study[1] and recommended reading the end of this chapter.

In this chapter we identify and discuss a number of managerial skills you will need to be effective and efficient as a health promoter. However, it is important to emphasize that possessing these skills will not automatically make you effective and efficient. Other factors also influence this, including:

For further reading on ethics and values in health promotion, see Chapter 3.

For reading on how to become a more empowered person, see the suggestion at the end of this chapter.

- how well you integrate ethical principles into your basic everyday work. How you exercise your **responsibility** as a health promoter. ('Response-ability' is your ability to choose your response and is a product of your conscious choice, based on values, rather than a reaction to your circumstances.) A fundamental aspect of health promotion is that it involves empowering ourselves, and others, to have more control over our health and our lives, and this in turn empowers us to each fulfil our unique potential.

- the people you work with. Your effectiveness and efficiency is limited or enhanced by the competencies and motivation of those you work with – receptionists, secretaries and colleagues within and outside your organization, for example;

■ your organization. Both the structure and culture of your organization will influence what you are able to achieve;
■ the wider world. The state of the economy, government legislation, the organization of local government and the impact of social trends are just a few examples of factors in the world outside your organization which influence how effective you can be.

This book is designed to increase your awareness of these wider influences on your work, as well as to develop your own skills, both of which will help you to improve your competencies.

We now discuss some key aspects of personal effectiveness which will help you to manage health promotion.

Managing Information

It is easy to be swamped by paper, so only keep paperwork that is essential for your job and cannot be kept by someone else or in another existing system.

Think about who else collects information in your workplace and how they store it. Is there a central filing system? Does it work? Which things could you keep in it? Has a computer information system been introduced at your work base? Have you access to it and have you had training in how to use it? Familiarity with what computers can do will not only enhance your career prospects, it can also help with planning your health promotion work. For example, a computer system could be used to collate and analyse any survey work you undertake; data on health surveys can be retrieved using computer packages.[2]

| Exercise 8.1 | **What information do you need to store?** |

Make a list of all the types of information you collect at present and analyse it by asking yourself the following questions about each one.

1. Do I need to keep this information?
2. How easy is it for me to find the information when I need it?
3. Could someone else, or another information system, keep the information for me?
4. Who else might need access to this information? How easy would it be for them to find it?
5. How could this information best be stored?

Principles of Effective Information Systems

When reviewing or setting up your information system, it is useful to keep reminding yourself of three basic principles:

1. Keep it simple! Systems are only as effective as the people who put in and take out the information. The simpler the system the more likely it is that busy people will use it correctly.

2. Do not devise any more systems than are absolutely necessary.
3. Organize systems so that anyone who might want to use them can easily understand them.

Writing Reports

Important information is often conveyed through written reports. For example, you are likely to need to write a report on plans for health promotion, or an evaluation report on a specific project. You may need to write reports for your manager, or formal reports for committees. With written reports like these, they are likely to be read when you are not there, so there is no immediate feedback to provide information about whether your key points have been understood. To reduce the danger of being misunderstood, good skills in preparing and writing reports are essential.

See Chapter 10 (section on written communication skills).

Work through the following stages each time you prepare and write a report:

Stage 1. Define the purpose. To help to clarify the purpose, complete the following sentence: 'As a result of reading this report, the reader will. . . .' What?

The purpose could be to inform, to influence decision-making, to initiate a course of action, or to persuade. Whatever it is, keep it clearly in mind throughout all the later stages.

Stage 2. Define the readers. Identify the readers and consider them at all stages. Direct the report to the needs and interests of the readers. What do they already know about the subject? How much time do they have for reading? What kind of style is appropriate, for example formal or chatty?

Stage 3. Prepare the structure. Decide on the structure of the report. The usual parts of a report are:

- **title** – this should accurately describe what the report is about.
- **origins** – for example the author's name, occupation, work base and date.
- **distribution list** – it is a great help to readers if they know who else has seen the report. They may detect that someone vital has not received a copy.
- **contents list** – a long report will need a contents list, showing the main sections of the report and the pages on which the reader can find them. This is not necessary for short reports.
- **summary** – this is vital for all except the very shortest of reports (less than a single page). It helps the reader if the summary is easy to find at the beginning of the report. Remember that busy people will often only read the summary (and perhaps the conclusions and recommendations), or at least read the summary first in order to decide whether it is worth spending time reading any more. So the summary needs set out the essence of the report clearly and concisely.
- **introduction** – this sets the context for the report, for example why the work was done.
- **the 'body' of the report** – this will be bulk of the report. You need to break up the content into sections and subsections, all with clear headings. Headings should be helpful signposts so that the reader can see a route through the document, and can get an overview just by skimming through the headings.

Sections need to be ordered in a way which will be logical for the reader. It may help to organize material into sections by writing headings on index cards, then grouping them into a logical sequence. This can also be done on a computer: write all the possible headings down, then move them around until you are satisfied that they are in the most logical order.

- **conclusions** – summarizes the conclusions which can be clearly drawn from the information in the report.
- **recommendations** – these relate to the future, and summarize any changes which the author thinks are needed.
- **references** – putting any references at the end makes the report easier to read.
- **appendices** – a much misused feature of many reports, to be avoided unless really necessary. Ask yourself 'What information will most of my readers need the first time they read this report?' If they need this information straight away, put it in the main body of the report.

Stage 4. Write the report. Tackle the various sections in the order that makes it easiest. For example, it may be easiest to write the detailed body of the report first, then summarize the information, then discuss the information, then draw your conclusions, then set out your recommendations, then write the summary of the report and lastly finish it off with the title, contents list, origin, distribution list and other essential details.

Stage 5. Review and revision. After the report has been typed, review it and revise as necessary. Make sure pages are numbered and check that sections and subsections are correctly numbered. It is a good idea to show the report to one or two colleagues, preferably those who have good report writing skills and who will give constructive comments.

Stage 6. Final check. Always do a final check for writing and typing errors, spelling mistakes, etc. It can be helpful to ask someone who has not seen the report before to check it for typing and layout errors.

Using Time Effectively

How well organized and effective are you at your work? The following paragraphs should give you some ideas about how to improve your effectiveness by looking at how you use your time. Time is an expensive resource, and the one that many health promoters find hardest to manage. First of all, you need to know where your time goes, so we look at ways of analysing and improving the use of your time. Then we outline an approach to scheduling your work.

Time Logs and Time Diaries

A time log involves keeping a record of how you spend your time at regular intervals, which may be as often as every five or ten minutes. It is useful if you wish to know exactly how you are using your time on an activity which seems to be taking longer than you think it should. It can then help you to pinpoint the source of the problem. But it is time-consuming itself, so is really only worthwhile if a particular activity is causing you problems.

If you want to know more about how you generally use your time you can keep a time diary. This records how you have spent your time day by day and you can take a few minutes to fill it in at the end of each day. If you have a short memory you may find it better to fill it in more frequently, say at the end of the morning and at the end of the afternoon, or at any other convenient break between blocks of work.

Scheduling Your Work

See Chapter 6.

Health promoters generally find that they want to do far more than their time permits, and that they are faced daily with an almost bottomless pit of requests and demands. This means that, first and foremost, they must be very clear about what their priorities are. Secondly, they must be assertive about saying 'no' to requests to take on non-priority tasks. Thirdly, they need to develop skills of organizing time to ensure that work which should get done actually does get done, that is, scheduling work.

Scheduling work into the time available involves three steps:

1. Identify how long you need to spend on a job. This depends on:
   (a) the nature of the activity. For example, whether it is possible to cut corners without endangering people or the outcomes;
   (b) how important it is. If it is unimportant it does not merit a large investment of your time. Ask yourself, what am I employed for? Will doing this job contribute to my main aims and objectives? If not, it is unimportant. If it is important it merits a large investment.
2. Identify how soon you need to have the job completed. This depends on: how urgent it is. Urgent jobs are ones that have imminent deadlines. If an urgent job can be completed quickly, deal with it right away. That means it will not interfere with you getting on with the most important jobs.
3. Plan when the work will be done. This involves:
   (a) breaking the job down into manageable parts. If the job is big or difficult, or parts of it are boring, try setting aside regular, but small, amounts of time to complete specific bits. Using this 'salami' method (dividing it into thin segments), will help you to see that you are progressing.
   (b) estimating how long each part will take to complete. It can be difficult to estimate how long it will take you to complete a particular task, but an informed guess will at least help you to be more realistic in future! Here are some suggestions which may help:
   - ask someone you know who has experience in doing the job;
   - use your experience from similar jobs;
   - consult colleagues;
   - build in some contingency time;
   - keep a note of how long it actually takes, so that you can make a better estimate next time.
   (c) Scheduling in your diary or organizer when the work will be done. You may find that you need to re-schedule daily, to take account of changing priorities. The important thing is to ensure that the key tasks you need to undertake are scheduled to allow enough time for their completion.

Exercise 8.2   **Analysing and improving your use of time**

1.   Devise a recording format that suits you, based on the example below.

Then photocopy a supply of the sheets. Use as many sheets as necessary each day. Remember to include any work you do away from your base, for example at home.

   If you discover that a particular activity, for example telephone interruptions, is causing you a problem, then make a detailed log of what happens each time. *Do this immediately* – do not leave it till the end of the day. Keep the diary for at least a week. If none of your weeks is 'typical' you will need to keep it for several weeks.

   Using codes will save you time. For example, you could use M for meetings, I for interruptions, P for phone calls, IP for phone interruptions.

Time diary

Day _____   **Date** _____   **Page no.** _____

Activity   **Time spent**   **Comments**

_____   _____   _____

_____   _____   _____

_____   _____   _____

2.   Now analyse how you used your time.

Each week, analyse your use of time by asking the following questions:
- How did you actually use your time compared with how you planned to use it?
- How much of your time do you spend on different activities? Does this reflect the importance of the different activities? Important activities are those that help you to achieve your objectives.
- Which jobs did not get done? Does it matter? Did you finish all the *important and urgent* jobs?
- How much time do you lose through interruptions? What sort of interruptions do you get?
- How much of your time is spent on other people's work?
- Do you do the right job at the right time? Most people have a time of day when they work best. Do you use this time for your most important work?

3.   Now plan how to improve your time management.

Some of the changes you could make will be obvious. For example:
- You discover that jobs started early in the morning tend to get completed quickly. So you decide in future to do your most important work at this time.
- You discover that you spend about eight hours each week handling interruptions. You decide to experiment with techniques to cut down this time.
- You discover that urgent jobs are generally done but important long-term projects tend to be neglected. You decide to make realistic plans to ensure that these jobs will be done.
- What else can you do?

Managing Project Work

First, we need to know what a 'project' is, and why planning and managing it is different from other managerial activities you undertake. When you are first given responsibility for a project, it can seem rather daunting. It is for you to turn something which does not yet exist into reality, and to control its progress so that it delivers effectively and efficiently.

The most obvious thing about a project is that it has a particular (unique) purpose, which may be encapsulated in its name, such as 'Bromley Active Lifestyles Project' or 'Portsmouth Needle Exchange Project'. It is probably most useful to think of a project as an instrument of change, which, when it is successfully completed, will have made an impact as defined in its aims and objectives. Another key aspect of projects is that they are time-limited: they have clearly identifiable start and finish times. Projects vary enormously in their scope. Small projects can last only a few days and involve activities by a single person; large projects can involve many people, and indeed many agencies and last for several years.

All projects, however, have the same basic underlying structure and go through a number of stages, as set out in Box 8.1.

Box 8.1.	The stages of a project

1. Start.
2. Specification.
3. Design and planning.
4. Implementation.
5. Evaluation, Review and Final Completion.

The **start** is the most important stage of any project and covers areas such as setting the overall aims, gaining approval, and the allocation of a budget. It will set the foundations for the rest of the lifetime of the project.

Specification involves defining the detailed objectives of the project, i.e. what the outcomes will be and what the targets are for delivering these outcomes in terms of quantity, quality and timing.

The **design** stage is when the 'what' is translated into 'how'. It may take the form of detailed plans.

The **implementation** stage is when the plans are put into operation. It is important to note that the end of implementation is not the end of the project.

The **evaluation, review and final completion** stage will be marked by the delivery of a final report, which includes evaluation findings and the details of a post-implementation review. This review should take place some time after the end of the implementation stage, so that it is possible to include data on the long-term outcomes of the project.

These stages are, of course, very similar to the basic planning and evaluation cycle which we described in Chapter 5 and the present section should therefore be read in conjunction with Chapter 5. The difference is that when you are delivering

an on-going service, rather than a one-off project, the cycle repeats itself over
See Chapter 5. and over again.

Because projects vary so much, in terms of their scale and length of life, it is
particularly important that they are planned systematically. It is also vital to
See Chapter 7 for a discussion
of health promotion strategic
planning. understand how the project contributes to the wider strategic plans of the
organization concerned.

Starting a Project

The start of a project will be a proposal or written document, which can take a
number of guises, such as 'terms of reference' or 'report of a feasibility study'. The
key elements which must be described in this document include the following:

- Who is proposing to carry out the project, for example, an NHS Trust or
  voluntary organization.
- Who is the purchaser or commissioner of the project, for example, a local
  authority.
- The aims and outcomes of the project.
- The scope of the project, for example who will use or receive the project, the
  setting in which it will be delivered, which departments, agencies and people
  will be affected.
- The costs of the project, in terms of staffing, buildings, equipment and other
  resources.
- The project stages and time scales.
- Methods and standards: the use of any particular techniques or methods and
  the adoption of any recognized quality standards.
- Roles and responsibilities of participants in the project (especially important
  when the project is commissioned by an alliance of a number of agencies).

Detailed Planning

For anything but the very smallest of projects, you will need to develop a
detailed plan of each stage, immediately before you enter it. Typically planning
the next stage will be one of the last tasks in the planning of the previous stage.
The bar chart (also known as the Gantt chart after the man credited with
inventing it) is the primary tool which you can use for scheduling the project
tasks and subsequently controlling its progress (Fig. 8.1).

The Gantt or bar chart is made up of a task information side (on the left) and
a task bar side (on the right). The task information side sets out the nature of
each task and who is responsible for it. The task bar is a line which graphically
represents the period in time during which the task will be carried out. The
precise content of a Gantt chart should be determined by what you intend to use
it for. A bar chart is easy to draw and it presents the plan in a visual form which
is easily understood by most people.

It can be used at every level in the planning process from initial outline
planning down to the detailed planning of individual tasks. For complex projects
any single bar on the master chart for the whole project might have to be broken
down and represented by a more detailed bar chart for that particular task or
stage of the project.

| Case study 8.1 | Using a Gantt chart in project planning |

This small pilot 8-month project aimed to explore the feasibility of using community pharmacists (retail chemists) to promote physical activity with customers. Its objectives included identifying barriers and opportunities, and seeing whether training helped.

The plan was to recruit ten volunteer pharmacists, interview them to ascertain their attitude towards promoting physical activity with customers and their current practice, and then work with them in a training session. After the training, the pharmacists had a six-week period to implement the training, followed by another interview to see if their attitude and actions had changed.

A project manager had responsibility for planning and managing the project; a researcher was employed to design and carry out the interviews and help with the final report.

Figure 8.1 shows the Gantt chart drawn up by the project manager. It was useful for clarifying what needed to be done when, and for seeing when possible timing difficulties could arise. For example, would pharmacists' or researcher's holidays interfere with the schedule? Were there too many tasks to be completed at one time (for example, recruiting pharmacists and appointing the research worker in February and March)? The Gantt chart also showed which stages required the research worker, so that the project manager could negotiate appropriate numbers of hours worked at appropriate stages.

One major benefit of Gantt charts is that they highlight critical points, for example where progress in X is dependent on Y already being completed.

It pays to remember that planning tools such as Gantt charts are only aids to help you to achieve your purpose. Sticking slavishly to your plan will not necessarily bring success; you may have to alter your plan because of unforeseen circumstances. However, without systematic planning you are unlikely to be able to keep your project on course at all. An example of a Gantt chart is set out and described in Case Study 8.1 and Figure 8.1.

Controlling Implementation

For more discussion about quality, see the section on 'Working for Quality' later in this chapter.

In addition to detailed plans any project needs to have built in control procedures: controlling projects is about identifying problems as soon as they arise, working out what needs to be done to ameliorate them, and then doing it. Things which need to be controlled include time, the budget (i.e. costs) and quality. Methods for control include progress reports and one-to-one and group progress meetings. Large projects will need to use all of these methods. Progress reports can sometimes be best presented in a standardized form, which compares progress with the Project Plan.

Some problems will be outside the immediate control of the project. For example a project could be influenced by the training policies of an organization or other factors deeply embedded in the structure and culture of an organization. In these cases project managers should do what they can to reduce the impact of these issues on the project, but should also remember that they have a duty to highlight these issues in reports, and not cover them up.

Fig 8.1   **Gantt chart.**

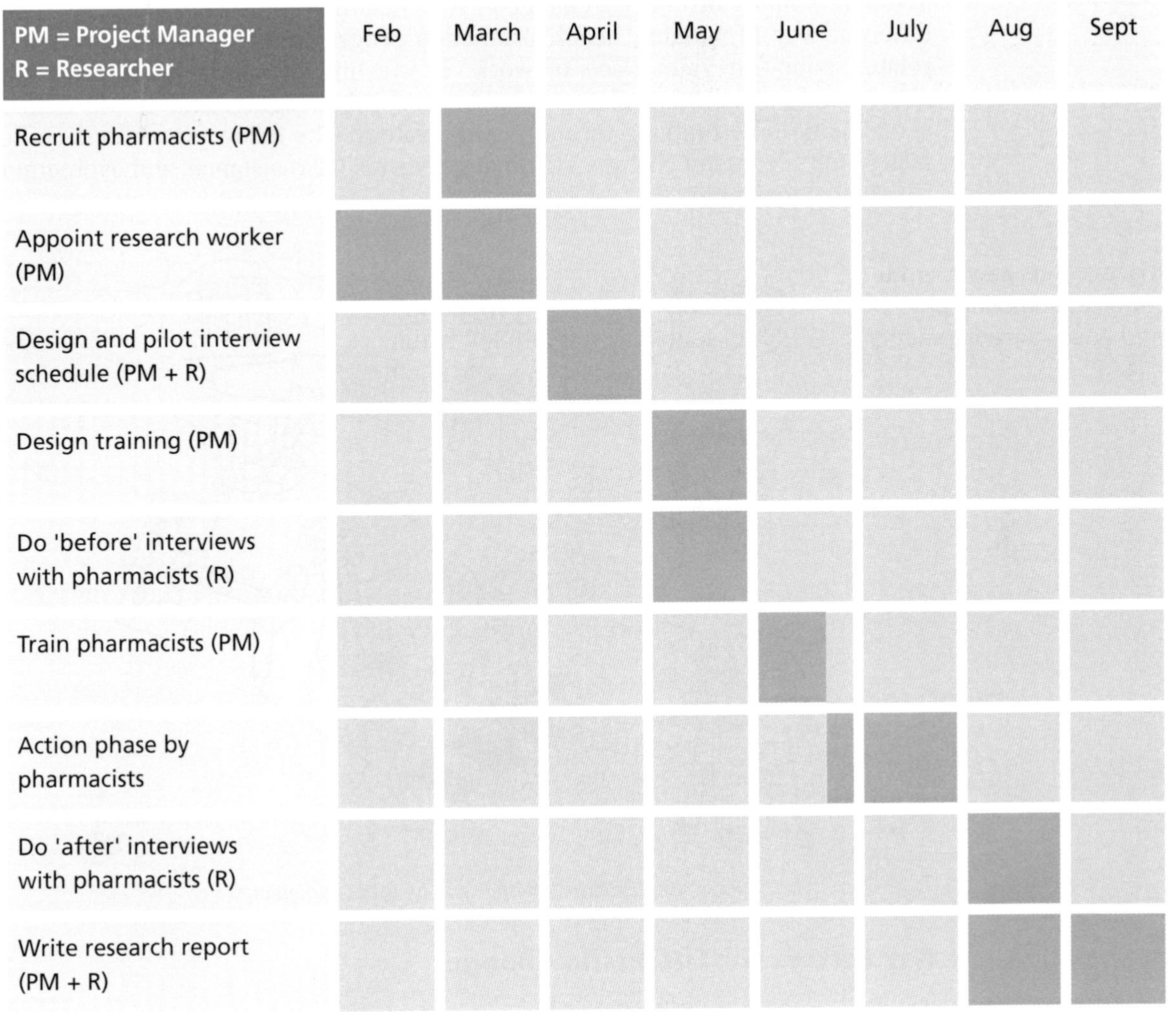

PM = Project Manager R = Researcher	Feb	March	April	May	June	July	Aug	Sept
Recruit pharmacists (PM)		■						
Appoint research worker (PM)	■	■						
Design and pilot interview schedule (PM + R)			■					
Design training (PM)				■				
Do 'before' interviews with pharmacists (R)					■			
Train pharmacists (PM)						■		
Action phase by pharmacists						■	■	
Do 'after' interviews with pharmacists (R)							■	
Write research report (PM + R)							■	■

Managing Change

Health promoters may experience change in two ways: one is being a part of an organization which is undergoing change itself – in other words, finding yourself being reorganized, with your job and your location within your organizational structure changed. The second way is by being a change agent yourself, by implementing changes in health promotion policy or practice.

The first way, experiencing organizational change, has been common in statutory agencies in the late 1980s and 1990s, as reform and reorganization affect NHS and local authorities in particular. The topic of understanding and surviving organizational change, and feeling positive about it, is outside the scope of this book. However, thinking about the second way – how to implement change successfully – may also help you to understand and cope better with being part of an organizational change.

Suggestions for further reading about organizational change are made in the Recommended Reading Section at the end of this chapter.

Implementing Change

You may want to introduce a change in your health promotion practice, such as a different way of running health promotion programmes, introducing a health-related policy at your place of work, or starting off new health promotion activities. Implementing change can be very challenging, and it will help to spend some time thinking through your strategy. The following sections on key factors for successful change, identifying reasons for resistance, and overcoming resistance, may help.

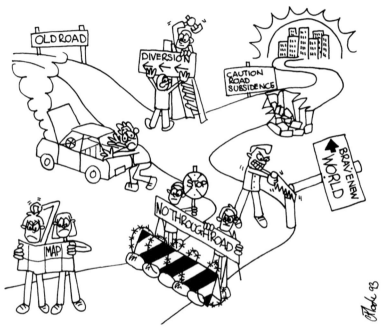

Implementing change can be very challenging

Key Factors for Successful Change

The key to gaining commitment to change, and overcoming resistance to change, lies in understanding the motivation of all the people who could be affected by the change and how they feel about it. Overall, do they feel positive or negative about the proposed change? The balance between positive and negative factors can be expressed as follows in Box 8.2, in a 'change equation' developed as a tool to help analyse the key factors involved.[3]

The basis of the equation is the simple assumption that people are rarely interested in change unless the factors supporting change outweigh the costs. As a change agent your job is to either reduce D, the perceived costs, or to increase the sum of A, B, and C. We shall now examine each of the elements in the equation briefly in turn.

A: Dissatisfaction with the way things are. If we are dissatisfied, we may wrongly assume that others are too. If people are comfortable with the way things are they are unlikely to support change.

Box 8.2.	**The Change Equation**

A = the individual's or group's level of dissatisfaction with things as they are now;
B = the individual's or group's shared vision of a better future;
C = the existence of an acceptable, safe first step;
D = the costs to the individual or group.

Change is likely to be viewed positively, and be implemented successfully, if:

$$A + B + C \text{ is greater than } D$$

B: A shared vision of a better future. If a vision of a better future does not exist, or is unclear, people will not strive to achieve it. If there are several competing visions, energy will be dissipated in arguments. Few people would buy into a vision which threatens their livelihood or other cherished aspects of their lives. A vision which threatens important aspects of an individual's or a group's life is almost bound to fail.

C: An acceptable, safe first step. The size of the change and the risks involved can seem overwhelming. Many of us could share a common view of what better health for all would mean. But where do we begin? First steps are acceptable if they are small, are likely to be successful or, if they fail, do not cause too much damage and the situation is retrievable.

D: The costs to the individual or group. What is important here is how people *perceive* the costs, not how they actually are. There will always be costs; change is often painful and unfair. Costs can be tangible things like time, money, resources, or more intangible costs like stress or loss of status.

Reasons for Resistance

We now look more closely at some of the main reasons why people resist change. Different people react differently to change for a variety of reasons. While one person passively resists a change, another may actively try to sabotage it, whereas a third may not be resistent and may actually bring it about.

Whether you are campaigning for a change, or implementing a change in policy or practice in your work, you will need to deal with the fact that many people resist change for a number of reasons, including:

Self interest. While a change may be in the interest of most people, it may not be in everyone's best interest. For example while most people, including some smokers, may support a smoking policy, others may see it as an infringement of personal liberty and not in their interest.

Misunderstanding. People can easily misunderstand what is being proposed. For example people may misunderstand an alcohol policy and think that it is letting people with drinking problems 'off the hook', so that they do not have to meet the same standards of work performance and behaviour as everyone else.

Case study 8.2 **Change in a district general hospital[4]**

An example of significant change originating from a few people started in the physiotherapy out-patients' department of a district general hospital. One of the physiotherapists found that, in addition to giving instructions verbally, it was useful to write down instructions for patients who needed to do exercises at home. She enlisted the help of the Medical Illustration Department in designing and printing some leaflets based on these instructions. A second physiotherapist had begun to collect a small library of books, such as those produced by the Arthritis and Rheumatism Council. Meanwhile the receptionist had taken another initiative. A friend had told her about a local support group for arthritis sufferers, and she pinned up a poster, giving information about it, in the waiting area.

The superintendent physiotherapist in charge encouraged the staff to share their ideas. As a result a departmental strategy to improve the provision of information to patients was launched, and patients were asked about their needs and preferences.

Other out-patients' departments in the hospital heard about the venture and expressed interest. As a result, a number of other initiatives took place across the hospital to improve patient information. Plans are now underway for a Patient Education Centre to be located in the foyer of the main hospital entrance, and this has the support of the Community Health Council and the Friends of the Hospital.

This case study illustrates the factors in the 'change equation':

A. The individual's or group's level of dissatisfaction with things as they are now: two of the physiotherapists and the receptionist, and through them their supervisor and the rest of the department, saw that there was room for improvement.

B. The individual's or group's shared vision of a better future: the idea of improved help for patients was shared and spread through an increasing number of people in the hospital.

C. The existence of an acceptable, safe first step: this change was built on a number of small successes, and did not present any major hurdles which could have induced resistance. If the *first step* had been to propose a Patient Education Centre, people may well have perceived major difficulties.

D. The costs to the individual or group: these were small in the first instance, just a little time and effort. By the time major investment was required for the Patient Education Centre, everybody was committed.

Misunderstandings are particularly frequent in organizations where there is a lack of trust between the managers and the workforce.

Belief that a change is not in the interest of the people it is intended to benefit. People may believe that the costs of a change will outweigh the benefits, not only to themselves, but to other people or to a whole organization. For example, people may feel that the introduction of ethnic monitoring as part of an equal opportunities policy could actually increase discrimination against black and minority ethnic groups.

Awareness of these opinions is important for the policy-maker, because they may be based on knowledge of what goes on in parts of the organization with which the policy-maker has little contact. Policy formation must be based on an accurate analysis of the situation; this is particularly relevant in large organizations, like the Health Service and County Councils.

Low tolerance for change. People may resist change because they are anxious about new demands which will be made of them. For example, there may be demands to provide separate rest rooms for smokers, or to provide health counselling for people with alcohol problems. Organizational change can require people to change too much, or fail to provide them with the time and support they need.

Methods for Overcoming Resistance to Change

In order to overcome resistance to change it is vital to select the best approach, or combination of approaches, for the situation and the people involved. Five possible options are:

1. **Education and communication.** This involves educating people about a change before it happens and communicating with them in a variety of ways: one-to-one, group discussion, written documents, etc. An educational and communication approach is indicated when resistance to change is based on inadequate or inaccurate information. The limitation is that it can be time-consuming, especially if a lot of people are involved.

2. **Participation and involvement.** Resistance to change may be forestalled if those initiating the change identify the people that they think will be resistant, and actively involve them in the process of designing and implementing the change. The initiators of the change must genuinely be prepared to listen and learn. A token effort is liable to provoke more resistance, because people will feel tricked if their advice is not heeded.

Participation and involvement is indicated when people need to be committed to a policy change in order to make it work; policies work when people feel ownership for them because they have been involved in their development. This approach is also useful when the initiators do not have full information about the implications of the change for certain groups of people or certain departments. It could also be the preferred option where the initiators of change have little power, because it harnesses the power of others as a force for change.

Nevertheless, this approach does have limitations. It is very time-consuming and demands a high degree of coordination. It can lead to a poor outcome if it tries to please everybody.

3. **Facilitation and support.** This involves helping people to identify what changes are required and providing them with support to plan and manage the change themselves. This could be done, for example, by providing 'time out' for people to reflect on the situation, and to identify their own objectives and how to meet them. Support could include emotional support to cope with stress and 'burn out', and the development of 'mentoring' or 'facilitator' schemes, where more experienced people help others with their managerial or professional development. This approach works best where anxiety and fear lie at the heart of resistance. The limitation of this approach is that it, too, can be time-consuming and expensive (for example, if it is necessary to employ counsellors for a large workforce).

4. **Negotiation and agreement.** This involves offering incentives to actual or potential resisters, for example, through negotiating with trade unions about the effects of the change on their members' pay. This is particularly appropriate when

it is obvious that some people will lose out as a consequence of the changes. It can be effective if there are specific pockets of resistance, but could be expensive if everyone leaps on the bandwagon and tries to argue that they are also losing out.

5. Political influencing. This approach can be useful where one, or a few, powerful individuals are the source of resistance. It can be relatively quick, but has the drawback that it can lead to problems in the future if people feel that they have been manipulated.

See also Chapter 16, section on The Politics of Influence.

Working for Quality

There is now a lot of emphasis on the *quality* of services, that is, looking at the nature of the service, and assessing how 'good' it is when judged against a number of criteria.

Criteria for Quality

What are the criteria for quality in health promotion work? We suggest that the following checklist may be helpful in identifying aspects of quality in your health promotion work. The checklist can be applied to your work overall, or to a particular health promotion programme.

| Box 8.3. | **Checklist: criteria for quality in health promotion[5]** |

1. **Appropriateness**: is it relevant and acceptable to clients – the individual, group or community concerned?
2. **Effectiveness**: does it achieve the aims and objectives you set?
3. **Social justice**: does it produce health improvement for all concerned, not for some people at the expense of others? In other words, is it 'fair'?
4. **Equity and access**: is it provided to all people whatever their racial, cultural or social background on the basis of equal access for equal need? (This may mean, for example, unconventional clinic times, wheelchair access, leaflets in Braille and ethnic minority languages, information on audio- and video-cassettes, etc.)
5. **Dignity and choice**: does it treat all groups of people with dignity and recognize the rights of people to choose for themselves how they live their lives? Is it non-judgmental, accepting that people have the right to withdraw from, or reject, health promotion if they so wish?
6. **Environment**: does it ensure an environment conducive to people's health, safety and well-being? Does it recognize that people feel at home in different environments, and may feel uncomfortable or intimidated in some settings? Is the social environment friendly and welcoming?
7. **Participant satisfaction**: does it satisfy all those with an interest in the outcomes of the health promotion work, such as commissioners, managers, clients and other interest groups, acknowledging that the views of clients should be paramount?
8. **Involvement**: does it involve all those with an interest, including clients, in planning, design and implementation? Does it avoid 'tokenism', with client's views genuinely sought and incorporated in a non-patronizing way?
9. **Efficiency**: does it achieve the best possible use of the resources available, and provide value for money?

Improving Quality

Initiatives to improve quality are usually successful if people work together to pool ideas. This could be a group of people authorized by management to examine a particular issue or problem, such as improving the quality of patient information literature, the way in which antenatal advice is being given to prospective parents, or the way a GP practice is tackling helping patients to stop smoking.

Sometimes such groups are called **quality circles**. These are 'natural work groups' of between about three and twelve employees who do the same or similar work, who meet regularly to address work-related problems. The issues to tackle are selected by the group itself and the outcomes are presented to management. In many cases the group is also involved in implementing the solutions. Management commitment to taking account of the outcomes and implementing recommended changes is crucial to success.

Typically, a quality circle will:

- begin by drawing up a list of issues for consideration, using techniques such as brainstorming;
- select the issue to be addressed;
- gather information about the nature of the problem, and analyse the causes;
- generate a range of solutions, and establish the best options or combination of options;
- prepare a report on their findings for management decision.

An example of a quality circle might be a group of nurses working in a coronary care unit looking at how to improve the quality of the patient education programmes which are run for discharged patients. The activities of such a group are described in the case study below.

Case study 8.3	**Bloggsville Royal Hospital: Coronary Care Unit**

Improving the Quality of Patient Education

A group of four nurses in the Coronary Care Unit have been meeting regularly as a quality circle, and have decided to investigate how to improve the quality of education for discharged patients. At present a course of six group sessions is provided for patients after discharge, and nurses take turns to organize and run the courses.

The group first looked at the data for attendance at the group sessions. They discovered that, over the last year, 60% of discharged patients have attended at least one session, but of these, only 20% attended 3 or more sessions.

They conducted a series of interviews with discharged patients to investigate the reasons for attendance or non-attendance, and to find out patients' preferences about how they would like the education to be provided. They discovered that some patients do not like attending a group under any circumstances, and some strongly dislike coming back into the hospital environment. But some of these would like one-to-one opportunities for guidance from specialists such as a dietitian (on healthy eating), a physiotherapist (on exercise and fitness) and a psychologist (on how to stop smoking, stress management and relaxation).

They discovered that other patients would prefer to have written information, audiotapes (for relaxation and self-hypnosis) and videotapes (of appropriate exercise routines), rather than come back to the hospital. Other patients would like more information about community groups and facilities for exercise tailored to their needs; for example, free trials of fitness classes, swimming sessions for elderly people. Others are interested in knowing if there are self-help or voluntary groups they could join, such as clubs for people who are being rehabilitated following heart disease. Some patients, especially those who are socially isolated, have particularly valued the opportunity to meet as a group and to exchange experiences.

After analysing these findings, the group of nurses produced a report for their manager recommending that a range of educational opportunities is provided for the education of discharged patients including:

- putting patients in touch with local self-help and cardiac rehabilitation schemes;
- setting up a video- and audio-tape library providing appropriate material for discharged patients on free loan;
- offering opportunities for counselling by specialists (dietitian, physiotherapist, psychologist) prior to discharge;
- selecting or producing appropriate written material, and making it available to patients prior to discharge;
- inviting all patients to return for an open evening, with information and demonstrations about facilities and activities available locally. This would include local authority exercise and leisure facilities, alternative medicine practitioners, community and self-help groups and commercial leisure organizations.

The report includes a financial breakdown, which demonstrates that the recommendations will have additional costs, primarily related to the proposed services to be provided by the paramedical professions. However, savings will be made on the nursing staff time currently devoted to running the courses and through financial sponsorship of written material by approved 'ethical' commercial sponsors.

This case study shows how the quality of the patient education programme could be improved on a number of criteria:

- **Appropriateness**: clients would find the new approach more acceptable and relevant.
- **Effectiveness**: more clients would gain from the programme.
- **Equity and access**: clients could access advice and help in different ways, and those who disliked group meetings, or found attendance difficult, would have their needs met in other ways.
- **Environment**: it was recognized that some people disliked the hospital environment.
- **Participant satisfaction**: clients and nurses would be more satisfied with the results.
- **Involvement**: clients were involved in redesigning the programme, with their views taken into account.
- **Efficiency**: it would be a better use of resources because it would reach the people intended, and avoid wasting resources on a programme which reached very few.

Developing Quality Standards

It may be helpful to look at improving quality by setting specific quality standards to aim for. A quality standard can be defined as:

an agreed level of performance negotiated within available resources.[6]

See Chapter 16 (section on The Voice of the Consumer in the NHS).

Examples of standards are those set out in the Patients Charter. For example, a quality issue for an ambulance service is that it reaches the scene of an accident quickly. A quality standard is the specified maximum length of time this takes.

Quality standards in health promotion work have been developed.[7] For example, quality standards can be set for health promotion materials, and the criteria listed in Chapter 11 could be developed as a list of quality standards for health education leaflets:

See Health Promotion Materials: Criteria for Choice, in Chapter 11.

- appropriate for achieving your health promotion aims;
- content consistent with your values and approach;
- relevant for the people you are working with;

■ not racist or sexist;
■ easily understood by the people the leaflets are intended for;
■ accurate, up-to-date information;
■ free of inappropriate advertising.

A further challenge is to develop standards which are *quantifiable* in some way. This is a difficult task, but you could, for example, develop a 5-point scale for assessing the quality of your leaflets, so that you score them out of 5 for the extent to which they fulfil each quality standard. Another example could be that you decide that a quality management issue is to respond quickly to requests from your clients. You could develop this by setting a standard such as returning telephone calls within 24 hours, and written requests within 3 days.

Setting, monitoring and reviewing quality standards can involve a great deal of time and effort. The benefit comes from seeing clearly identified improvements in service. There is considerable literature on developing quality in services, and suggestions for further study are given.

PRACTICE POINTS

■ To implement health promotion work successfully you need to develop management skills, including information management, report writing, time management, project management, managing change and developing quality.

■ Managing information: only keep paperwork which is essential and cannot be kept by someone else or in another information system (for example, on a computer). Store information in the simplest possible way, easily understood by everyone who might need access to it.

■ Writing a report: be clear about its purpose and who will read it; decide the structure and outline content; write the sections in the order you find easiest; allow time for what you have written to 'sink in' and then review, edit and change it as necessary; and always get your report checked at the final stage by someone else.

■ Managing time: know more about how you spend your time through using time logs and diaries. Schedule your time by thinking about how long a job is likely to take (usually longer than you think); when it must be completed by; and when you can devote time to it.

■ Planning your project work: even the smallest project is unlikely to succeed without detailed and systematic planning. A Gantt chart is a useful tool. Planning tools are aids to success, but good management means that plans may be subject to change.

■ Managing change: change is more likely to be successful if people believe that the factors in favour of the change outweigh the costs. A shared vision of a desirable future and a small, safe, first step forward help to make change acceptable. It is important to identify reasons why people resist change and design an effective change strategy.

■ Working for quality: working to improve quality is best achieved through groups of people working together and pooling ideas. Management support and involvement is essential for success, but the staff who do the job are in the best position to know what is practical and feasible.

Recommended Reading

On Personal Effectiveness

➤ Covey S R (1992) *The Seven Habits of Highly Effective People: Powerful lessons in personal change.* London: Simon and Shuster. (A highly acclaimed book on a principle-centred approach to personal effectiveness, which argues that highly effective people integrate ethical principles into their basic character.)

On Management

➤ DuBrin A J (1997) *Essentials of Management*, 4th edn. Cincinnati, Ohio: South-Western College Publishing.
➤ Francis D and Woodcock M (1996) *The New Unblocked Manager: A practical guide to self-development.* Aldershot: Gower.

On the Management of Health Services

➤ Harrison S (1996) *Managing Health Services: A basic text.* Buckingham: Open University Press.
➤ Iles V (1997) *Really Managing Health Care.* Buckingham: Open University Press.
➤ Clark J E & Copcutt L (eds) (1997) *Management for Nurses and Health Care Professionals.* London: Churchill Livingstone

On the Management of Voluntary Organizations and Other not-for-Profit Organizations, such as NHS Trusts

➤ Hudson M (1995) *Managing without Profit: The art of managing third-sector organizations.* London: Penguin/Directory of Social Change.

On Writing Reports and Proposals:

➤ Seraydarian P and Pywell S (1994) *Successful Business Writing.* London: Cassell.
➤ Jay R (1994) *How to write proposals and reports that get results.* London: Pitman/Institute of Management Foundation.
➤ Burnard P (1996) *Writing for Health Professionals: A manual for writers*, 2nd edn. London: Chapman and Hall.

On Time Management

➤ Croft C (1996) *Time Management.* London: International Thomson Business Press.

On Project Management

➤ Lock D (1996) *The Essentials of Project Management.* Aldershot: Gower.
➤ Burton C & Michael N (1992) *A Practical Guide to project management: how to make it work in your organization.* London: Kogan Page.
➤ Brown M (1992) *Successful project management in a week.* London: Hodder & Stoughton/Institute of Management Foundation.

On Organizational Change

➤ Sadler P (1995) *Managing Change.* London: Kogan Page.
➤ Blair G & Meadows S (1997) *A Real-Life Guide to Organisational Change.* Aldershot: Gower.

On Developing Quality

➤ Ellis R & Whittington D (1993) *Quality Assurance in Health Care: A handbook.* London: Edward Arnold.
➤ Joss R and Kogan M (1995) *Advancing Quality: Total Quality Management in the National Health Service.* Buckingham: Open University Press.
➤ Ovretveit J (1992) *Health Service Quality: An Introduction to Quality Methods for Health Services.* Oxford: Blackwell Science.
➤ Gatiss G F (1996) *Total Quality Management: A Total Quality Approach.* London: Cassell/Institute for Supervision and Management.

On Quality Assurance in Health Promotion, with Examples of Quality Standards

➤ Evans D, Head M J & Speller V (1994) *Assuring Quality in Health Promotion: Developing Standards of Good Practice.* London: Health Education Authority.

Notes and References

1 The Open University Business School provides a comprehensive distance learning course in management – The Effective Manager. For further details contact The Open University, Open Business School, Walton Hall, Milton Keynes MK7 6AG. Tel: 01908 274066.

The NHS Training Directorate (NHSTD) (now the Institute for Health and Care Development) (IHCD) has commissioned a comprehensive open learning scheme for health service managers – the Management Education Scheme by Open Learning (MESOL). It comprises two programmes: Managing Health Services (MHS) for first line managers in the health service; and Health and Social Services Management (HSSM), for middle and senior managers in health and social services (including statutory, voluntary and private sectors). These are available through the Open University and locally through some Health Authorities and colleges. For further information on the availability of MESOL programmes contact The Open University (address above) or the IHCD (address below).

The NHS Training Directorate (now the Institute for Health and Care Development) has also commissioned Health Pickup. This is a modular training programme to develop the non-clinical skills of health service professionals including nurses, midwives, health visitors, dietitians, physiotherapists, occupational therapists, speech therapists, clinical psychologists and chiropodists. It includes modules on setting objectives and standards, assessing needs and priorities, managing caseload and time, and effective team working, plus modules on Information Management and Technology aimed at a wider range of health service staff. For further information on the availability of Health Pickup contact the IHCD, St Bartholomews Court, 18 Christmas Street, Bristol BS1 5BT. Tel: 01179 291029.

2 For example, the Health Education Authority produced a package in March 1997 on CD-ROM: *Health and Lifestyles National Surveys Guide*. It gives information on 44 national quantitative health and lifestyle surveys of sound methodological design carried out since 1989.

3 The change equation was developed by David Gleicher as a pseudomathematical tool. For further information see:

Open Business School/Institute of Health Services Management/NHS Training Authority (1990) *Managing Health Services*, Book 9, pp 36–37, *Managing Change*. Milton Keynes: The Open University.

4 This case study is based on case material described in:

Spurgeon P & Barwell F (1991) *Implementing Change in the NHS*. London: Chapman & Hall/ Health Services Management Centre.

5 This checklist draws on the main principles of the WHO Health For All Movement (see Chapter 1 section Addressing the Determinants of Health) and the White Paper Working for Patients:

WHO Regional Office for Europe (1985) *Targets for Health For All*. Geneva: WHO.

Secretaries of State for Health (1989) *Working for Patients*. London: HMSO.

6 Wessex Regional Health Authority (1991) *Using Information in Managing the Nursing Resource – Quality*. Macclesfield: Greenhalgh & Co.

7 A useful quality assurance framework for health promotion, and examples of quality standards, is:

Evans D, Head M J & Speller V (1994) *Assuring Quality in Health Promotion: developing standards of good practice*. Wessex Institute of Public Health Medicine/London: Health Education Authority.

9 Working Effectively with Other People

SUMMARY

In this chapter we focus on developing skills of working effectively with other people and organizations in order to implement health promotion plans. We discuss the following key aspects: communicating with colleagues; coordination and teamwork; participating in meetings; effective committee work; and working in health alliances with other organizations. We include practical exercises and case studies.

You may plan and undertake your health promotion work entirely on your own, but more likely you will be working with other people:

- colleagues who may be your peers or your managers or people that you manage;
- colleagues in other parts of your own organization;
- people in different organizations but who are working with you on a health promotion activity of mutual interest.

A key aspect of success will be how well you work with other people, and in this chapter we discuss the knowledge and skills needed. First we look at the basics of your communication with your own colleagues.

Communicating with Colleagues

See Chapter 10 Some fundamentals of good face-to-face and written communication are dealt with in Chapter 10. Whilst these are presented primarily with health promoter: client contact in mind, they are also, of course, applicable to contact between health promotion colleagues. We suggest that the following factors are particularly important to ensure effective working relationships:

- working in a partnership with colleagues which recognizes and builds on colleagues' strengths, developing their self-confidence and mutual trust;
- actively listening to colleagues, so that you understand clearly their opinions, thoughts and feelings.

A considerable proportion of your time may be taken up by communications with working colleagues, including telephone conversations, face-to-face dialogues and written communications on paper and via computer (e-mail). Try the following exercise in order to increase your awareness of how you communicate with colleagues, and how your communication might be improved.

| Exercise 9.1 | How you Communicate with Colleagues |

Record all the types of communication with colleagues that you carry out over one working day, by making a tally of all the occasions in three categories, as set out below. Then add up your total for each category, and your grand total for the day.

You might like to compare your results with those of some colleagues.

	Face-to-face verbal	Telephone	Written
	_____	_____	_____
	_____	_____	_____
	_____	_____	_____
	_____	_____	_____
	_____	_____	_____
	_____	_____	_____
	_____	_____	_____
TOTALS	_____	_____	_____

Think about whether there is anything you would like to change or improve; for example:

- if you spend a lot of time on the telephone, could you improve your telephone skills?
- could you use your time more efficiently if you used less time-consuming methods of communications, for example, phone or e-mail instead of write letters or have meetings?
- do you need to selectively spend more time face-to-face in order to understand colleagues and establish a closer working relationship?

Coordination and Teamwork

Health promotion often involves different professions and disciplines working together, including working with colleagues from other departments, and even from different agencies. Therefore it requires good coordination and teamwork.

Poor coordination can result in dramatic losses in efficiency and even the total breakdown of programmes; it is especially difficult when big bureaucracies like health authorities, NHS Trusts and local authorities are working together. There are several ways of coordinating, and it is important to use the one best suited to the situation.

Appointing a Coordinator

The problem for coordinators is that they do not directly manage the people they are trying to coordinate and therefore cannot control them in the same way as a manager can; they must convince people that any requests they make are legitimate. Often coordinators are at a modest level in a hierarchical organization. A diabetic nurse trying to coordinate the production of a patient information leaflet, for example, might find that it is difficult to get the commitment of the consultant. The very word *coordinator* may provoke resistance in some people, because they think they will be 'organized' by someone else.

Although resistance to coordination cannot be magically spirited away, there are several tactics which can help.

Your reputation. People will find it difficult to turn down any reasonable requests if your work is well known and well thought of locally and you are respected by those who work with you. So you need to publicize your work and seek to establish a good reputation.

Good relationships. There is no substitute for building and maintaining good relationships, and there is no denying that this requires a lot of continuing effort. It may be tempting to think that this is not 'getting on with the job' but it is an essential investment for every coordinator.

Bargaining. It may be possible to bargain with individual people or departments – could you offer something in return for cooperation?

Out-ranking. This could be used, but only in extreme circumstances. It means getting a senior manager from your hierarchy to request cooperation through the other person's manager. While the other tactics build trust and goodwill, this one endangers it and may give you even more headaches in the future.

Discussion and negotiation. Talking to all involved could result in a clarification of responsibilities and more mutual understanding, leading to you being given more legitimate authority by the group. This could mean first discussing the issue with individuals, and later convening a meeting when you have got sufficient commitment to solving the problem.

Policies, Rules and Procedures, Protocols

Policies are discussed further in Chapter 16

Policies are an increasingly important way of coordinating health promotion work. Rules and set procedures are a way of coordinating routine tasks. Protocols are agreed written procedures which everyone follows, which ensure that everyone carries out that particular task in the same way. For example, there may be a protocol in a GP surgery about how to deal with helping a patient to stop smoking. The protocol ensures that whoever is dealing with the patient (the doctor, the practice nurse, the district nurse or the health visitor) will offer the same range of help and follow the same follow-up procedures.

Joint Planning

In this approach the parties involved not only agree objectives but meet regularly to develop and implement a joint plan. This may minimize the need for one individual to be given the job of coordinator and prevent the problem of one agency or department being perceived as telling another what to do. However, it can be a major headache to get all the people involved together on a regular basis, and make sure that communications are always clear to all those involved.

Joint Working Through Creating Teams

A particular team is given the authority, training, money, staff, premises and equipment to carry out the programme. The team are autonomous and get the satisfaction of 'running their own show'. There is no need for a coordinator, since the whole team are working together from the same base. Joint working of this kind is not suitable for short-term programmes, but can be excellent for long-term projects, such as a community development project.

Creation of Lateral Relations

This type of coordination depends on strengthening relationships between individuals in broadly equivalent jobs in different departments or agencies. This can be done by setting up project teams, which are dissolved once the particular project is completed. Or it can be done by forming interdepartmental or multidisciplinary teams, who are given more authority for making decisions 'at the sharp end', without having to refer them up the different hierarchies. This can lead to conflict with the existing vertical lines of command, and works best where there are also good links between the various managers.

Exercise 9.2   **Improving coordination and teamworking**

In the health promotion work you do which involves working with other people, can you think of any ways by which you could improve coordination and teamworking?

- **What steps could you take to enhance the reputation of your health promotion work?**
- **Whom could you build a better relationship with to improve coordination or teamwork?**
- **What have you got to offer if you are bargaining?**
- **Can you think of any health promotion activities that you undertake routinely together with other people, which could be more efficient with a set procedure?**
- **Are there any ways by which you could develop stronger links with other staff at your level in different departments or agencies, to facilitate joint working in health promotion?**
- **Have you any opportunities for joint objective-setting or joint planning which could help to coordinate health promotion in your situation?**
- **Can you think of anything else? Discuss this with colleagues who are also involved in health promotion.**

Characteristics of Successful Teams

There are different sorts of teams – some are competitive, like sports teams; others are associations of people with a common work purpose, for example a primary health care team. Successful teams have the characteristics set out in

For more discussion about working with people in groups, see Chapter 13. the box below. If you experience a team which does not seem to be working well, it can be helpful to consider this list together, to identify the roots of the difficulties.

Box 9.1.　Characteristics of Successful Teams

- A team consists of a group of identified people.
- The team has a common purpose and shared objectives which are known and agreed by all members.
- Members are selected because they have relevant expertise.
- Members know and agree their own role and know the roles of the other members.
- Members support each other in achieving the common purpose.
- Members trust each other, and communicate with each other in an open, honest way.
- The team has a leader, whose authority is accepted by all members.

Participating in Meetings

The detailed planning and organization of meetings is beyond the scope of this book, but we offer you some guidance, below, on how to be an effective participant at meetings. As a participant there are a number of constructive things you can do:

- Encourage the chair into good practices, for example, ask for clarification on the purpose of the meeting, ask for a summary of what has been agreed at the end.
- Come prepared and arrive on time. Insist on ending on time too!
- Acknowledge the authority of the chair.
- Agree what to do about taking notes: does each person take their own, or does one person take them and circulate a copy to everyone else? Do you want detailed notes of everything you discussed, or just action points?
- Do not speak for more than two minutes at a time.
- Actively contribute to the meeting – express your views, keep an open mind and listen to other people's opinions.
- Encourage everyone to participate – draw in quieter people by referring to their relevant experience or expertise.
- Only make commitments that you are genuinely able to fulfil, and make sure you do so on time. Say 'no' clearly and non-defensively if you are unable or unwilling to do something.
- Remember that discussion and argument about ideas will help decision-making but personal rivalries will not.

Effective Committee Work

A committee is a group of people appointed for a specific purpose accountable to a larger group or organization; examples are the management committee of a voluntary organization or the health committee of a local authority. There are many common routines and procedures which help to oil the wheels of committees, and it is useful to be familiar with these. The details will vary from committee to committee, although principles remain the same. Some committees start their life with recommendations from a steering group which include proposals for the interim committee rules. These are then approved at the first committee meeting. After review and modification, a set of rules will be agreed which become the accepted rules for the committee.

Officers

The officers are servants of the committee and carry out its instructions. In practice, these are powerful positions which can be abused and a good chair will work for the active involvement of all committee members. Many committees have three key officers – the chair, the secretary and the treasurer. As committees grow the officers often need help with their work and additional appointments may be necessary, for example, a minutes secretary.

Chair. Much of the work of the chair may be done between meetings, but at the meetings she is most visible, and is responsible for ensuring that the committee successfully completes its tasks. It is vital for the chair to project her voice during meetings, so that all the committee can hear and be involved. Good chairs delegate as much as possible, to ensure active involvement of all members. The chair also has the responsibility of preparing or 'grooming' the next chair and must ensure that opportunities are provided for the vice-chair to develop.

Secretary. The secretary is responsible for all the non-financial papers and reports, for general planning and organization, often in collaboration with the other officers, and for seeing that the committee's work is coordinated and nothing is forgotten. Typing ability and skill in the use of words are extremely helpful. Good organization and coordination skills are needed.

The secretary is responsible for compiling the agenda for the committee meetings. This is the list of things to be done or agreed during the meeting. It will often include standard items such as 'apologies for absence', 'minutes of the previous meeting', 'matters arising from the previous meeting' and 'any other business'. The important point is that the agenda acts as an advance organizer for everyone attending the meeting, so that they are able to prepare. The members need to receive the agenda in good time before the meeting.

The secretary is also responsible for the final version of the minutes, and for agreeing these with the chair, even if a minutes secretary takes the notes at the meetings. Minutes are accurate records of the meeting, and should always precisely identify who has responsibility for what action by what date, and when a report back will be made to the committee.

Treasurer. A treasurer will be necessary if the committee is responsible for any financial undertakings. Treasurers are expected to report on the financial position quickly and precisely at any time. This is achieved by recording and summarizing every transaction as it happens, so that it is easy to see the current situation. At the end of the financial year all financial transactions are summarized in an annual statement – a clear one-page summary.

Quorum

In the real world it is unlikely that all committee members will be able to attend all meetings. The rules usually state the minimum number of members who must be present for the meeting to be considered representative of members' views and to have the authority to make decisions. This is called a quorum and is usually one-third or one-half of the total voting membership.

Committee Behaviour

Committees tend to be more informal nowadays than they were in the past. Nevertheless, it is good to bear in mind the reasons for various formal behaviours. For example the 'rule' that only one person speaks at a time, and is not interrupted, is meant to ensure a fair hearing for everyone. The chair should not allow a vociferous few to dominate the meeting.

The rule of everyone speaking by addressing the meeting through the chair helps to prevent a number of subdiscussions developing at the same time. On the other hand, it may seem more natural and helpful to address another committee member directly. Ultimately it is the job of the chair to set the tone which encourages all members to participate whilst keeping the meeting under control.

For further information, including conduct of elections of officers and annual general meetings, see the suggestions at the end of this chapter.

Understanding Conflict

In itself, conflict is not bad. Conflict is inevitable at times in any group because of differences in needs, objectives or values. The results of conflict will be positive or negative depending on how the group handles it. Handled well, conflict can be a creative source of new ideas and can help a group to change and develop. It can also strengthen the ability of group members to work together. Conflict is badly handled when it is either ignored (burying your head in the sand) so that negative feelings are left to fester, or approached on a win/lose basis (one person only can win, the rest of the group lose).

Working in Health Alliances with Other Organizations

Health promotion programmes and projects often require people from different organizations to work together: when these organizations link up it is often called a 'health alliance'. The term came into prominent use because it featured in the *Health of the Nation* national strategy for health in England[1], but it is a way of working which has been recognized in health promotion for many decades.

Generally the term 'health alliance' is used to mean formally-recognized working partnerships between two or more organizations such as health authorities or NHS trusts, local authorities, and voluntary or community groups. These organizations are usually called 'partners' or 'members'. In practice, the

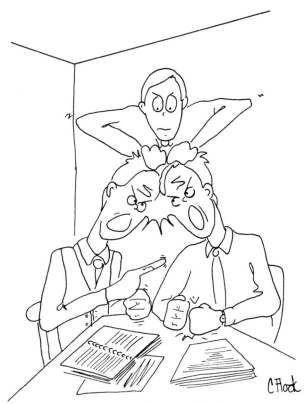

What's your conflict resolution style?

| Exercise 9.3 | **Your conflict resolution style** |

When confronted with conflict in a group you work in, assess which of these styles you use:

Style	Characteristic behaviour
Avoidance	Ignores the problem; avoids raising the issue; denies that there is a problem
Accommodating	Attempts to cooperate with everyone, even at the expense of not meeting personal or team objectives
Win/lose	Fights to win at any cost, even if it means alienating colleagues or causing the rest of the team to fail in meeting their objectives
Compromising	Suggests a compromise which would meet everyone's basic needs and maintain good relationships
Problem-solving	Openly confronts the problem and encourages everyone to face the disagreements and to express fully their opinions and ideas. Searches for a new solution which meets everyone's needs as fully as possible

Review this chart with other members of groups you work in. Can you think of situations in which these different approaches to conflict resolution were used? Discuss what worked and what did not. What could have been done differently that might have improved the outcome?

working links may be at different levels from chief executives to field workers. Alliances may be formally structured, with, for example, a written constitution and terms of reference, or they may be fairly informal arrangements. They may be long term, or set up for a time-limited period to work on a specific project.

The main reasons for setting up an alliance are:

- to harness a range of complementary skills and resources to work towards common goals;
- to avoid duplication and fragmentation of effort;
- to avoid gaps in services or programmes.

Alliances can work in different ways, and vary in terms of how closely members work together. It is useful to think of three main ways of working, spanning a range of degrees of involvement between partners:[2]

Networking — Cooperating — Joint working

Networking means coming together with other people from different agencies, and exchanging information and ideas on activities and plans.[3] This is useful for coordinating activities, avoiding duplication and sharing knowledge of mutual interest. Members meet and talk, but they do not actually work together. This has the lowest degree of involvement between partners.

Cooperating means that member agencies help each other in ways which are compatible with their own goals. They meet, talk, and agree to participate in each other's work when this is helpful for their own work plans. For example, in an accident prevention alliance, people who work in an accident and emergency (A&E) department of a hospital may cooperate with a local alcohol advisory service (a voluntary organization) to ensure that patients brought in with a drink problem know that they can go to the alcohol agency for help. This cooperation helps the alcohol agency to reach needy potential clients, and helps the A&E department to fulfil its role of helping patients with their health problems, possibly even preventing patients from coming back again in a similar state. This way of working in an alliance means a moderate degree of involvement between partners.

Joint working means coming together to agree a mutually acceptable plan, and working together to carry it out. This necessitates a high degree of involvement between partners. For example, the police, the probation service, road safety officers from the local authority, and a local alcohol advisory service may all work together to plan, implement and evaluate a joint programme of work on drink/driving.

Alliances operate in one, two or all of these ways. Sometimes joint working is thought to be the 'gold standard' of alliance work, but networking and cooperating can be useful in themselves. It is not always feasible or worthwhile to aim for full joint working.

Factors for Success[4]

See earlier sections in this chapter on coordination and teamwork.

Successful health alliances do not 'just happen': they are usually the result of investing a considerable amount of resources, skill and time in order for alliances members to work well together. Key factors for success are:

■ all partners need to be working towards the same thing: a shared vision of what the alliance should achieve, with an agenda and goals which all partners agree to;

■ all partners need to feel a sense of ownership of the alliance, and not that one partner dominates, with others as 'second class' fringe members;

■ commitment from the highest level of member organizations is vital to ensure that membership fits with the organization's strategic aims and that there will be management support for input of time and other resources;

■ there must be commitment of sufficient time and resources and realistic expectations; alliance working is time-consuming, and it may take months or years to develop a shared understanding and joint plans, let alone achieve results from joint health promotion activities. On the other hand, there must be demonstrable achievements; otherwise the alliance will be regarded as a mere 'talking shop';

■ someone acceptable to all partners needs to take responsibility for running the alliance (for example, setting up, chairing and servicing meetings) and coordinating action. A full-time coordinator can be extremely helpful;

See section on coordination earlier in this chapter

■ there must be mutual respect between partners; all partners need to feel that others value their input;

■ working relationships need to be characterized by openness and trust;

■ there needs to be an agreed framework for reviewing the alliance, changing the way of working if necessary, and even bringing it to an end if the alliance has outlived its usefulness or is unproductive.

Potential Difficulties

Alliances can face many difficulties. Major problems are:

■ organizational change, which blights long-term commitment and planning;

■ competition between member agencies for contracts in the market-place of health promotion provision, between, for example, NHS trusts and voluntary organizations;

■ lack of resources, both money and person-power;

■ lack of top-level commitment from agencies on the alliance;

■ individual personalities who can dominate an alliance (for good or bad);

■ an imbalance of input from different agencies which can lead to resentment, issues of ownership of joint activities and who takes the credit for success;

■ professional jealousy and unwillingness to share expertise and information;

■ differences between agencies and individuals in terms of different goals and values; different organizational cultures and ways of working; different levels of expertise and experience.

It is worth bearing in mind that not all alliances are successful. Many may fade out or be wound up. Alliances are not an end in themselves; they are a means to an end, and there may be circumstances where the end is better achieved by an organization working alone.

Avon Sexual Health Promotion Alliance (ASHPA)[5]

ASHPA originated in 1987, when a public health physician from a health authority convened a meeting for senior people from neighbouring health and local authorities around the Bristol area to discuss what to do in response to the new threat of AIDS and HIV.

The agencies agreed to set up a multiagency group called Avon HIV/AIDS Prevention and Education Group. The first meeting was convened by the District Health Promotion Officer from one of the health authorities, when people agreed to meet quarterly with the remit:
to co-ordinate activities, exchange information, and advise parent organisations on issues of HIV/AIDS prevention and education.

Ten years later, in 1997, the alliance is now called Avon Sexual Health Promotion Alliance (ASHPA) and is still active. Its remit is:
to co-ordinate activities, exchange information and advise parent organisations on issues of promoting sexual health through education and preventive activities.

Membership includes the health authority, several NHS trusts, various departments of four local authorities, and three voluntary organizations. People and disciplines actively involved include health promotion specialists, public health medicine, genitourinary medicine (GUM), family planning, environmental health, social services, education; and voluntary organizations concerned with contraceptive services for young people, people living with HIV/AIDS, and services for drug users.

ASHPA meets quarterly, chaired and serviced by the health authority, and attracts an attendance of ten to sixteen people at each meeting. Many more are linked in through wider networking and subgroups which focus on particular client groups or activities.

The alliance has gone through several changes. NHS reforms and local government reorganization meant that none of the NHS or local authority member agencies remained in the same configuration as when the alliance was set up in 1987. During almost continuous reorganization, membership fluctuated and there have been long periods of uncertainty about organizational commitment.

During its lifetime, the alliance has reviewed its membership and way of working several times. Significant changes and milestones were:

- the first production of a joint action plan in 1993, with a commitment to systematically review action in key target groups;
- a decision to widen the remit from HIV/AIDS prevention to promoting sexual health in 1996. This meant focusing on preventing unwanted pregnancies and the spread of sexually transmitted diseases in addition to HIV/AIDS issues;
- production of a revised action plan in 1996.

ASHPA works at all degrees of involvement: **networking**, **cooperating**, and **joint working**. **Networking** is fostered by the meetings themselves which provide a focus for making contacts; an opportunity for people to inform others about current work and future plans; and to share information on, for example, teenage pregnancy rates or evidence for changing patterns of sexual behaviour. Members **cooperate** on issues such as publicizing each others' services to clients.

There is **joint working** on activities such as: a coordinated programme of local activities to support World AIDS Day; production of a regular newsletter called *ASHPA News*, to which many members contribute; and a sexual health helpline scheme piloted in 1996/97.

The history of ASHPA illustrates some factors for success and some of the difficulties identified above.

Factors which have contributed to its success include:

- shared commitment to preventing the spread of HIV and AIDS, and (later) to preventing other sexually transmitted diseases, unintended pregnancies and to promoting sexual health;

- a range of complementary expertise from related fields of health promotion, family planning, GUM, public health, and from people with expertise in working with young people, the gay community, workers in the sex industry, people in custody and other key population groups;
- members with commitment to aspects of sexual health as their fulltime work. This is partly possible because of ring-fenced government money dedicated to HIV prevention;
- a few key individuals who have given time and energy to the alliance consistently over its life span, so that there is a stable core membership;
- a member acceptable to all agencies who chairs and services alliance meetings; other members who willingly take responsibility for leading joint projects and running subgroups;
- ability to review the alliance openly and honestly and change plans and ways of working.

Difficulties include:

- constant organizational change, which causes policy vacuums in 'new' agencies, uncertainty about top-level commitment, inability to make long-term commitment to plans, and people threatened by possible redundancy or job changes;
- patchy support, with some NHS trusts and local authorities more involved than others;
- tensions caused by the contractual relationship between different member agencies, and competition for funds;
- controversial policy decisions by member agencies which have been opposed by other members, e.g. health authority decisions about changing contracts for provision of family planning services.

PRACTICE POINTS

- A key aspect of successfully implemented health promotion programmes is how well you and other health promoters work together.
- You need to think about how you communicate with colleagues: the channels you use, how well you use them, and the quality of your relationships.
- Health promotion often involves different professionals and disciplines working together; there is a range of ways in which you can encourage good teamwork and coordination.
- For effective meetings and committee work, you require knowledge of how people behave in meetings, the roles and responsibilities of committee members, and skills of making the most use of meetings and committees.
- Health alliances are working partnerships between two or more organizations, which work at varying levels of involvement with each other, from networking to full joint working. Think about the many factors which contribute to success, and the potential pitfalls to avoid.

Recommended Reading

On Teamwork

➤ Rolls L (1992) *Team Development: a manual of facilitation for health educators and health promoters*. London: Health Education Authority.

A classic text on team building is:
➤ Adair J (1987) *Effective Teambuilding*, 2nd edn. London: Pan.

See also:
➤ Woodcock M (1989) *Team Development Manual*, 2nd edn. Aldershot: Gower.

On Running and Taking Part in Meetings

➤ Stanton N (1996) *Mastering Communication*, 3rd edn. Chapter 9. Basingstoke: Macmillan.
➤ Williams D (1997) *Communication Skills in Practice – a practical guide for health professionals*. Part Three: Professional Meetings. London: Jessica Kingsley Publications.

On Health Alliances

For a succinct overview of alliance working see:
➤ Naidoo J & Wills (1994) *Health Promotion: Foundations for Practice*. Chapter 8, Healthy alliances – working together. London: Baillière Tindall.

For a more detailed look at different alliances in action, and aspects of alliance working, see:
➤ Scriven A (ed.) (1998) *Alliances in Health Promotion: Theory and Practice*. Basingstoke: Macmillan.
➤ Naidoo J & Wills (1998) *Practising Health Promotion: Dilemmas and Challenges*. London: Baillière Tindall.

For a practical framework to use when planning, evaluating or developing an alliance, see:
➤ Funnell R, Oldfield K & Speller V (1995) *Towards Healthier Alliances: a tool for planning, evaluating and developing alliances*. London: Health Education Authority/Wessex Institute of Public Health Medicine.

Notes and References

1 Secretary of State for Health (1992) *The Health of the Nation: a Strategy for Health in England*. London: HMSO.

Department of Health (1993) *Working Together for Better Health*, London: HMSO.

2 Based on:

Powell M (1992) *Healthy Alliances: a report to the HealthGain Standing Conference*, pp. 31–32. London: Office for Public Management.

3 Although in this chapter we focus on local networks of people, there are many wider networks in health promotion. They may be organized on a regional or national basis. For example, the Health Education Authority has set up a Young People's Health Network, which publishes a regular newsletter on issues affecting young people's health. It provides a means of exchanging of information on research, news,

projects, events and useful contacts. Contact: Young People's Health Network, Health Education Authority, Trevelyan House, 30 Great Peter Street, London SWIP 2HW.

4 These factors are drawn from our own experience, and from:

Department of Health (1993) *Working Together for Better Health*, London: HMSO.

Powell M (1992) *Healthy Alliances: a report to the HealthGain Standing Conference*. London: Office for Public Management.

Naidoo J & Wills J (1994) *Health Promotion: Foundations for Practice*. Chapter 8, Healthy alliances – working together. London: Baillière Tindall.

5 This case study is a real-life alliance chaired by one of the authors (Linda Ewles).

3 DEVELOPING COMPETENCE IN HEALTH PROMOTION

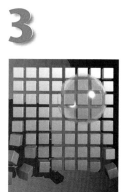

Part 3 aims to provide you with guidance in how to assess, develop and improve your competencies in health promotion.

Competencies are the combination of knowledge, attitudes and skills needed to perform work of a satisfactory standard in health promotion. As a health promoter, you need competencies to plan, evaluate, and implement health promotion activities, in different settings and with different goals, which we discussed in Part 2. You will also need to develop other core competencies of health promotion: communicating and educating, marketing and publicizing, facilitating and networking, and influencing policy and practice. We address these in Part 3.

Some chapters of Part 3 will be more important to some professions or disciplines than others. So you may wish to start by studying the chapters most relevant to you, rather than going through them in sequence. We have provided cross-referencing to help you to identify which sections of other chapters may also be relevant to your particular needs.

In Chapter 10 we address the fundamentals of communication, including establishing relationships, promoting self-esteem and assertiveness, identifying communication and language barriers, and basic communication skills.

In Chapter 11 we look at how to produce and use communication tools, including displays, audiovisual resources, written materials and statistical information. We discuss how mass media can be used effectively in health promotion, including practical help about working with the local press, radio and television. We include an introduction to the use of information technology in health promotion.

In Chapter 12 we outline the principles of adult learning and how you can help people to learn. We include guidelines on giving talks, and on patient education.

Chapter 13 is about working with clients in groups.

Chapter 14 is about how to help people to change their behaviour towards healthier living. We include information on models of behaviour change, and how you can relate strategies to the stages and processes of change. We outline skills of counselling to help people to make decisions and we discuss techniques to help people to change behaviour.

In Chapter 15 we focus on community-based work in health promotion, including community participation, community development and community health projects.

Chapter 16 is about the politics of influencing policies and practices, how to develop and implement policies, and how to campaign for changes.

10 Fundamentals of Communication

SUMMARY

We start this chapter by exploring relationships with clients and discussing the links between self-esteem and communication, and follow with a case study on relationship skills. We continue by identifying communication and language barriers. Discussion on four basic communication skills follows: understanding non-verbal communication, listening, helping people to talk, asking questions and obtaining feedback. We end with a section on written communication. Exercises are provided on overcoming communication barriers and on each basic communication skill.

Good communication between people is fundamental to successful health promotion, whether it happens in the context of a consultation with a patient, a conversation with a colleague or a request to a manager. By 'good communication' we mean clear, unambiguous two-way constructive exchanges, without distortion of the message between when it is given and when it is received.

This chapter discusses some fundamentals of relationships with clients, communication barriers and basic communication skills. The application of these skills often will be in one-to-one situations, though they may apply when working in groups and when teaching as well as in more formal situations. These skills will help to develop better communication, but they should not be expected to provide a blueprint for every situation, or a quick and easy route to being a good communicator. They are a start, but improving communication is a life-long developmental process.[1]

Exploring Relationships with Clients

We start by asking health promoters to look at some fundamental (and possibly uncomfortable) questions. For example, what is your basic attitude towards the people you work with? Do you accept them on their own terms or do you judge them by your own standards? Do you aim to encourage people to be independent, make their own decisions, take charge of their health, solve their own problems? Or are you actually encouraging dependency, solving their problems for them and thereby decreasing their own ability and confidence to take responsibility for themselves? We suggest that you work through the following questions, thinking about how you relate to the people you work with.

Accepting or Judging

Accepting people means:

- recognizing that people's knowledge and beliefs emerge from their life experience, whereas your own have been modified and extended by professional education and experience;
- understanding your own knowledge, beliefs, values and standards;
- understanding your clients' knowledge, beliefs, values and standards from their point of view;
- recognizing that you and the people you work with may differ in your knowledge, beliefs, values and standards;
- recognizing that these differences do not imply that you, the professional health promoter, are a person of greater worth than your clients.

Judging people means:

- equating people's intrinsic worth with their knowledge, beliefs, values, standards and behaviour. For example, saying of someone who drinks 'people who get drunk are stupid' judges (and condemns) that person, and takes no account of life experience and cultural background. 'Drunkenness can result in people getting hurt' does not judge the person.
- ranking knowledge and behaviour. For example, 'I'm the expert so I know better than you' is judgmental; 'I know more than you about this particular thing' is not – it is a statement of fact. 'My standards are higher than yours' is judgmental; 'my standards are different from yours' is not.

Autonomy or Dependency?

There are a number of ways in which you can help clients to take more control over their health.

Autonomy can be helped by:

- encouraging people to make their own decisions, and resisting the urge to 'take over' the decision-making;
- encouraging people to think things out for themselves, even if this takes much longer than simply telling them;
- respecting any unusual ideas they may have.

Autonomy can be hindered if:

- you impose your own solution on your clients' problems;
- you tell them what to do because they are taking too long to think it out for themselves;
- you tell them that their ideas are no good and won't work, without giving an adequate explanation or opportunity to try them out.

We suggest that the appropriate aim is to work towards as much autonomy as possible. By doing this, you are helping people to increase control over their own health, which is a basic aim of health promotion. Obviously, there are times when people are dependent on a health promoter, and rightly so; for example, they may be ill, confused or likely to put themselves or other people in danger. There is also the very real problem that working towards autonomy is time-consuming. However, in the long run, it is time well spent.

A Partnership or a One-way Process?

Do you think of yourself as working in partnership with people in pursuit of health promotion aims, or do you see health promotion as your sole responsibility, with yourself as the 'expert'?

A partnership means:

- there is an atmosphere of trust and openness between yourself and your clients, so that they are not intimidated;
- you ask people for their views and opinions, which you accept and respect even if you disagree with them;
- you tell people when you learn something from them (e.g. 'I never thought of it that way before')
- you use informal, participative methods when you are involved in health education, drawing on the experience and knowledge which clients bring with them;
- you encourage clients to share their knowledge and experience with each other. People do this all the time, of course (for example, knowledge and experience is discussed between patients in a hospital ward and parents in a baby clinic) but do you deliberately foster and encourage this?

A one-way process means:

- you do not encourage clients to ask questions and discuss problems;
- you imply that you do not expect to learn anything from your clients (and if you do, you don't say so);
- you do not find out what people already know and have experienced;
- you do not encourage people to learn from each other, only from you;
- you use formal methods when you are undertaking health education, such as lectures, rather than participative methods.

Clients' Feelings – Positive or Negative?

A change in people's health knowledge, attitudes and actions will be helped if they feel good about themselves. It will rarely be helped if they are full of self-doubt, anxiety or guilt.

Clients will feel better about themselves if:

- you praise their progress, achievements, strengths and efforts, however small;
- the consequences of 'unhealthy' behaviour (e.g. smoking) are discussed without implying that the behaviour is morally bad;

See Chapter 14 Helping People towards Healthier Living.

- time is spent exploring how to overcome difficulties (e.g. practical strategies to help a client stop smoking). This will help to minimize feelings of helplessness.

Clients will feel bad about themselves if:

- you ignore their strengths and concentrate on their weaknesses;
- you ignore or belittle their efforts;

- you attempt to motivate them by raising guilt and anxiety (e.g. 'if you don't stop smoking you'll damage your baby' or 'you're killing yourself with what you eat'.)

To sum up, we suggest that the health promotion aim of enabling people to take control over, and improve, their health is best achieved by working in a non-judgmental partnership. This should seek to build on people's existing knowledge and experience, move them towards autonomy, empower them to take responsibility for their own health and help them to feel positive about themselves.[2]

Self-esteem, Self-confidence and Communication

The ability to communicate is closely linked to how people feel about themselves. People with a low sense of self-esteem tend to be over-critical of themselves and to underestimate their abilities. This lack of self-confidence is reflected in their ability to communicate. For example, they may lack assertiveness and thus may either fail to speak up for themselves, or react with inappropriate anger and even violence.

By 'assertiveness' we mean saying what you think and asking for what you want openly, clearly and honestly. It does not mean being aggressive or bullying, but it is in contrast with hiding what you really feel, saying what you don't really mean or trying to manipulate people into doing what you want.

Assertiveness helps people to create win–win situations (situations where everyone involved feels that they have done all right) through direct and open communication and through avoiding aggressive behaviour (win–lose situations, where one party feels that they have won and the other party feels they have lost) or manipulation (lose–lose situations, where, for example, one party in a negotiation walks out). It builds the self-esteem of all concerned. Successful negotiations are a good example of how assertiveness can work. In a successful negotiation both parties come away with the following thoughts:[3]

- This is an agreement which, whilst not ideal, is good enough for both of us to support.
- Both of us made some compromises and sacrifices.
- We shall be able to have successful negotiations with each other in future.

Many clients with low self-esteem will need to learn how to feel better about themselves before they can communicate better with professionals and others. This requires opportunities for 'life skills education', by which we mean education in the key skills necessary for living. These skills include how to improve self-esteem, and how to communicate and relate to others in a morally responsible manner, with respect for oneself and others, and with sensitivity towards the needs and views of others. Unfortunately, we are often expected to 'catch' these skills automatically, without any proper learning process to help us. Furthermore, the time allotted to personal and social education in schools has decreased with the advent of the National Curriculum.[4]

One way to develop these life skills is through relationships with people who are 'healthy' role models and there is a body of research on the characteristics of the psychologically most healthy people.[5] However, we cannot choose our parents and many people have little choice of workmates or employers, so health promoters need to find opportunities for 'life skills education'. For further reading on how to develop life skills and assertiveness and improve self-esteem, see the suggestions at the end of the chapter. The following case study illustrates how parents can learn to develop the self-esteem of their children and ensure that their children understand the rights of other people. While the case study refers to parents and children, and we have used this example because it is supported by research evidence, the same principles can be used by health promoters with their clients.

See also the section on Working for Client Self-empowerment in Chapter 14.

Case study 10.1

Relating Skills – Lorraine and Jack

Lorraine is late for work and tries to coax her three-year old son, Jack, into his coat so that she can take him to nursery school. Jack starts to cry. Lorraine hugs him but tells him that he's got to go to school. She is at a loss about what else to do, and when she reaches nursery school Jack is still crying. One of the nursery nurses notices his distress and manages to calm him. When Jack has recovered, the nurse talks to Lorraine about what she's learnt from a book about good parenting which is based on up-to-date research.[6]

A week later in a similar situation Lorraine tries out what the nurse suggested. She starts in the same way as before, by empathizing with Jack, but this time she goes further and provides him with guidance on what to do with his uncomfortable feelings. The conversation goes something like this:

Jack: 'It's not fair. I don't want to go to school'. (Starts to cry.)
Lorraine: 'Come here Jack'. (Takes him on her knee.) 'I'm sorry but we can't stay at home. I have lots to do at work. Does that make you feel sad?'
Jack: (nodding) 'Yes'.
Lorraine: 'I feel a bit sad too. It's OK for you to cry.' (Hugs him while he cries.) 'I know what. Let's think about what to do on Saturday when I don't have to go to work and you don't have to go to school. Can you think of anything special you would like to do on Saturday?'
Jack: 'Can we go to the park and feed the ducks?'
Lorraine: 'Yes. That would be great.'
Jack: 'Can Nick come too?'
Lorraine: 'Perhaps. We'll have to ask his Mum. But right now it's time to get going.'
Jack: 'OK.'

Lorraine has gone through five steps:

1. She becomes aware of Jack's feelings.
2. She recognizes the opportunity for helping Jack to learn about how to handle emotions.
3. She listens to Jack, tries to understand his feelings, and lets him know it is OK to feel bad and upset sometimes, and that she has these feelings too.
4. She helps Jack to find the words to label the emotion he is having.
5. She sets limits while exploring strategies to solve the problem.

Studies show[6] that children whose parents consistently practise these five steps have better physical health and score higher academically than children whose parents do not. They also get along better with friends, have fewer behaviour problems and are less prone to acts of violence.

So, when working with clients with low self-esteem, you may find it helpful to:

- be aware of the client's feelings;
- recognize the opportunity to help the client to learn about how to handle difficult feelings;

For guidance on how to listen effectively and help people to talk, see sections later in this chapter.

- listen and acknowledge that you have these feelings too;
- label the feelings;
- set limits for the interaction while exploring strategies to solve the problem.

Communication Barriers

As a health promoter, you may encounter numerous difficulties in communicating. Recognizing that communication barriers exist is the necessary first stage before work can begin on tackling the problems. There are no easy solutions, but increased awareness and skill can go a long way towards improvement.

Common communication barriers may be categorized into six groups:

1.   Social and Cultural Gaps

A number of factors can cause gaps, among which are:

- different ethnic background;
- different social group, which may be apparent in dress, language or accent;
- different cultural or religious beliefs, for example about hygiene, nutrition or contraception;
- different values, reflected in a different emphasis on the importance of health issues;
- different gender or sexual orientation, reflected in different approaches, interests or values.

2.   Limited Receptiveness

You may want to communicate, but the reverse is not always true: people may not want to be communicated with. They may be unreceptive for many reasons, including:

- learning disability or confusion;
- illness, tiredness or pain;
- emotional distress;
- being too busy, distracted or preoccupied;
- not valuing themselves, or not believing that their health is important.

3.   Negative Attitude to the Health Promoter

Some people may be 'anti' you, even before you have met. This may be caused by:

- previous 'bad' experiences;
- lack of trust in 'them' – that is, anyone seen as an authority figure or part of 'the establishment';
- lack of credibility of the health promoter (perhaps you set a poor example of good health yourself?);
- perceiving you as a threat, coming to criticize or pass judgement;
- believing that 'I know it all anyway', and you will be 'teaching your grandmother to suck eggs';
- believing that advice will be given which cannot be complied with because of financial or social constraints, or being asked to give up the 'few pleasures in life';
- not wishing to confront unpleasant issues such as results of medical tests, or the need to change policies and practices.

4.   Limited Understanding and Memory

There may be difficulties because people:

- understand and/or speak little or no English;
- have limited education or learning difficulties, and may be unable to read and write;
- are being confronted with technical words, jargon or medical terminology which they do not understand;
- have poor or failing memories and cannot remember what was discussed previously.

5.   Insufficient Emphasis by the Health Promoter

Communication may fail because you do not give it sufficient time and attention. The reasons may be:

- it was given a low priority in basic training, so it is given low priority in practice;
- lack of confidence, skills and knowledge which may be the result of inadequate training;
- being too busy with other things, and just unable to find the time;
- managers not being supportive about time spent on health promotion;
- reluctance to 'demystify' and share professionally-acquired health knowledge.

6.   Contradictory Messages

Communication barriers are erected when people get different messages from different people. For example:

- different health professionals give different advice;
- family, friends or neighbours contradict health promoters;
- 'the experts keep changing their minds' as information is updated.

Exercise 10.1   **Identifying communication barriers**

This exercise can be done alone, but it is best carried out in pairs or small groups so that ideas can be shared.

Consider the six kinds of communication barriers discussed.

1.   How many of them can you identify in your own experience?
2.   What other communication barriers can you add to this list?
3.   What communication barriers cause you the most problems?
4.   What suggestions can you make for helping to break down communication barriers? (Share examples from your own experience and make additional suggestions.)

Overcoming Language Barriers

There is more about concepts of health and illness in ethnic minority groups, and the different health experience of ethnic minority groups, in Chapter 1.

Language is only one facet of the gulf which may exist between people of different ethnic backgrounds. The root of many communication problems is racism; this is a huge topic, largely outside the scope of this book, but we recommend all health promoters to take time out for racism awareness training when working with people from different ethnic groups. We make suggestions for further reading at the end of this chapter.

However, when we focus solely on the question of language barriers, learning a few key words and phrases in the person's language may help. Words such as hello, goodbye, hot, cold, food and money may be useful. Help with learning the language may be available from multicultural education centres run by local education authorities.

When faced with a language barrier, there are some useful guidelines which you can follow to help someone with limited English to understand what is being said.[7]

Box 10.1   **Guidelines for communicating with someone who speaks little English**

1. Speak clearly and slowly, and resist the temptation to raise your voice in an effort to get through.
2. Repeat a sentence if you have not been understood; repeat it using the same words. This gives the listener more time to 'tune in' and understand, whereas if you use different words you are likely to cause more confusion by introducing even more words which are not understood.
3. Keep it simple. Use simple words and sentences. Use active forms of verbs rather than passive forms, so say 'The nurse will see you' rather than 'You will be seen by the nurse'. Do not try to cover too much, and stick to one topic at a time.
4. Say things in a logical sequence: the sequence in which they are going to happen. So say 'Eat first, then take the tablet' rather than 'Take the tablet after you eat'. If the listener does not pick up the word 'after' correctly, he will take the tablet first, because that is the order in which he heard the instruction.
5. Be careful of idioms. Being 'fed up', 'popping out' and 'spending a penny' may be totally incomprehensible.
6. Do not attempt to speak pidgin English. It does not help people to learn correct English, and sounds patronizing.
7. Use pictures, mime and simple written instructions which may be read by relatives or friends who understand written English. Be careful of symbols on written material; ticks and crosses, for example, may not convey what you intend.

See section on Asking Questions and Getting Feedback later in this chapter.

8. Check to ensure that you have been understood, but avoid asking closed questions that require a one-word answer such as 'Do you understand?' A reply of 'Yes' is no guarantee that your client really has understood.

Exercise 10.2   **Overcoming language barriers**

The following five extracts come from the district nurse's side of a conversation with a patient whose English is very limited.

'Hello – Oh, we are looking brighter today!'

'Have you been visited by the doctor today yet – did he give you a new prescription?'

'I'll see about your insulin after I've seen how your leg's getting on'.

'The doctor says you should take one of these tablets three times a day … I don't think you understand – I'll say that again … We want you to take one of these tablets three times a day … Oh dear … (louder) … DOCTOR SAYS YOU TAKE TABLET THREE TIMES A DAY'.

'I'll leave this list of foods for you. There are ticks and crosses on it to show you what you can eat and what you should not eat. Do you understand? Your son can read English, can't he?'

Using the guidelines that have just been described:

- identify what is unhelpful about the way the district nurse speaks to the patient;
- suggest better alternatives.

Non-verbal Communication

Non-verbal communication includes all the ways by which people communicate with each other except the words they use, and is sometimes called body language. The main categories of non-verbal communication are as follows:

Bodily Contact

Bodily contact is people touching each other, how much they touch, and which parts of the body are in contact. Shaking hands, holding hands, or putting an arm around someone's shoulders, for example, all convey a meaning from one person to another.

Some health promoters, such as nurses, obviously touch patients frequently in the course of their work, whereas others, such as environmental health officers, may rarely do so. Touching people is surrounded by 'rules' dictated by cultural expectations and taboos, and by expectations of 'professional distance', which may be barriers to the positive use of touch. For example, a handshake can say 'I'm glad to see you – welcome' and touching a distressed person can say 'I'm here for you'.

Proximity

Proximity is how close people are to each other. Consider the different messages being conveyed to a bed-ridden patient by someone who talks to him from 6 feet away at the foot of the bed and someone who comes closer and sits on the bed or a chair. However, people vary in the amount of 'personal space' they need, and feel uncomfortable when others come too close.

Orientation

How individuals position themselves in relation to other people and objects is known as orientation. A useful example is to consider the messages conveyed by the lay-out of a room where a small group of people are meeting. Chairs in rows facing one separate chair (perhaps with a table in front of it) imply that one person will dominate and control the meeting, whereas chairs placed in a circle without a table to act as a barrier imply that everyone is encouraged to join in, and that no one individual is expected to dominate.

Level

This refers to differences in height between people. Generally, communication is more comfortable if people are on the same level; so it feels better to bend down or sit down to talk to a child or a person in a wheelchair, for example. Talking to someone on a different level can leave one or both parties feeling disadvantaged, and sometimes this is done deliberately; not offering a chair to someone entering an office conveys a message that the visitor is not welcome to stay.

Posture

Posture is how people stand, sit or lie. For example, are they upright or slouched, arms crossed or not? Posture can convey a message of tension and anxiety, for example, by being hunched up with arms crossed, or one of welcome by being upright with arms outstretched.

Physical Appearance

All kinds of messages may be conveyed by physical appearance, such as a person's social standing, personality, tidy habits or concern with fashion. Physical appearance may be very important to health promoters because of the messages it conveys. A uniform may convey an impression of professional competence, but it may also convey an unwelcome image of authority. Casual dress in a formal committee may convey the impression (perhaps a false one) that the committee's work is not being taken seriously.

Facial Expression

Facial expression can obviously indicate feelings, such as sadness, happiness, anger, surprise or puzzlement.

Hand Movements and Head Movements

Movements of the hands and head can be very revealing. Nods and shakes of the head obviously convey agreement and disagreement without the need for words. (But beware of the fact that movements of the head may not convey the same meaning in different cultures.) Clenched fists, fidgeting hands (and some-

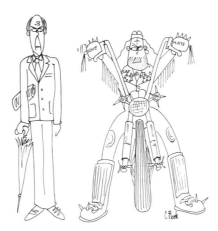

All kinds of messages can be conveyed by physical appearance

times tapping feet) reveal stress and tension, whereas still, open hands usually denote a relaxed frame of mind. Mental discomfort, such as confusion or worry, is often shown by putting hands to the head and playing with hair, stroking a beard or rubbing the forehead.

Direction of Gaze and Eye Contact

Whether people are 'looking each other straight in the eye' is significant. As a general rule, a speaker looks away from the listener for most of the time when talking (because she is concentrating on what she is saying), and she looks directly at the listener when she wants a response. For the listener, the general rule is that he will look the speaker straight in the eye while he is paying attention to what she says, but will look elsewhere if his attention has wandered.

This is particularly important if you work with people on a one-to-one basis: a person who is talking to you will infer that you are not listening if you are looking anywhere other than at the speaker. This is particularly important when counselling someone in distress; the counsellor needs to be giving the client full attention, and if the client looks up and sees the counsellor gazing elsewhere the implication is that the counsellor is not listening.

Non-verbal Aspects of Speech

Consider how many ways a word like 'no' can be said. The way in which it is said can convey meanings such as anger, doubt or surprise. Tone and timing are two non-verbal aspects of speech which convey messages to the listener.

See the suggestions at the end of the Chapter 7.

Raised awareness of non-verbal communication can help you to improve communication between yourself and the people you work with. For example, a person who says 'Yes, I understand' in a doubtful tone of voice, with a puzzled frown or with clenched fists clearly requires further help. Words alone are only part of a message, and can be misleading. Non-verbal communication is an area worth further study.

Exercise 10.3   **Non-verbal communication in your work[8]**

Work through the following questions and exercises with a partner.

1. **When do you touch people at work, if at all?**
    What 'rules' govern when it is acceptable/unacceptable to touch them?
    Would people you work with be helped if you touched them more?

2. Carry on a conversation with your partner, first standing too close for comfort, then standing too far away.
    What does it feel like? What is the most comfortable distance?
    What implications does this have for your work?

3. **When you talk to an individual in the course of your work, where do you sit or stand in relation to that person? For example, is furniture a barrier between you?**
    If you talk to people in groups, how do you seat them?
    Do you think communication could be improved by making changes? If so, what changes?

4. Have a conversation with your partner when one of you is sitting and the other is standing. Both describe your feelings.
    Do you ever work with people who are on a physically different level from you? What are the implications?

5. Practise tense and relaxed postures, then welcoming and rejecting postures.
    Which do you normally adopt with people?

6. Identify a few people you work with whom you know fairly well. Think back to your first impressions of these people.
    Do you think that your first impressions were right?
    What were the important features of their appearance which led to your first impressions?
    What is the importance of physical appearance in your health promotion work?
    If you wear a uniform, or a white coat, how do you think it affects your relationships?

7. Look around at other people in the room.
    What can you infer from their facial expressions, hand and head movements?
    What is the importance of noticing facial expression, hand and head movement in your job?

8. Hold a conversation with your partner while staring into each other's eys all the time, and then without looking at each other at all.
    Describe your feelings.
    Watch two people talking. **Do they look directly at each other or do they frequently look away?**
    Do they look more at each other when speaking or listening?
    How important is eye contact in your job?

9. Say 'I don't know' in as many ways as possible, trying to convey a different feeling each time, such as despair, confusion and irritation.
    How important is it for you to pick up on non-verbal aspects of speech in your health promotion work?

Listening

As a health promoter, you need to develop skills of effective listening, so that you can help people to talk and identify their needs and feelings.

Listening is an active process. It is not the same as merely hearing words. It involves a conscious effort to listen to words, to the way they are said, to be aware of the feelings shown and of attempts to hide feelings. It means taking note of the non-verbal communication as well as the spoken words. The listener needs to concentrate on giving the speaker full attention, being on the same level as the speaker and adopting a non-threatening posture.

It is easy to allow attention to wander. Some of the things you may find yourself doing instead of listening are planning what to say next, thinking about a similar experience, interrupting, agreeing or disagreeing, judging, blaming or criticizing, interpreting what the speaker says, thinking about the next job to be done or just plain day-dreaming.

The task of a listener is to help people to talk about their situation unhurriedly and without interruption, helping them to express their feelings, views and opinions, and to explore their knowledge, values and attitudes. This reinforces the speakers' responsibility for themselves and is essential for helping them towards greater responsibility for their own health choices.

Exercise 10.4   **Learning to listen**

Work in groups of from three to six people. Appoint someone as a timekeeper.

1. Person A speaks for two minutes, without interruption, on a subject of her choice to do with work or other interests (e.g. sensible drinking guidelines, keeping fit and active, pets, holidays). Everyone else in the group listens, without interrupting or taking notes.
2. Person B repeats as much as she can remember, without anyone else interrupting. B may *not*:
   - add anything extra to what A said;
   - give interpretations (e.g. 'It's obvious from what she said that …');
   - give comments (e.g. 'She's just like me …').
3. A, and the rest of the group, identify what was inaccurate, forgotten or added.
4. Repeat, with a different topic, until everyone has had a turn at being A and B.
5. **Discuss the following questions:**
   - **What helped me to listen?**
   - **What helped me to remember?**
   - **What hindered my listening?**
   - **What hindered my remembering?**
   - **What did I learn about myself as a listener?**

Helping People to Talk

As we have said, the main task of the listener to help someone to talk. There are several useful techniques, as follows.

Giving an Invitation to Talk

To get someone started it may be helpful to give out a specific invitation to talk. Examples are:

'You don't seem to be your usual self today. Is something on your mind?'

'Can we talk some more about that matter you raised briefly at yesterday's meeting?'

'You look worried – are you?'

Giving Attention

This means listening closely to what is being said, and being fully aware of all the channels of communication, including non-verbal behaviour. It requires effort and concentration to listen hard and give full, undivided attention.

Encouraging

This means making the occasional intervention to encourage someone to carry on talking. It tells the speaker that you really are listening, and wanting to hear more. Such interventions include noises like 'mm mm', words such as 'yes …' and short phrases such as 'I see …' or 'And then …?' or 'Go on …'

Another useful intervention is the repetition of a key word which the speaker has just used. For example, if the speaker says 'My work's getting on top of me' you could repeat the word 'work …?'

Paraphrasing

This means responding to the speaker using your own words to state the essence of what the speaker has been saying. Use key words and phrases, for example, 'So you're not sure whether to have the baby vaccinated or not?' or 'So you think some people will be very angry if you ban smoking in the office?'

Reflecting Feelings

This involves mirroring back to the speaker, in verbal statements, the feeling he is communicating. To do this it helps to listen for words about feelings, and to observe body language. Examples are 'You seem pleased' or 'You are obviously upset about this'.

Reflecting Meanings

This means joining feelings and content in one succinct response, to get a reflection of meaning:

'You feel … because …'

'You are … because …'

'You're … about …'

For example:

'You feel pleased about your progress'

'You're depressed because your children have grown up and left home'

'You're angry about all the rubbish and dumped cars left lying in this neighbourhood'

Summing-up

This is a brief re-statement of the main content and feelings which have been expressed throughout a conversation. Check back with the speaker to ensure that the statement is accurate. For example, say 'It seems to me that the main things you've been saying are. ... Does that cover it?'

| Exercise 10.5 | **Helping people to talk** |

Work in pairs.
Each person chooses a topic she feels strongly about (which might be a personal experience or topic of general concern such as sex education, traffic jams, cuts in the health service or violence on television). Stay with the same topic for all three stages of the exercise.
(The whole exercise takes about 45 minutes.)

Stage 1. Giving attention

One person speaks for two minutes, and the other listens, giving only non-verbal feedback. Then swap roles. After both of you have had your turn, spend 10 minutes discussing these questions:

When you were listening:

- **what did you find difficult about listening?**
- **did your mind wander?**
- **did you maintain eye contact?**
- **what did you notice about the speaker's non-verbal communication?**

When you were speaking:

- **what did the listener do which helped you to talk?**
- **did the listener do anything which made it difficult for you to talk?**

Stage 2. Encouraging

One person speaks for two minutes. The other listens and gives encouraging interventions (such as 'mm mm'), words ('yes ...') and non-directive comments ('I see ...') or repeats key words. Then swap roles. Then spend five minutes discussing these questions:

When you were listening:

- **what sort of interventions did you make?**
- **how did you feel about making them?**

When you were speaking:

- **what interventions did you notice?**
- **did you find them helpful?**

Stage 3. Paraphrasing, reflecting back and summing up

One person speaks for five minutes and the other listens. The listener makes encouraging interventions as in Stage 2, but *also* paraphrases, reflects feelings and reflects meaning when she feels it is appropriate. At the end, she makes a brief statement summing up the main content and feelings of the speaker, checking with the speaker that her summing up is accurate. Then exchange roles, followed by 10 minutes discussing these questions:

When you were listening:

- **what sort of interventions did you make?**
- **how did you feel about making them?**

When you were speaking:

- **what interventions did you notice?**
- **did you find them helpful?**

Asking Questions and Getting Feedback

Skilful questioning will help people to give clear, full and honest replies. It is useful to distinguish different types of questions.

Types of Questions

Closed questions are questions which require short, factual answers, often only one word.
Examples are:
'What is your name?'
'Is this address correct?'
'Are you able to see me again next Tuesday?'
Closed questions are appropriate when brief, factual information is required. They are not appropriate when the aim is to encourage talking at more length. So 'did you get on OK with your healthy eating plan last week?' which could be answered by 'yes' or 'no', is not the best way to encourage people to express their experiences of trying to change what they eat. A better question would be 'How did you get on with your healthy eating plan last week?' This is an open question.
Open questions give an opportunity for full answers. Examples are:
'How did you get on at the meeting yesterday?'
'How do you feel about introducing a non-smoking area in the pub?'
'What do you think about trying to take a short brisk walk every day?'
Note that words like 'how', 'what', 'feel' and 'think' are useful for encouraging a full response.
Biased questions indicate the answer which the questioner wants to hear, or expects to hear. In other words, biased questions (sometimes called 'leading questions') are likely to bias the response by leading the person who answers in a particular direction. Examples are:

'You're feeling better today, aren't you?' (This is biased because it would be easier to answer 'yes' than 'no'.)

'You have been doing what we discussed last time, haven't you?'

'Surely you aren't going to do that, are you?'

Multiple questions contain more than one question. Multiple questions are likely to confuse, because the listener will not know which question to answer, and probably will not remember all of them. Examples are:

'Is this a serious problem for you – when did it start?'

'Does your store have a policy on promoting healthy foods – do you stock low-alcohol drinks and did you promote displays of low-fat products during the special campaign last September?'

'What are you going to do to get the Council to take all this rubbish away and are you going to get more bottle banks and newspaper recycling bins?'

'Are you sure you know what to do or would you like me to explain it again?'

Getting Feedback

After people have been given some information, or have been taught a skill, it is very important to check to make sure that they really have understood what was said, and remembered it, or mastered the skill. This is especially important when there is any doubt about how much has been understood, perhaps because, for example, someone is in a state of anxiety or has a limited command of English. There are two key points to note about getting feedback.

It is *your* responsibility to ensure that the communication has been received and understood. It is not the fault of the listener if he tried but did not understand, and he should not be blamed or made to feel small or stupid.

It can be helpful to ask questions in a way which shows that it is your responsibility as a health promoter to 'get it across'. For example, say 'I'd like to make sure I've explained this properly, so could you please tell me what you're going to do about it tomorrow?' or 'May I check to make sure I've covered everything – could you just recap what you understand so far?' Avoid questions such as 'Let's see if you've learnt it yet – could you show me?' or 'I don't think you've totally understood – tell me what you think the main points are'.

Ask open questions. Closed questions such as 'do you understand?' are not an adequate way of getting feedback. People may answer 'yes' because they are embarrassed, intimidated or afraid of making a fool of themselves by admitting that they do not understand. Or they might just want to draw the conversation to a quick conclusion. Ask open questions, such as 'Could you please tell me what you're going to do …'

Written Communication

See sections on Writing Reports in Chapter 8 and Writing Leaflets in Chapter 11 – including writing plain English and non-sexist writing.

Writing is a craft, as well as an art, which all health promoters need to develop. The 12-point guideline in Box 10.2 may help.[9]

Exercise 10.6   **Asking questions**

Work in groups of about 10 people.
Decide on a topic on which it is easy to think of questions – such as pets, holidays, my job, or my family.
Person A volunteers to answer questions.
Person B observes the length of A's response to questions.
Person C observes A's non-verbal behaviour (body language).
Everyone else has the task of asking questions.

Firstly, everyone in turn asks a *closed* question on the topic.
Secondly, everyone in turn asks an *open* question on the topic.
Thirdly, everyone asks *biased* questions on the topic.

After these three rounds of questions:
Person A says how she felt about having to answer the three different kinds of questions (e.g. clear? muddled? irritated? angry? confused?).
Person B says what she observed about the length of A's responses to the three kinds of questions.
Person C says what she observed about A's non-verbal behaviour when answering the three different kinds of questions.

Discuss the application of what you found out to your work.

Box 10.2.   **Guidelines on Writing**

1. The point of writing is clear communication, not showing how clever you are. On the whole, the more simply and briefly you write, the more effective your writing is likely to be.
2. Think about what kind of document you are writing. For example, is it a paper for a formal committee, a memo to your manager, or a letter to a client? This will help you to know what style to write in: formal in a set lay-out for a committee, brief and to the point for a manager, business-like but friendly to a client.
3. Think about who is reading what you write, and what sort of communication they will welcome: how long should it be, how detailed, how formal or chatty, first person or third person?
4. Use clear, simple language, and avoid long or obscure words if you can find shorter or more familiar ones.
5. Avoid technical terms if you can. If you must use them, explain them in the text or a footnote the first time you use them.
6. Keep sentences short.
7. Break the text up with paragraphs. A paragraph should usually deal with one point and its immediate development. A new point needs a new paragraph. In formal papers and reports use heading and subheadings to break up the text and guide the reader through.
8. Use active rather than passive verbs where possible, and this sounds stronger and simpler. For example, write 'the nurses covered the patients with bedclothes' rather than 'the patients were covered with bedclothes by the nurses'.
9. Make sparing use of adjectives and adverbs. The sparer your writing the more striking it will be. For example, 'the patient was really very upset, cried and sobbed a lot and said she would never, ever come back to the clinic again' (23 words) could be better expressed 'the patient was in tears and said she would never return to the clinic' (14 words).

10. Use language accurately. If in doubt check with a guide to English Usage[10]. A common inaccuracy is to confuse *it's*, which is a shortened form of 'it is' ('it's raining'), and *its*, which is the possessive of 'it' ('the cat had its flea collar on'). Another common inaccuracy is to confuse apostrophes around the letter *s*. *Cats* is plural ('two cats'), *cat's* is possessive ('the cat's flea collar'), *cats'* is the plural possessive used instead of saying 'cats's' ('both the cats' flea collars were lost').

11. If you have difficulty with spelling and punctuation, use a spell and grammar checker on a word processor or ask someone to check your writing for you.

12. If you have the time, finish a piece of writing and then put it aside for a few days. This gives your subconscious mind a chance to think about it, and you can take a fresh look and edit it. Check for clarity, simplicity and structure.

PRACTICE POINTS

- The quality of your relationships with your clients is at the heart of your helping role. It is important to review and consider how your attitudes and values are reflected in your relationships.

- Good communication is fundamental to these relationships. It is not just a matter of common sense but involves specific skills such as active listening.

- Words, whether verbal or written, are only a small part of communication, and it is important to consider all aspects of a communication.

- You are responsible for communicating effectively with your clients and it helps if you make it clear to them that you accept this responsibility (through asking *them* to help *you* by giving you feedback).

- Skills of written communication are important in health promotion, and need to be reviewed and developed.

Recommended Reading

On Communication and Counselling Skills

➤ Evans M & Learmonth A (1990) *Working One-to-One: a training course for health and related professionals*. A Vital Communication. Available from: TACADE, 1 Hulme Place, The Crescent, Salford M5 4QA.

➤ Burnard P (1994) *Counselling Skills for Health Professionals*, 2nd edn. London: Chapman and Hall.

➤ Burnard P (1992) *Effective Communication Skills for Health Professionals*. London: Chapman and Hall.

➤ Nelson-Jones R (1993) *Practical Counselling and Helping Skills: How to Use the Lifeskills Helping Model*, 3rd edn. London: Cassell. (Communication and facilitation skills including group facilitation and life skills training; includes exercises for self and group teaching.)

➤ Ellis R & McClintock A (1990) *If you take my meaning – theory into practice in human communication*. London: Edward Arnold. (Includes chapters on verbal and non-verbal communication, listening, communication in groups and within organizations.)

See also Chapter 12 on Helping People to Learn which discusses communication and education between health promoters and patients, and Chapter 14 for the section on Strategies for Decision Making which discusses counselling skills.

➤ Hargie O D W (1997) *The Handbook of Communication Skills*, 2nd edn. London: Routledge. (Includes one-to-one and group communication, non-verbal communication, questioning and listening.)

➤ Bull P and Frederikson L (1995) in Argyle M and Colman A M (eds) *Social Psychology*. Chapter 5 on Non-verbal communication. London: Longman.

➤ Williams D (1997) *Communication Skills in Practice – a practical guide for health professionals*. London: Jessica Kingsley Publishers. (Practical advice and guidance on developing communication skills for the health professional. Includes verbal and non-verbal behaviours; clinical interviews; working with interpreters.)

➤ Katz J and Peberty A (eds) (1997) *Promoting Health: Knowledge and Practice*. Part 2: Communicating and Educating for Health. Basingstoke: Macmillan/The Open University.

On Assertiveness

➤ Townend A (1991) *Developing Assertiveness*. London: Routledge.

➤ Ferguson J (1996) *Perfect Assertiveness*. London: Arrow Books.

Introducing the Skills Needed to Develop and Maintain Personal Relationships

➤ Nelson-Jones R (1996) *Relating Skills: A Practical Guide to Effective Personal Relationships*. London: Cassell.

On Child Development

Explaining how children can learn emotional lessons which will enable them to communicate their feelings and have flourishing relationships:

➤ Goleman, D. (1996) *Emotional Intelligence: Why it can matter more than IQ*. London: Bloomsbury.

➤ Gottman J with DeClaire J (1997) *The Heart of Parenting: How to raise an emotionally intelligent child*. London: Bloomsbury.

Practical Help with Life Skills Education

➤ *Living Skills 2* (1994) St Leonards-on-Sea: Outset Publishing. (Available from Outset Publishing, Conqueror Industrial Estate, Moorhurst Road, St Leonards-on-Sea, East Sussex TN38 9NA).

On Racism and Working with People from Different Ethnic Backgrounds

➤ Douglas J (1995) Developing anti-racist health promotion strategies. Chapter 6 in Bunton R, Nettleton S & Burrows R (eds) *The Sociology of Health Promotion*. London: Routledge. (Outlines, reviews and provides a critique of health promotion approaches to promoting health with back and minority ethnic communities in the UK.)

➤ Douglas J (1997) Developing health promotion strategies with black and minority ethic communities which address social inequalities. Chapter 27 in Sidell M, Jones L, Katz J & Peberdy A (eds) *Debates and Dilemmas in Promoting Health*. Basingstoke: Macmillan/Open University Press. (Explores the role of health promotion in opposing the impact of race and racial discrimination and discusses lessons learnt from health promotion work in Smethwick and Sandwell.)

➤ Peberdy A (1997) Communicating across cultural boundaries. Chapter 10 in Sidell M, Jones L, Katz J & Peberdy A (eds) *Debates and Dilemmas in Promoting Health.* Basingstoke: Macmillan/Open University Press.

➤ Ahmad W (ed.) (1994) *'Race' and Health in Contemporary Britain.* Buckingham: Open University Press.

➤ Balarajan R and Raleigh V S (1993) *Ethnicity and Health: A Guide for the NHS.* London: Department of Health.

On Written Communication

➤ Burnard P (1996) *Writing for Health Professionals: a manual for writers,* 2nd edn. London: Chapman & Hall.

➤ Maslin-Prothero S (ed.) (1997) *Baillière's Study Skills for Nurses.* Chapter 12. London: Baillière Tindall/Royal College of Nursing.

➤ Jay R (1994) *How to Write Proposals and Reports That Get Results.* London: Pitman/Institute of Management Foundation.

➤ The Plain English Campaign produces information and runs courses on writing plain English. Contact: The Plain English Campaign, PO Box 3, New Mills, Stockport SK12 4QP. Tel: 01663 744409. Fax: 01663 747038.

Notes and References

1 For reading which aims to develop awareness of the ways we communicate in order to lead to changes for the better, see:

Hargie O D W (1997) *The Handbook of Communication Skills,* 2nd edn. London: Routledge.

2 For a discussion of the concept of self-empowerment, see:

Tones K and Tilford S (1994) *Health Education: Effectiveness, efficiency and equity,* 2nd edn. Chapter 1. London: Chapman and Hall.

Many of the ideas in this section are adapted from:

Habeshaw T (1983) *Empowering the Learner.* Bristol Polytechnic (unpublished).

3 Faulkner M (1996) Negotiating a Contract. Chapter 6 in *Managing Health Service Contracts.* Hodgsan K, Hoile RW (eds) London: Saunders.

4 National Foundation for Educational Research (1993) *A Survey of Health Education Policies in Schools.* London: Health Education Authority.

5 See:

Skynner R and Cleese J (1993) *Life and How to Survive It.* Chapter 1. London: Methuen.

Beavers R (1990) *Successful Families.* New York: Norton.

6 Gottman J with DeClaire J (1997) *The Heart of Parenting: How to raise an emotionally intelligent child.* London: Bloomsbury.

7 Material in this section is largely based on:

Henley A (1979) *Asian Patients in Hospital and at Home.* King Edward's Hospital Fund for London, Chapter 12. (Reproduced by permission of King Edward's Hospital Fund for London.)

8 Adapted from teaching materials produced by Sue Habeshaw, Bristol Polytechnic. (Reproduced by kind permission of Sue Habeshaw.)

9 These are adapted from a number of sources:

Legat M (1986) *Writing for Pleasure and Profit.* London: Robert Hale.

Maslin-Prothero S (ed.) (1997) *Baillière's Study Skills for Nurses.* London: Baillière Tindall/Royal College of Nursing.

10 Such as:

Greenbaum S and Whitcut J (1991) *Longman Guide to English Usage.* London: Longman.

11 Using Communication Tools

SUMMARY

In the first part of the chapter we suggest some principles governing the choice of health promotion communication tools and a summary of the uses, advantages and limitations of the main types of teaching and learning resources. In the next section we outline points for making the most of display materials, for producing written materials (including guidance on non-sexist writing), and for presenting statistical information. The following section is about mass media: identifying the key characteristics of mass media; the variety of ways in which mass media are channels for health issues; what mass media can be expected to achieve; how they can be used effectively. We give practical guidelines for health promoters working with radio, television and local press. We include a case study on the use of mass media advertising, and exercises on writing plain English, preparing and presenting material on television and radio, writing a press release and writing a letter to the editor. We finish the chapter with an introduction to using information technology for health promotion.

In this chapter we look at a range of communication tools used by health promoters in their work: written materials such as leaflets and hand-outs; and audiovisual materials such as posters, displays, and videos. These materials are often collectively referred to as **health education or health promotion resources**. We also discuss the use of mass media in health promotion: television, radio and newspapers.

These communication tools are used extensively but are they always used effectively? In this chapter we aim to give you information and guidelines to help you to choose and use them with maximum effectiveness, and create your own where appropriate. Throughout, it is vital to bear in mind that these tools will only be useful if they are used with skill; *how* they are used is as crucial as the quality of the resources themselves.

First we look at how to select health promotion resources such as leaflets, posters or videos which can be used for displays, group teaching or for use with individual clients.

Health Promotion Resources: Criteria for Choice

There is a huge range of material available, with a constant turnover as items become out of date or out of print and new ones come on the market. So you find yourself with the task of selecting a leaflet, poster, display or video from a range of possibilities. Or you may find that there is very little available, and you have to decide whether the one item you have found is suitable.

The following guidelines are designed to help you to select the most appropriate and useful resources. The guidelines apply to selecting any kind of material, such as leaflets, posters or videos, and can also be used when you are producing your own.

Guidelines for Selecting and Producing Health Promotion Resources

Is it appropriate for achieving your aims?

See Chapter 14 (section on stages of change).

Think about the item in the context you intend to use it: for example, if you are working with a group of young smokers who are not motivated to stop, a leaflet or video on 'How to Stop Smoking' is unlikely to be helpful at this stage; materials to trigger discussion with the aim of challenging attitudes might be better.

Is it the most appropriate kind of resource?

Will something else be cheaper and just as effective (e.g. photographs instead of a video?) Could the real thing be used instead of being portrayed via a teaching aid (e.g. parents in person talking about their experiences of a new baby instead of appearing in a video, a real baby instead of a doll, actual foods instead of pictures or models?)

Is it consistent with your values and approach?

See the section on Exploring Relationships With Clients in Chapter 10.

If your approach is to work in a non-judgmental partnership with your clients, the materials you use should reflect your values. So you need to avoid material which is patronizing, authoritarian or scaremongering, for example.

The resource should not be 'victim blaming'. That is, it should not attribute blame to individuals experiencing ill-health when that ill-health is rooted in their social circumstances, for example low income, poor housing.

Is it relevant for the people you are working with?

Does it reflect the values and culture of your clients? Does it reflect their concerns? Does it take into account their age, ethnic group, sex and socioeconomic circumstances? Does it reflect local practice and conditions and health services available?

Obvious examples of irrelevance are videos portraying American lifestyles, or homes of affluent middle-class families, which are unhelpful if you are working with people in the UK who are not well-off. Another example is that materials designed for one ethnic group may not be appropriate for another, not just because of language but because some aspects (such as sexual behaviour or attitudes to bereavement) may be seen differently in different cultures.

Is it racist or sexist?

All resources should be non-racist. Racist material is that which stereotypes people into racial types, attributing certain roles or character attributes on the basis of ethnic group alone. Implicit in this are the assumptions that one ethnic group (usually white, Caucasian or European) is superior to another, and one ethnic group (usually white), represents the desired 'norm'.[1]

Guidance on non-sexist writing is provided later in this chapter.

All resources should be non-sexist. Sexist material is that which stereotypes men and women into certain roles or character attributes on the basis of gender. In particular, it is any portrayal of women as sex objects for the gratification of men, any trivialization or demeaning of women as second class citizens, dependent on their relationships with men for social status, and any assumption that male equals desirable norm, whereas female equals undesirable deviant. Resources should also not make assumptions about sexual orientation.

Resources should reflect the fact that we live in a multi-racial society where the roles of men and women have changed and continue to do so. Strong, positive messages and images should be provided of people of all ethnic groups and both sexes.

Will it be understood?

There is more about writing plain English later in this chapter.

Is it written in plain English which people will readily understand? Are there any incorrect assumptions about the level of literacy or existing knowledge? Does it need producing in other languages, to make it accessible to people from minority ethnic groups? Do leaflets need producing in other formats so that they are accessible to people with disabilities, such as in large type or Braille, or (for videos) with a sign language insert on the screen?

Is the information sound?

Is information in the materials accurate, up-to-date, unbiased and complete? Or does it contain half-truths, one-sided information on controversial issues, and out-of-date or incomplete messages?

Does it contain advertising?

Much material is produced by commercial companies such as drug companies, baby food manufacturers or makers of safety equipment. Leaflets and posters, for example, usually carry the name of the company or its products, or include advertisements. Using these resources can imply that you (or your employer) are endorsing the product. It may also damage your image as a credible source of unbiased health information, and lead people to doubt the value of the information ('they're just trying to sell me something').

For these reasons, resources containing company names, products and advertising should be avoided whenever possible. However, the item may be just what you want, and there may be no alternative. In this case, we suggest that:

- the product or service advertised must be ethically acceptable as 'healthy' and 'environmentally friendly'. This excludes tobacco, alcohol and confectionery advertising, for example;
- the advertising content must be low key. The company name on the front or back cover is acceptable, but constant references to named brand products are not.

The Range of Health Education Resources: Uses, Advantages and Limitations

A wide range of resources is available for health education sessions with groups or individuals. Two points are worth emphasizing by way of introduction.

1. Educational resources are aids and not substitutes for the educator. Leaflets can be distributed by the thousand with no thought of targeting the audience or using in conjunction with face-to-face discussion.[2] Videos can be easily misused by being presented without introduction or follow-up discussion, but shown just because 'it's a good video'.

2. It takes time and practice to become familiar with all the teaching aids available, and it takes courage to try new things – but it is worth it.

See the section on Teaching and Learning in Chapter 12

Table 11.1 summarizes key points about the uses, advantages and limitations of the main types of teaching aids.

Table 11.1	**Resources to use in health education sessions**	
Type of resource	**Uses and advantages**	**Limitations**
Leaflets and handouts	Clients can use at their own pace and discuss with other people. Educator and client can work through together. Can be easy and cheap to produce basic written information. Can reinforce points in a talk, and add further detailed information.	Commercially produced leaflets can be expensive and may contain advertising. Mass-produced leaflets are not tailored to everyone's needs. Not durable, easily lost. Mass distribution can be wasteful.
Posters and display charts	Can raise awareness of issues. Can convey information and direct people to other sources (addresses, tel. no.'s, 'pick up a leaflet'). Simple posters and information displays can be cheap to produce.	High quality is expensive to make or buy. Gets tatty quickly unless laminated. Need to ensure any writing is big enough to be read at the distance most people will see it. Displays need changing frequently to attract attention.
Videos[3]	Can be used to convey real situations otherwise inaccessible (e.g. childbirth), convey information, pose problems, demonstrate skills, trigger discussion on attitudes and behaviour. Can be used for self-teaching. Can be stopped, started or replayed to allow discussion.	Normal TV-size screen too small for large audiences. Educator relies on equipment working properly. Equipment expensive and not easily transported. May need partially darkened room.
Slides	Useful in large halls or lecture theatres with a big screen. Complex information (such as graphs) can be seen clearly.	Needs slide projection equipment and screen, and blackout.

Audiocassette tapes	Good for certain skills development, e.g. relaxation, exercise routines. Equipment cheap, easy to use and transport.	Lack of visual material requires extra concentration to hold attention.
Overhead projector transparencies	Cheap and easy to produce. Can build up information by overlaying one or more transparencies. Use with large or small audiences. Equipment relatively cheap, and portable models easy to transport.	Educator dependent on equipment working properly. Need special sloping screen to avoid image wider at the top than the bottom, with uneven focus. The lens part of the projector, and the person using the projector, can obstruct the audience's view of the screen.
Projection of computer generated images[4]	Can enable text and sophisticated, complex images to be prepared in advance and produced on large or small screen. Can build up information on screen.	Requires sophisticated, expensive equipment and technical expertise with computer hardware and software. May need some blackout.
Blackboards and whiteboards	Good for building up information, explaining particular points. Cheap, re-usable.	Educator needs to turn back to audience to write on board. Image too small for large groups.
Flip-charts	Good for brainstorming and involving groups in producing ideas which can be stuck up round the room for discussion. Useful for recording notes to be written up later. Can be prepared in advance. Useful where no blackboard or white board available.	Educator needs to turn back to audience to write on board. Flip-chart paper easily torn and dog-eared.

Producing Resources

See Chapter 5.

Guidelines on written communication are given in Chapter 10 in the section on *Written Communication,* and there is more about written information for patients in the section on *Improving Patient Education* in Chapter 12.

Most resources, particularly posters, leaflets and audiovisual materials, come ready made, but you may want to work with a community group to help them to produce their own materials, or produce some yourself.

We have not attempted to give a comprehensive guide on how to produce materials, but approaching the task in a systematic way using the *Planning and evaluation flowchart* in Chapter 5 may be helpful. If you are producing a resource such as leaflet you will need to consider who will write the draft, who will edit it, whether and how to pilot the draft, what it will cost and whether you need the services of a desk top publisher, designer, illustrator, translator or printer.

We have identified some important points for making the most effective posters, displays and written materials as follows.

Making the Most of Display Materials

Posters, charts, display boards and stands.

Be brief and to the point. Keep the objective firmly in mind. Do not include material which is irrelevant – it will only serve to distract from the main message.

Emphasize the key point(s). Use size of lettering, style or colour to achieve this. Place them just above the centre of a display, which is the point of maximum visual impact.

Use language the audience understands. Explain any unfamiliar technical terms. If possible, express the message in both pictures and words. Test it out on a few people to ensure that you have no unexpected ambiguities in your message (e.g. does the phrase 'beating heart disease' refer to information about how to avoid getting heart disease, or is it information on a health problem known as beating-heart disease?)

Be bold. Words and pictures should be as large as possible.

Make the most of colour. It can create continuity; for example, a repetition of background colour can link a series of posters. Colour can be used to identify parts of a diagram or highlight important information. Choose colours with care, because responses to colour are emotional, e.g. blue is cool, green is soothing, and because colours may be associated with certain messages, images and places, e.g. red for danger, purple for funerals, white for clinical cleanliness.

Improve the display site. If all you have is a blank wall or a wall covered with a distractingly-patterned wallpaper, fix a rectangle of coloured card to the wall as a background display board. If a display board has a rough or marked surface, give it a coat of paint or a covering of coloured paper, hessian or felt.

Use the display site to best advantage. Busy corridors can only be useful sites for posters with immediate appeal and few words. More information can be conveyed in a waiting area and it may be possible to supplement displays with leaflets to take away. Ensure that writing on displays is at eye level and large enough to be read without having to move from the queue or the chair.

Be aware of lighting. Daylight is unreliable; spotlights directed on to a display are ideal.

Making Written Materials

Instruction sheets and cards, leaflets and booklets.

Always test materials on a sample of consumers. Do not *assume* that you know what they like, want or need – *ask them*.

Use colour, layout and print size to improve clarity. Large print may be helpful for older people.

Use plain English. Simple words and short sentences are vital. Use the active tense rather than the passive tense, e.g. say 'change the bandage ...' rather than 'the bandage should be changed ...'

Do a Gobbledygook readability test on your written materials.[5] The test is a rough measure of readability for adult readers based on the principle that, by and large, the combination of long sentences and polysyllabic words is harder to comprehend. It is nonetheless also important to note that many other factors which affect readability, such as sentence structure, print size and the educational background of the reader, are not taken into account.

| Box 11.1. | The Gobbledygook Test |

This test is based on R. Gunning's FOG (Frequency of Gobbledygook) formula and was adapted by the Plain English Campaign.

This is what you do:

- Count a 100 word sample.
- Count the number of complete sentences in the sample.
- Count the total number of words in the complete sentences.
- Divide the number of words by the number of sentences. This gives the average sentence length.
- Count the number of words with three or more syllables in the 100 words. This gives the percentage of long words in the sample.
  Numbers and symbols are counted as short words; hyphenated words are counted as two words; a syllable, for the purposes of the test, is a vowel sound. So 'advised' is two syllables; 'applying' is three.
- Add the average sentence length to the percentage of long words to give the test score: the higher the score, the lower the 'readability'.

It is usual to do this three times to three different samples, one from the beginning of the text, one from the middle and one from near the end. These scores can then be added and divided by three to give the average score.

Tests carried out in 1980 by the National Consumer Council showed that the following publications had these scores:

Woman magazine	25
The Sun	26
Daily Mail	31
The Times	36
The Guardian	39

Try doing Gobbledygook tests on a range of current publications such as *The Sun* and *The Independent* and see what range you get.

Non-Sexist Writing

We have already discussed the importance of material being non-racist and non-sexist, but using language in a non-sexist way presents particular challenges. One is the use of 'man' as a generic term for 'human being'. For example, people talk about 'manning' an exhibition stand when it is as likely to be 'manned' by a woman. And 'manpower resources' are assumed to include both men and women, with the hidden assumption that women are second class resources. Many job titles end with 'man' and date from the time when only men performed these duties, for example postman, ambulanceman. So it is important that, today, we choose words which reflect the reality of our situation. For example, instead of 'housewife' we can say 'houseworker'. Table 11.2 provides some more suggestions.

Exercise 11.1   The Gobbledygook Test

Do the Gobbledygook test on the following 100-word samples.

Sample 1

From now on, measures of alcohol will be stated in terms of beer, remembering that the alcohol content of all the following measures is roughly the same, so that statements made about, say, three pints of beer are also true of three doubles of spirit, or six glasses of wine, six glasses of sherry or two pints of special lager (which happens to be half as strong again as ordinary beer).

One has to consider, when trying to link intake of alcohol to the effects it has on individuals, that it is not only the amount of drink involved, but the . . .

Sample 2

We know that whooping cough vaccine works. The fact that there was so little whooping cough around when most children were immunized is one sign of how effective the vaccine is.

Remember that there are many different causes of brain damage in your children – many very much more common than whooping cough vaccine. In fact, the part played by whooping cough vaccine in causing any sort of brain damage at all is very tiny indeed.

Remember, too, that when doctors talk about brain damage, they do not necessarily mean severe mental handicap but usually something much less serious from which . . .

Exercise 11.2   Writing plain English

Write 'plain English' versions of the following. The first three are very similar to the instructions found on the packages of medication bought over the counter in chemist shops. The last three are very similar to passages in health education leaflets.

1. *Wheezoff* paediatric syrup is specially formulated for children. It is indicated for the relief of cough and its congestive symptoms and for the treatment of hay fever and other allergic conditions affecting the upper respiratory tract. Contraindications, warnings, etc. Hypersensitivity to any of the active constituents. If symptoms persist consult your doctor.
2. *Notwinge* cream – directions for use.
   Apply a sufficient quantity of balm to the part affected. Massage lightly until penetration is complete.
3. *Soothe* vapour rub – how to apply.
   Rub on chest, throat and back. Then spread it thick on chest. Repeat at bedtime. Leave bedclothes loose around the neck so that the decongestant antiseptic vapours may be inhaled freely. For severe nasal catarrh, head colds, coughs and bronchitis, melt some *Soothe* in boiling water and inhale the intensified decongestant antiseptic vapours.
4. If the room has a solid fuel, oil or gas-burning appliance ensure adequate ventilation.
5. The baby lies curled up in what is called the fetal position. It lies in a bag of water and the membranes which make up this fluid-filled balloon are enclosed in the womb.
6. Vitamin B1, also called thiamin, is required for the functioning of the nervous system, digestion and metabolism. Insufficient vitamin B1 can cause anorexia and fatigue.

Table 11.2	Non-sexist writing	
Change from:	**To:**	
Foreman	Supervisor	
Salesman	Sales associate, salesperson	
Repairman	Repairer	
Manpower	Workforce, staff, personnel	
Manning	Staffing	
Ambulancemen	Ambulance staff	
Newsman	Newscaster, reporter	

When *man* comes in the middle of a word, finding a one-word alternative can be difficult. Fortunately synonyms can usually be found; for example, instead of 'the carpenters did a workmanlike job,' say 'the carpenters did a skilful job'.

Another problem is the generic use of the pronoun 'he'. For example 'each doctor presented a case from his own practice', assumes that all the doctors are men. While it may seem clumsy to say 'he or she', it can sometimes usefully emphasize that both sexes are involved. An alternative is to turn the singular into a plural and use the words 'they' or 'their': 'The doctors presented cases from their own practices'. Similarly, instead of: 'A health promoter must be a fluent communicator. He must also be a good listener.' say: 'Health promoters must be fluent communicators. They must also be good listeners.'

It may be possible to rephrase a passage to eliminate the pronouns altogether. So, instead of 'Information given to a social work agency is confidential in the same way as communications between a doctor and his patients' say 'in the same way as communications between doctors and patients.'

Another way is to use 'you' instead of 'he' or 'she' or a noun which implies male or female. For example, in a leaflet on parenting, you could change 'A mother often finds difficulty in persuading her two-year-old to eat' to 'You may find difficulty in persuading your two-year-old to eat' or 'Parents may find difficulty …' This avoids the implication that it is only mothers (not fathers) who have a parenting role.

Another way to avoid 'he' is to find another noun. Thus, in 'You may find difficulty in persuading your two-year-old to eat. He may prefer throwing his food around instead' you could say '… A child at this age may prefer throwing food around instead.'

Sometimes, though, it seems impossible to avoid saying 'he' because the alternatives are clumsy or unclear. When we have found that to be the case in this book, we have chosen to use 'she' to denote a health promoter rather than 'he'. Many writers do this, thus challenging the tradition of using 'he' when meaning 'he or she'.

It is also important to avoid sexism when speaking as well as writing. So, for instance, a consultant who refers to the women who attend for breast cancer screening (mammography) as 'the ladies' and the female radiographers as 'the girls' may intend no insult, but it could affront both groups. It is far better to refer to the radiographers as 'the staff' ('girls' are women who have not yet grown up) and to the women who attend as 'women', 'patients' or 'clients'. A test is to think how it would seem to use male equivalents (would you refer to men attending a clinic for testicular cancer as 'the gentlemen' and the staff attending them as 'the boys'?).

Fur further discussion of language barriers, see the section on *Overcoming Language Barriers* in Chapter 10.

Presenting Statistical Information

Numbers are useful for answering questions which begin how much? how many? how long? what's the risk? But numbers can be indigestible and meaningless unless they are carefully presented in a visual way. The increasing availability of desk-top publishing and computer graphics means that it is becoming easier to produce information in ways which are visually arresting and easy to understand. Health and local authorities are likely to have the equipment and expertise to do this quite easily.

Figures 11.1–11.4 show how to bring statistics to life.

The article from The Guardian (Fig. 11.1) is an example of concise and well-illustrated statistical information from a survey.[6]

Figures 11.2–11.4 show statistics from a health survey of over six thousand schoolchildren in England in 1995.[7]

Using Mass Media in Health Promotion

The mass media are channels of communication to large numbers of people: television, radio, magazines and newspapers, books, displays and exhibitions. Leaflets and posters are also mass media when they are used on a 'stand alone' basis, as opposed to use as a learning aid in face-to-face communication with an individual or a group. However, usually when people talk loosely about 'the media' they mean television, radio and newspapers.

Health promoters are most likely to become involved with mass media when undertaking health promotion programmes or campaigns with the public, or when a health issue becomes a news item. Probably most involvement will be with local newspapers and local radio or television. However, it is useful to put this into a wider context, and appreciate the range of ways in which health issues and messages are portrayed via mass media.

Mass Media as Channels for Health Issues

Health messages and information are sent through the mass media in a number of different ways.

- Planned, deliberate health promotion, e.g. displays and exhibitions on health themes, Health Education Authority advertisements on television and in newspapers, Open University community education programmes on health. In discussion about using mass media in health promotion, people are generally thinking of this kind of promotion, mainly advertising on television and radio, or via posters or advertisements in newspapers and magazines;
- Health promotion by advertisers and manufacturers of 'healthy' products and services, e.g. advertisements for wholemeal bread or for toothpaste, educational leaflets on 'feeding your baby' or guides to 'healthy eating establishments' which also promote relevant products or services.
- Books, documentaries and articles about health issues, e.g. television programmes and magazines about food, AIDS, pollution or physical fitness. Often issues will feature in the media because of new research reports or

Fig 11.1   **Effective use of graphics to illustrate statistical information.[6]**

Junk food 'winning war'

What's for tea?

Children's food markets sales by sector, 1995

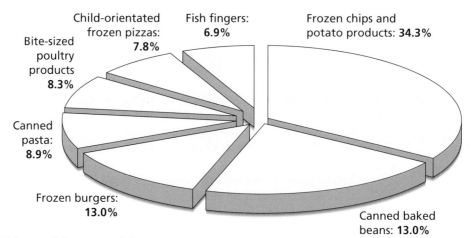

Child-orientated frozen pizzas: **7.8%**

Fish fingers: **6.9%**

Frozen chips and potato products: **34.3%**

Bite-sized poultry products **8.3%**

Canned pasta: **8.9%**

Frozen burgers: **13.0%**

Canned baked beans: **13.0%**

Chips with everything

Changes in children's food markets, current prices, 1991 – 95

Frozen chips and potato products	39%
Bite-sized poultry products	28%
Canned pasta	No change
Frozen beef burgers	-2%
Fish fingers	-13%
Canned baked beans	-21%
Child-orientated frozen pizzas	-36%

Source: Mintel

Fig 11.2 **This figure uses bar charts to show the proportions of all children, then boys and girls separately, who assess themselves as 'very healthy', 'quite healthy', or 'not very healthy'.[7]**

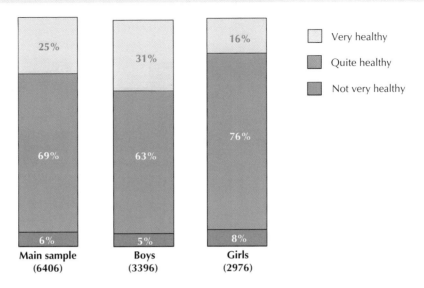

Fig 11.3 **This figure uses a graph to show what proportion of boys and girls desire to change their physical appearance, and how this desire increases with age. (Base: all main sample–6406).[7]**

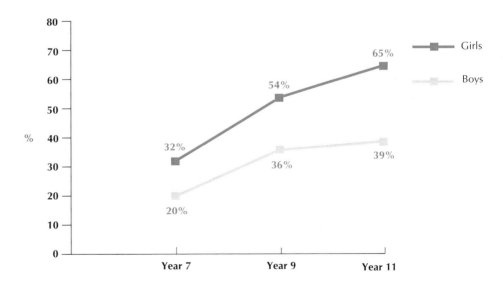

Fig 11.4   **This figure uses a bar chart to show which topics children wanted more lessons on, with drugs and sex education being the most common requests, and smoking and food/diet the least requested.[7]**

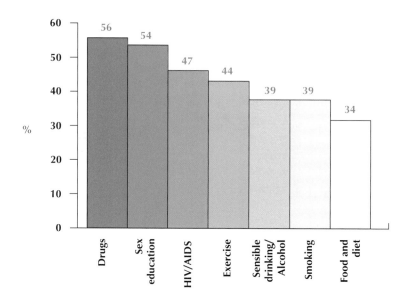

government publications, and may be distorted with attention-grabbing headlines (Fig. 11.5).

- Discussion of health issues as a byproduct of news items ('Rock star dies from drugs overdose') or entertainment programmes, notably soap-opera series where a character has a health problem, such as being abused as a child or suffering from cancer.
- Health (or anti-health) messages conveyed covertly or incidentally, e.g. well-known personalities or fictional characters refusing cigarettes or, conversely, chain smoking. The portrayal of alcohol on television, for example, conveys a norm of heavy drinking and associates consumption of alcohol with benefits rather than costs.[8]
- Planned promotion of anti-health messages (probably denied or rationalized as not anti-health!), e.g. advertisements for tobacco, sweets and chocolates.
- sponsorship of health promoting events and services by organizations or commercial companies, such as sponsorship of sporting events by cigarette manufacturers or health promotion events by commercial companies. By associating with a health promoting event or service, the sponsor's product or service is brought to the public eye with an implied stamp of approval and a sense that it is somehow associated with health.

Using Mass Media for Effective Health Promotion[10]

The fact that the message is sent via a medium (such as radio) makes it difficult to obtain immediate feedback and modify communication to be responsive to the

Fig 11.5

Often issues will feature in the media because of new research reports or government publications, sometimes distorted with attention-grabbing headlines.[9]

FEBRUARY 1997   VOLUME 3   NUMBER 1   ISSN: 0965-0288

Effective
Health Care

Bulletin on the effectiveness of health service interventions for decision makers

NHS Centre for Reviews and Dissemination, University of York

CHURCHILL
LIVINGSTONE

Preventing and reducing the adverse effects of unintended teenage pregnancies

■ Teenage pregnancy is associated with increased risk of poor social, economic and health outcomes for both mother and child.

■ A factor strongly associated with deferring pregnancy is a good general education.

■ The health and development of teenage mothers and their children has been shown to benefit from programmes promoting access to antenatal care, targeted support by health visitors, social workers or 'lay mothers' and provision of social support, educational opportunities and pre-school education.

■ School-based sex education can be effective in reducing

teenage pregnancy especially when linked to access to contraceptive services. The most reliable evidence shows that it does not increase sexual activity or pregnancy rates.

■ Contraceptives when used properly are highly cost-effective and can result in significant savings.

■ Increasing the availability of contraceptive clinic services for young people is associated with reduced pregnancy rates.

■ Contraceptive services should be based on an assessment of local needs and ensure accessibility and confidentiality.

When this research report was published, *The Times* ran an article with the following headlines:

Target the young, say NHS advisers

Birth control urged

for 11-year-olds

needs and characteristics of the audience. Audience phone-ins are a way of ensuring some two-way communication, and exhibitors may involve a minority of people attending an exhibition, but the majority are only subjected to one-way communication. This characteristic of one-way communication has major implications. For example, it is not possible for the sender to repeat, clarify or amplify the message, so in general the mass media are best used for conveying simple, rather than complex, messages.

Many research studies have now shown that the direct persuasive power of mass media is very limited.[11] Expectations that the mass media alone will produce dramatic long-term changes in health behaviour are doomed to disappointment. A particular problem is that mass media campaigns can be an easy response to many health problems, with the characteristic of being high-profile. Many health campaigns in the media are driven by the need to be doing something, and to be seen to be doing it, even though there is evidence that a media campaign on the issue is likely to be useless.

So it is important for you to know what success you can realistically expect when you use mass media in your health promotion work. We can summarize the research evidence which tells us how mass media can be used effectively, and what it cannot be expected to achieve, as follows.

Mass media *can* be an effective health promotion tool if it fulfils the following criteria:

1. The information is perceived as relevant ('for people like me').
2. The information is backed up with other methods such as one-to-one advice.
3. The information is new and presented in an emotional context.
4. The aim is to:
    (a) raise awareness of health and health issues (for example, to raise awareness that the budget for running the NHS is not bottomless and difficult choices about what to spend it on have to be made; or to raise awareness about the link between over-exposure to the sun and the risk of skin cancer);
    (b) deliver a simple message (for example, that babies should sleep on their backs not their tummies; that there is a national helpline for people who want to stop smoking);
    (c) change behaviour if it is a simple one-off activity (for example, phone for a leaflet) which people are already motivated to do and which it is easy to do. (Phoning for a leaflet is more likely if you are at home with a phone than if you're at a friend's house or if the nearest phone is a broken public one two streets away.)
5. The use of mass media is part of an overall strategy which includes face-to-face discussion, and personal help, and attention to social and environmental factors which help or hinder change. For example, mass media publicity is just one strand in a long-term programme to combat smoking.[12]

What mass media *cannot* be expected to do is:

1. convey complex information (for example, about transmission routes of HIV);
2. teach skills (for example, how to deal assertively with pressure to have sex without a condom or take drugs);

3. shift people's attitudes or beliefs. If a message challenges a person's basic beliefs, he is more likely to dismiss the message than change his belief (for example, 'My dad drank six pints a night till he died at 80, so saying I shouldn't have more than two pints a day is rubbish');

4. change behaviour unless it is a simple action, easy to do, and people are already motivated to do it (for example it will not change the eating, drinking or exercise habits of people who do not want to change them or find it difficult to change).

Exercise 11.3   Using mass media to stop young people taking drugs

A Department of Health mass media campaign in 1985/86 costing £2 million directed at heroin misuse was widely criticized.[13] Although it was very successful at penetrating the market (young people aged 13–20), and thus demonstrated the effectiveness of the mass media in raising awareness, it had little or no influence on drug-related behaviour.

Ten years later, in 1995, the tragic death of Leah Betts from taking one Ecstasy tablet on her 18th birthday led to a charitably-funded poster campaign. Many experts believed this to be a well-meant but ineffective approach.

The Independent, on 8th December 1995, put it this way in an article entitled 'Drugs: ads are not the answer':[14]

All will sympathise with the Betts family's attempts to use their daughter's awful death to warn others. But Mark Gilman, director of research at the drugs organisation Lifeline, doubts whether the campaign (like many others) will work. 'These posters may make some people feel like they're doing something, but all they do is compound the fears of parents and serve to reinforce those young people who have decided to say no already. It won't put anyone else off'.

Talking to young regular users of Ecstasy about the Betts case, Gilman found that they saw it as undeniably sad 'but a tragedy like any other – like a friend being killed in a car crash'.

Fear has been the main weapon in the long and losing ad and media war against drugs over the last two decades. ... In the meantime, drug use among the young has become almost the norm ... 16-year-olds ... know that the use of soft drugs such as cannabis or – for the vast majority of users – Ecstasy does not result in death. ... 'When you're young, you think you're immortal. You know that having sex can kill you, that driving over the speed limit can kill you, that almost everything else your parents disapprove of can kill you. But you do it anyway – because it's fun.

This has now been tacitly acknowledged by the Department of Health, which has passed on the responsibility for its antidrugs crusade to the Health Education Authority. Its new campaign is designed primarily to promote the National Drugs Helpline, a daytime phone line staffed by trained counsellors offering non-judgmental advice.

What does this example tell you about how mass media can be used effectively and ineffectively?

What does *The Independent* article illustrate about the role of newspapers in health promotion?

Creating Opportunities

Even though most health promoters are motivated to use the mass media they may have misgivings and identify the need for further training.[15] For example you may feel apprehensive of interviews with reporters from the local news media (local newspapers, radio and television). You may feel that 'They'll misquote me', 'I'll dry up if I'm interviewed', 'They'll sensationalize the issue' or 'I'll get into trouble with my manager'.

There may be more than a grain of truth in these fears, so what can be done to overcome them and make useful alliances with journalists? Firstly, many health authorities, NHS trusts and local authorities now employ public relations specialists, with a background in journalism, and employees can enlist their help.

Another way forward is to establish personal contact with local journalists. Do not wait for them to ring you – you ring them. Establish an informal, personal relationship: get to know how they work and what their special areas of interest are, which will help to establish mutual trust and understanding. You can then approach them if you wish to give exposure to a particular topic, or if you wish to discuss how the media are portraying a current issue. The benefits are mutual; journalists will be more likely to approach you to get help with an item of health news.

Also, remember that it is in both your interests that you have good skills in communicating via the mass media, so why not ask for help with training needs? Many local radio and television journalists are happy to help with training. Short courses on using the media also may be available at local colleges and polytechnics.

Keep a record of what you find out about local media, and update it regularly. Include information on names and special interests of journalists and the 'copy dates' for each of the media in your area. The 'copy date' is the deadline for submitting written information ('copy'). For example, note the last day for submitting copy to a regular fortnightly magazine or local weekly paper. The daily newspapers should be able to respond immediately to a press release; radio often needs a few days to prepare coverage; television may need longer advance notice to allow time for booking a film crew. This information will help you to be prepared when opportunities for useful media coverage arise.

The following sections give practical guidelines on working with radio, television and local newspapers. Having this information may also help to overcome fear of working with the news media.

Working with Radio and Television

Using a spot on radio or television effectively requires research, preparation and skill. The following checklists are prepared to help you to get your health promotion story to the right person and have the best chance of getting coverage. You need to listen to your local radio and watch television to see which programmes might be interested in your kind of news.

Basic Information

- What hours do they broadcast?
- What region do they cover?
- Who are the listeners? Does the profile alter according to the time of day?

The Programmes

- What is covered on the news items?
- How many minutes of current affairs and local interest items?
- Are interviews used or straight reporting?
- What are the different kinds of programmes, and what is the proportion of time they occupy (news, current affairs, weekly events, phone-ins, music, etc.).
- Which programmes use guests or 'experts'?
- Is there any local programme that regularly covers health issues?
- Is there a round-up of 'Events in the week ahead' – what is the deadline for information?
- How much detail do they give? What sort of events get covered?

Interviews

- Which programmes use interviews?
- How many minutes?
- What is the tone (bland, chatty, aggressive)?
- How long is the average answer before the next question? Time it!
- Are they on location or in the studio?
- Are they recorded or live?
- Who are the presenters or interviewers on the programmes who might be interested in health? What is their style?

Finding Out About a Specific Programme

- What programme is it? What sort of approach does the programme have? How long is it? When is it to be transmitted? What kind of audience does it have?
- Why is your topic of interest *now*: is there some local or national controversy or news item which sparked off interest? If so, do you know all about it?
- How are you going to be presented: an information spot, an interview or a discussion panel?
- If it is an interview, who will do it? Will it be in the studio, on location (perhaps in your workplace or outdoors) or 'down the line' (where you are in one studio and the interviewer in another)?
  If it is to be a discussion, who else will be taking part?
- Will it be broadcast live or recorded first?
- How much time are you likely to have on the programme?
- When and where is the broadcast or recording to take place?

Preparing the Message

- Do your homework. You may know a lot or a little about the subject, but in either case you need to identify exactly what it is you want to get across, and to have this very clearly in your mind *before* you are 'on the air'.
- Be positive. Emphasise the good news, *not* a series of don'ts. Tell people what they *can* do and emphasize the benefits.

- You should have two or three key points to put across, and *no more*. You can expand on these and describe them in different ways but do not overload your audience with too much detail or too many points. They will not remember the additional information anyway, and may even forget the key points.
- Use anecdotes and analogies to illustrate what you mean; simple messages do not have to be bald and boring. Tell stories (short ones!) and use real-life experiences. Put complex points over with everyday analogies, e.g. 'Use too much fertiliser and you'll kill the plants – use the right amount and they'll grow strong and healthy. The same applies to food and people.'
- Avoid technical terms (unless these are essential, in which case use them and explain them) and jargon, but do not be patronizing. It helps to pitch the level right if you imagine that you are talking to an intelligent 14- to 15-year-old whom you have never met before.

Presenting Your Message

- Accept that you are nervous and regard it as a good thing because it means that you will be keyed up to do your best. Remember that the interviewer is there to help you tell your story and to put you at ease.
- Perform with more than 100% liveliness and conviction. Be alert and (if you are on television) look alert at all times. Always assume that the camera is on you even when you are not talking. Make sure your eyes look convincing and involved.
- Speak with your normal voice; if you have a regional accent this will make you more interesting to listen to. Speak clearly and distinctly, and (especially on radio) vary the pitch and speed.
- Make sure you say what *you* want to say. You do not have to follow the line of the interviewer's questions if, for good reason, you do not wish to. Provided you stick to the broad framework of agreed subjects, you have every right to steer the interview or discussion in such a way that you get over what you want to say. Regard the questions as springboards from which to make your points. For example, if you do not like a question you can say:

  'I can't really answer that question without explaining first that ...'
  'The real problem behind all this is ...'
  'We don't know the answer to that at the moment, but what we do know is ...'

- When the interview is over, sit still, keep alert and keep quiet until you are *told* it is over.
- On television, wear what makes you feel comfortable and good. Avoid wearing blue or bright red, predominant stripes, small patterns or flashing jewellery. As you will appear as a 'talking head' for most of the time, pay special attention to what you wear in the neckline area.

Working with the Local Press

Local newspapers are an excellent medium for health promotion in a local community. Local journalists will be interested in newsworthy health issues and it is worth studying the newspapers to see who writes about health topics. This is a checklist of what to look for when researching a paper.

Exercise 11.4   Looking good and sounding good on television and radio

1. Prepare your message

Select a health promotion topic that you are familiar with, e.g. slimming, eating health-giving food, sensible drinking, feeding your baby, keeping fit, avoiding home accidents, living with stress.

Identify *three* key points you would want to put across in a five-minute radio or television interview. Be clear in your mind:

- what the three key points are;
- how you will explain them in an interesting way – what illustrations, analogies or anecdotes you could use;
- how you will develop your points further if you have time.

2. Practise your presentation

Get a partner to act as your interviewer, and record your interview on an audio or a videotape. Ask a third person to be an observer. Play the tape back and assess your performance:

- Did you sound/look lively, alert and convincing?
- Was your voice clearly understandable? What did it sound like for speed and pitch?
- Did you get your key points across? Did you do so in an interesting way?
- Were you able to deal with 'difficult' questions?

Basic Information

- When is it published?
- What are the deadlines for copy?
- What locality does it cover?
- How many readers and who are they?

The Copy

- What is the style (bright, sober, campaigning, etc.)?
- What is the average length of articles (often different for news, business, features)?
- What percentage of articles have photos?
- How many photos per page?
- How are photos used generally?
- How are quotes used?

The Subjects

- What sorts of stories are used (local, jolly, controversial, educational) and how are they treated?
- What is the ratio of coverage for news, features, business, diary, etc.?
- How long and how full is the 'events ahead' section?
- Are there special sections or supplements on health, education, women, etc.? How long and on what day?
- Are there regular columnists? What are their special interests?

The Language

- What is the average length of sentences?
- What is the average length of paragraphs?
- What kind of language is used (multisyllabic, slangy, turgid, lively, short and simple)?

Your Special Interests

- Anything in the papers that may be of special use to you or to your organization?

This may seem a lot to cope with, especially if you have a number of local and regional newspapers. Gradually build up expertise, with a fact sheet on each one. This will be indispensable for targeting your press releases.

How to Write a Press Release[16]

To write a press release (sometimes also called a 'news release') you need:

A good text. Use a title to grab attention. The guts of the story must be in the first short paragraph. However complex the subject there will be one outstanding thing which makes it newsworthy. Start with a bang by spelling this out. Make your points in order of importance. (A story gets cut from the bottom up.) Use short sentences and easy language, with no abbreviations or jargon. Using quotes can bring a piece to life. Don't be afraid of making up things which you or your group might have said (but check first with the persons concerned). For example, Mrs Gloria Slim, the District Dietician, said 'I am delighted at the number of hospitals which now offer patients choices of vegetarian and traditional ethnic dishes on the menu.'

A short text. Keep it brief – one page if possible. If longer, type 'More follows. ...' at the bottom right hand corner. Don't carry over paragraphs or sentences to the next page. Type 'ends' after the last line of the release. Sentences must be short, paragraphs brief.

A local angle for a local paper. News is people and local news is local people. So focus on people rather than making generalized statements or quoting dry statistics. For example, say: Last week three Bloggsville children were admitted to the Royal Infirmary after accidentally swallowing weedkiller. This brings to over 100 the number of children who have been accidentally poisoned this year. Sister Florence Nightingale, in charge of the Accident and Emergency Department, said: 'It is heartbreaking to see the needless distress this causes ...'.

Good timing. Your news will not be newsworthy on the day of election of a new prime minister! Yesterday's news is dead, today's may still be of interest, but tomorrow's has the best chance of being printed. Alert newspapers a few days in advance so that they can send reporters to cover an interesting event. For example, contact on a Friday or Monday is usually best for a weekly paper published on the following Friday. If you want to launch a story at a particular time, use the 'embargo' system. This means writing, for example, 'Not for use until Wednesday July 3rd 1997' or 'Embargoed 6 p.m. July 3rd 1997' across the top of the press release.

Good presentation. A4 paper, headed with a logo if possible. Colour catches the eye, so a coloured heading or coloured paper will make your release stand out.

Good technique. Journalists work at speed, so make their task easier by:

- using only one side of the page, placing the text centrally on the page;
- using a lay-out with double spacing;
- leaving at least one inch (2–3 cm) margin on either side;
- putting a release date or embargo date at the top;
- giving names and telephone numbers of people in your organization for further information (including an after-hours telephone number);
- sending it to a named journalist if possible;
- not underlining any words (because this gives printers instructions to use italics; use **bold** for emphasis instead).

A big photo. If you are sending a photo, a 7″ × 5″ or 10″ × 8″, generally black and white is preferred, with a full label on the back giving names and details. Don't forget to include the names of everyone on the photo ('the picture shows left to right June Bloggs and Sam Smith. ...') and explain what they are doing ('presenting Healthy Eating awards at 3 p.m. on Tuesday March 10th at Bloggsville Town Hall'). Never write directly on the back of a photo, as this will destroy its quality. Photos should be eye-catching and clear.

Good communication. Send a copy of the press release to everyone who will be affected, including your organization's press officer, and to everyone mentioned or otherwise involved in the story.

A final check. Before you send it, ask yourself if this would tell you:

- What?
- Who?
- When?
- Where?
- Why?
- How?

Writing Letters to the Editor

Another way of using the local paper as a medium for health promotion is by writing letters to the editor. This can keep an issue in the public eye for some time, and provides good opportunities for public debate of controversial issues. Letters to the editor should be short (some newspapers restrict length), to the point, and be on one topic only.

Using Information Technology for Health Promotion

We cannot end this chapter on *Tools of Communication* without including the newest developments in communication. The Internet is a world-wide network accessed via computers, which links in to a huge bank of information. Increasingly,

Fig 11.6   **Local news is local people.**

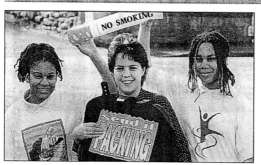

NEWS

Stub it out, pupils urged

SCHOOL nurses are marking No Smoking Week by urging children in Bath not to take up cigarettes.

Pupils have been entering anti-smoking poster competitions and a contest to see how many cigarettes they could pack away in suitcases.

Bath Health Promotion Unit runs anti-smoking training courses for health visitors, practice nurses and school nurses.

No Smoking Day events are continuing throughout the week. Health promotion spokesman Donna Smith said: "We teach the skills needed for people to give up smoking. The training is vital for one-to-one counselling or group work.

"And it also teaches how to recognise if a smoker is truly motivated to quit."

Pupils Debbie Russell, and Shanna Fields, both aged 14, were involved in an anti-smoking workshop held at Hayesfield School, Bath yesterday.

● PACK IN: Nurse Sam Shrubsole pictured putting the message across to Debbie Russell, left, and Shanna Fields.

Reproduced with kind permission of the Editor, Bristol Evening Post.

this includes information on health. The significance of this advance is that it is now possible for health promoters and the general public to gain access to, and exchange, health information which is available on 'web sites' (files of information accessible through the computer Internet). One of the important aspects of a web site is that it refers to other sites, so that the user can choose to follow paths to related information.

Web sites are increasingly used for health promotion, with information from organizations such as the national health promotion agencies and local health authorities. For example, the Health Education Authority and the Health Education Board for Scotland now have web sites.[17] Some sites are set up for specific health promotion themes or events, such as World Aids Day (accessed through the HEA's web site).

Most sites are 'read-only', that is, they are used to publish information for the user – a one-way process. But some also allow the user to interact. For example, users may supply information such as survey questionnaire responses or play 'games' on health themes.

There are ever-widening possibilities for the future, as more people have computers at home, and computers (some with 'touch screen' facilities) become available in schools, libraries and other public places.

Example 11.1   Press Release

KOFFCOUNTY DISTRICT HEALTH AUTHORITY
PRESS RELEASE 1st October 1997
SMOKERS HOTLINE LAUNCHED

Koffcounty's Smokers Hotline got off to a flying start this week, when Dr Jo Goodheart, a specialist in heart disease at Kofftown General Hospital, launched the service.

The hotline has been set up as part of Koffcounty Heart Week (2nd–9th October), to help people who want to stop smoking. Anyone ringing Kofftown 112233 will be sent a free pack of useful ideas to help them give up, including tips from ex-smokers and information about local stop-smoking groups.

'I smoked myself when I was younger and I remember what a struggle I had to stop. Many of my patients with heart trouble also find it incredibly difficult', said Dr Goodheart. 'That's why I'm delighted to launch this scheme. The pack has lots of useful information to help people over the difficulties.'

Smokers have a two to three times greater risk of having a heart attack than non-smokers. At least 80% of heart attacks in men under 45 are thought to be due to cigarette smoking. Stopping smoking could lead to 150 fewer deaths each year of men and women under 65 in Koffcounty.

For further information, please contact:

Sally Prohealth, Senior Health Promotion Officer, Central Health Clinic, People's Lane, Kofftown KT1 2YZ

Telephone Kofftown 456789 (day) or Nextown 123456 (evenings)

Exercise 11.5   Writing for the local paper

1. Write a press release about a health promotion issue you are currently concerned about (for example, school meals, uptake of antenatal classes, glue-sniffing or the local accident black spot).
2. Write a letter to the editor supporting a current health education campaign or drawing attention to a specific need for health promotion.

PRACTICE POINTS

- Communication tools useful for health promoters are written materials such as leaflets and hand-outs; audiovisual materials such as posters, displays and videos; and the mass media of television, radio and newspapers. You need to select and use them with skill in order to be effective.

- When you select materials such as leaflets and videos, ensure that you consider the criteria they should meet.

- Consider the range of advantages, uses and limitations of each kind of resource and audiovisual aid you are thinking of using.

- Create effective displays by considering factors such as site, colour, language and style.

- Make written materials in plain English, with attention to other issues such as non-sexist writing.

- Ensure that materials are accessible to everyone you want to reach by producing them in, for example, ethnic minority languages, large type or alternative formats such as audiotape instead of written materials.

- Present statistical information with appropriate use of graphics to bring it to life.

- Mass media of television, radio and newspapers are used to convey both deliberate and unplanned health messages, images and information. You can use mass media successfully to raise awareness of health issues, deliver simple messages and encourage one-off actions which are easy to do. You are unlikely to be successful if you try to use mass media to teach complex information or skills, or lead to shifts in attitudes, beliefs or lifestyle.

- In order to work effectively with local journalists on newspapers, radio and television, you need to research potential opportunities, and know how to prepare presentations and press releases.

- Consider the possibilities for using information technology as a means of communication in your work.

Recommended Reading

On Writing Plain English

➤ For information and training courses on writing plain English, contact The Plain English Campaign, PO Box 3, New Mills, Stockport SK12 4QP. Tel: 01663 744409. Fax: 01663 747038.
➤ Burnard P (1996) *Writing for Health Professionals; a manual for writers.* 2nd edn. London: Chapman and Hall. (Covers the basics of writing; buying and writing with a computer; keeping databases; writing essays, dissertations, articles, books and reviews.)

On Using Training Aids

➤ Flegg D & McHale J (1991) *Selecting and Using Training Aids.* London: Kogan Page.

On Using Mass Media in Health Promotion

➤ White S, Evans A, Mihill C & Tysoe M (1993) *Hitting the Headlines – a practical guide to the media.* Leicester: British Psychological Society Books.
➤ Tones K & Tilford S (1994) *Health education: effectiveness, efficiency and equity,* 2nd edn.

Chapter 6, The mass media in health promotion. London: Chapman & Hall. (A detailed review of the effectiveness of mass media campaigns in health promotion.)
➤ Reid D (1996) How effective is health education via mass communications? *Health Education Journal* **55**, 332–344. (Reviews effectiveness and cost-effectiveness of mass communications.)

On Information Technology

➤ Catford J (1997) The mass media is dead: long live multimedia. Chapter 34 in Sidell M, Jones L, Katz J & Peberdy A (eds) *Debates and Dilemmas in Promoting Health.* Basingstoke: Macmillan/ Open University Press. (Looks at new possibilities in the ever-expanding world of new technology in the mass media, and the challenges and opportunities this presents for health promotion.)

Two useful articles providing guidance on health promotion on the Internet:
➤ Beishon M (1996) Health Promotion moves beyond the final frontier. *Healthlines,* Issue 31, April, pp. 14–16.
➤ Beishon M (1996) The holes in the super-highway. *Healthlines,* Issue 32 (note: published with 'Issue 31' on the cover), May, pp. 18–19.

Notes and References

1   The issue of promoting health with black and minority ethnic communities is much wider than simply ensuring that materials are non-racist. See:

Douglas J (1995) Developing anti-racist health promotion strategies. Chapter 6 in Bunton R, Nettleton S & Burrows R (eds) *The Sociology of Health Promotion.* London: Routledge. (This chapter outlines, reviews and provides a critique of health promotion approaches to promoting health with black and minority ethnic communities in the UK.)

2   Murphy S & Smith C (1993) Crutches, confetti or useful tools? Professionals' views and use of health education leaflets. *Health Education Research* **8**(2), 205–215. (This study on the views and use of health education leaflets by health professionals showed that they thought leaflets were important and used them extensively, but at the same time they did not believe that they were particularly effective; there were contradictions between how

leaflets were used and their perceived effectiveness. For a full report, see: Murphy S & Smith C (1992) *Crutches, Confetti or Useful Tools.* Good Health Wales Technical Report Number 3, Health Promotion Authority for Wales.)

3   Eiser J R & Eiser C (1996) *Effectiveness of video for health education.* London: Health Education Authority. (Assesses 175 studies of video-based projects and considers the use of video to promote health in a training context, with people with learning disabilities and in patient education.)

4   At the time of writing (1997) there are two types of computer-generated ways of producing visual images on large screens, suitable for any size of audience. Both use special equipment which plugs into an ordinary computer (normal-sized PC or a portable model). The first type is a piece of equipment plugged into the computer and then placed on top of an ordinary overhead projector; this enables the

image on the computer to be projected on to a screen. The second type of equipment is similar to a slide projector. It plugs into the computer and throws the image directly on to a screen (no overhead projector is required). In both cases, the value is that the computer user can show what is on her small computer screen to a large audience. This can be text, diagrams, tables or whatever else she is generating, using any kind of software. The particular value of using computer generated images in giving talks is that special software programmes can be used to create highly professional sophisticated images in advance, such as sets of bullet points for a talk. The educator reveals these points on the screen one at a time during the talk at the touch of a computer button.

5   The Gobbledygook Test is reproduced by kind permission of the Plain English Campaign.

6   Article in *The Guardian* 6.8.96. (Reproduced with kind permission of *The Guardian*.)

7   Reproduced with kind permission of the Health Education Authority from Turtle J, Jones A & Hickman M (1997) *Young People and Health: the health behaviour of school-aged children – summary of key findings*. London: Health Education Authority.

8   Hansen A (1986) The portrayal of alcohol on television. *Health Education Journal* **45**, 127–31.

Institute for Alcohol Studies (1985) *The presentation of Alcohol in the Mass Media*. Report of a seminar, January 1985. Institute for Alcohol Studies, 12 Caxton Street, London.

9   Title of article from *The Times*, reproduced with kind permission of *The Times*. Front cover of *Effective Health Care Bulletin* reproduced by kind permission of Churchill Livingstone.

10   Some of this section is based on Naidoo J & Wills J (1994) *Health Promotion: Foundations for Practice*. Chapter 13, Part 4 Using the Mass Media in Health Promotion. London: Baillière Tindall.

11   Tones K & Tilford S (1994) *Health education: effectiveness, efficiency and equity*, 2nd edn. Chapter 6, The mass media in health promotion. London: Chapman & Hall.

12   Reid D J, Killoran A J, McNeill A D & Chambers J S (1992) Choosing the most effective health promotion options for reducing a nation's smoking prevalence. *Tobacco Control* **1**, 185–197. (This article reviews all the options for health promotion interventions to reduce smoking. It highlights the importance of creating unpaid publicity in the media, and that the effective use of mass communications is crucial to the success of the whole campaign.)

13   Tones B K (1986) Preventing drug misuse: the case for breadth, balance and coherence. *Health Education Journal* **45**, 223–230.

14   Reproduced by kind permission of *The Independent*.

15   Flora J A & Wallack L (1990) Health Promotion and Mass Media Use: translating research into practice. *Health Education Research* **5**, 73–80.

16   This section is based partly on:

Association of Community Workers (1986) Talking Point 74, June 1986.

Association of Community Workers, Colombo Street Sports & Community Centre, 25 Colombo Street, London SE1 8DP.

17   Health Education Authority:
http://www.hea.org.uk

Health Education Board for Scotland: HEBSWeb
http://www.hebs.scot.nhs.uk

12 Helping People to Learn

SUMMARY

In the first section of this chapter we discuss the principles of adult learning. We then use an exercise to analyse the qualities and abilities of a good teacher, and outline some principles of helping people to learn. Subsequent sections contain guidelines on giving talks, strategies for patient education and teaching practical skills. We include a role-play exercise on skills of patient education.

This chapter is about the skills and methods of helping people to learn, when the aims are primarily educational, concerned with helping people to acquire knowledge or skills. Examples are: giving a talk on a health topic to a large community group; teaching an adult education class in food hygiene and safety; running cardiac rehabilitation classes for patients recovering after heart attacks; giving information to a patient on a one-to-one basis about his diagnosis, treatment and self-care; or teaching a small group of colleagues about the techniques and procedures used in a screening programme.

Other chapters also contain relevant material, especially Chapters 10, 11, 13 and 14.

We have focused on selected aspects of education, teaching and learning which we identify as specially relevant for health educators and health promoters who are working with adults. This chapter is certainly not comprehensive, and further reading is recommended the end of this chapter.

Health promoters and health educators generally have credibility because of their training and expert knowledge. This is likely to be valued and respected by clients, but expertise alone does not make a good health educator. Effective educators get results in the form of measurable learning achievements by the individuals and groups with whom they work, such as greater retention of information, and better application of the learning in learners' own lives. To be effective, health educators need to understand key principles of adult learning which are based on extensive research. Authorities like Malcolm Knowles[1] and many others have been emphasizing for years that adult learners do best when they are involved and are treated with respect and dignity. They do not want merely to sit and listen, to be talked down to, to be bored, or to be bombarded with theory without opportunities for practical application. Effective educators therefore appreciate the importance of participative learning methods and use them. As Carl Rogers said[2]

> *I know I cannot teach anyone anything. I can only provide an environment in which he can learn.*

One of the most significant findings from research about adult learning is that when adults learn something naturally (as distinct from being taught in a formal way) they are highly self-directing. Furthermore, what they learn on their own initiative is learnt more deeply and permanently than what they are taught through traditional educational methods. Good educators also take account of recent brain research about the right and left brain which reveals that people are not only logical and rational (left-brain thinking) but also have the capacity to be spontaneous and creative (right-brain thinking). The basic principles of adult learning are summarized in Box 12.1

Box 12.1.   **Principles of adult learning**

- It is important for adults to direct themselves – they learn most effectively when they identify their own learning needs and set their own goals.
- The teacher's role is thus to enable or facilitate learning rather than to direct it. Teachers who adopt this approach often refer to themselves as 'facilitators'.
- Adult learners are generally most ready to learn things which they can apply immediately to existing problems or to their own situation. They do not, on the whole, learn for distant possibilities.
- Adult learners bring with them a wealth of life experience which should be seen as a resource and to which new learning should be related.
- Adult learners can help each other, because of their experiences, and should be encouraged to do so.
- Adults learn best by being active (not passive), by doing and experiencing, for which they need a safe environment where they feel accepted.
- Adult learners should be encouraged to carry out continuous evaluation of their own learning. Teachers should use this evaluation to fit the learning process to the learners' needs.

The next section is concerned with identifying the qualities and skills of a good educator.

What Makes a Good Teacher?

Every health promoter has spent many hours on the receiving end of other people's teaching, and this in itself is a useful learning experience. Exercise 12.1 will help health promoters to identify factors which have helped and hindered their own learning, and to assess their own qualities and abilities.

We do not suggest that health promoters set out to change their personalities. The aim of identifying strengths and weaknesses is to provide a basis for developing skills.

Some Principles of Helping People to Learn

Here we identify some basic principles which should be borne in mind in all health education teaching, whether working with individuals or groups.

Exercise 12.1   What helps and hinders learning?

Think of two occasions when you have been a learner, such as when you were a student in class, or in the audience listening to a talk, or when you were being taught on a one-to-one basis. These occasions need not have been connected with work (for example, listening to an art lecture or taking a driving lesson). One should be when you felt, overall, that the teaching session was *good* and the other when it was *bad*. The aim of the exercise is to identify the factors that made them good or bad for you.

In each of your two situations in turn identify factors which helped you to learn, and factors which hindered your learning. Think of these factors in three categories:

1. Those to do with the **environment** (e.g. too hot? noisy? hard chairs? a spacious, comfortable room?)
2. Those to do with the **qualities of the teacher** (e.g. sense of humour? appeared bored? contagious enthusiasm? seemed unfriendly?)
3. Those to do with the **presentation** (e.g. talked too long? used relevant illustrations? involved audience? muddled? used words you didn't understand? used audiovisual aids effectively?)

Enter these factors in on chart:

	Environment	Teacher	Presentation
Factors which helped			
Factors which hindered			

If you are working in a group, compare your chart with those of other people.

- **What have you learnt about the importance of the environment?**
- **What qualities of a good teacher do you think you already possess?**
- **What helpful points about presentation do you think you already use in your own teaching?**
- **What points about your own qualities or presentation would you like to improve?**

Plan Your Session

It is vital to put thought and time into preparation. It is an easy mistake to assume that you do not need to prepare a teaching session because you know your subject. Even if you are very skilled and knowledgeable, you still need to think through what you aim to achieve and prepare how you are going to introduce and develop your session, how you will involve your audience and so on. Preparation is especially important when teaching is new to you, but even the most experienced and self-confident teacher needs to spend some time in preparation.

It is also a fallacy to think that the educator can give less attention to planning if the learners are going to be active. Active participation is a more complex process and will require greater attention to planning.

Work from the Known to the Unknown

Your starting point is what people know already; this is obviously common sense, but frequently overlooked. The result is that time is wasted by teaching people what they already know, or by talking over their heads. You need to find out as much as possible about what your clients already know. If you cannot do this in advance, spend some time at the beginning of the session asking a few questions. If you have a mixed audience with varying degrees of knowledge, it may be best to acknowledge that some people know more than others, and you will have to make a decision about the level at which to pitch your information: 'Some of you will probably know this, but I'll talk about it briefly because it will be new to others ...'.

Your aim is build new information, or new skills, on to what is already known.

Aim for Maximum Involvement

People learn best if they are actively involved in the learning process, not just passively listening.

First, try to involve your clients in deciding the aim and content of the teaching. If you are running a course, such as a series of antenatal classes or one on food hygiene, you might begin by explaining your aims, asking for comments and suggestions, and then going on to discuss the content. This will help to increase motivation by including clients' own interests and, hopefully, stimulating them to think about new areas. It also helps clients to recognize that they are responsible for their own learning. The goals and content of one-to-one teaching can always be established by mutual agreement at the beginning of a session.

As a general rule, it is worth considering how much room for negotiation there is in your teaching, and spending time to find out what people really want. Ask yourself: 'Is what I teach what *I want to teach* or what *my clients want to learn?*'

Secondly, keep your clients involved as much as possible during teaching sessions. This is a challenge if you are giving a talk or a lecture to a large audience, but there are possibilities, such as asking people to respond to a question, e.g. 'I'd like you to put your hand up if you made a New Year resolution to take more exercise this year'. Or ask them to respond to a series of statements: for example, as an introduction to a talk on nutrition, ask the audience to stand up, then ask them to sit down if they: usually eat white bread ... add sugar to tea and coffee ... regularly eat fried food ... add salt at the table ... Most of them will be sitting down by now but they will feel alert and involved. Another way of keeping an audience involved is to give them time to talk. This can be done by having question-and-answer sessions, or by allowing short breaks when they can talk about something in groups of two or three for a few minutes. In a talk on passive smoking, for example, you could give your audience a couple of minutes to tell their neighbours how they are affected by other people's smoke.

You can also keep people involved with eye contact. Look members of your audience in the eye, and make sure that you look round at everybody, not just the people immediately in front of you.

Vary your Learning Methods

It is natural to consider teaching from the teacher's point of view but it may be more helpful to look at it from the client's point of view. For example, talking for half an hour demands concentrated effort and total involvement on your part; but all your audience is doing is listening, which only involves one of their senses and is highly unlikely to hold their full attention for that length of time.

Bringing variety into health teaching can be done in many ways, including strategies that can be used with individuals, groups, large audiences, children or adults (Table 12.1).

Table 12.1	Learning methods involving clients	
	Client involvement	**Materials and methods**
	Listen	Lectures, audiotapes
	Read	Books, booklets, leaflets, handouts, posters, black/white board, flipchart, overhead projector transparency
	Look	Photographs, drawings, paintings, posters, charts, material from magazines (such as advertisements)
	Look and listen	Films, videotapes, tape-slide sets, slides with commentary, demonstrations
	Listen and talk	Question-and-answer sessions, discussions, informal conversations, debates, brainstorming
	Read, listen and talk	Case studies, discussions based on study questions or handouts
	Read, listen, talk and actively participate	Drama, role-play, games, simulations, quizzes, practising skills
	Read and actively participate	Programmed learning, computer-assisted learning
	Make and use	Models, charts, drawings,
	Use	Equipment
For discussion of some of these methods, see Chapters 13 and 14; for discussion on the use of audio-visual aids, see Chapter 11.	Action research	Gathering information, opinions, interviews and surveys
	Projects	Making health education materials – videos, leaflets, etc.
	Visits	To health service premises, fire station, sewage works, playgroups, voluntary organizations
	Write	Articles, letters to the press, stories, poems

Devise your own Learning Activities

Activities are the means by which you help learners to think through what is being said and act on it, in their own way. Listening is passive; activities are active! It is not sufficient to ask a group of learners 'What do you think?' at the end of a talk or after viewing a video; planned activities are necessary to help people to explore ideas, feelings, attitudes and behaviour. It is important to have a mix. Activities specifically tailored for a particular group of learners will be most effective, so it is important to develop the skill of devising your own activities, rather than relying on learning aids made for general audiences. There is an almost infinite range of possibilities. Some of the more common types of activity are set out in Table 12.2. There are more ideas in the exercises we use in this book.

Table 12.2	Common types of learning activities
Type of activity	**Example**
Guidelines for discussions with particular people about particular topics	Guidelines on 'what to do if you think your child is offered drugs' for discussion at a parent–teacher meeting
Analysing and discussing diary records	Ask people to keep a diary or write down what they ate or drank in the last 24 hours. Ask them to talk about what they are pleased about and not pleased about.
Sentence completion	Ask people to complete a sentence such as 'I feel really stressed when…'.
Using checklists	Have a list of 'ways to be green' such as keeping a compost heap, recycling newspapers and bottles, using biodegradable detergents, and discuss how many you use.
Identifying your own thoughts/feelings/behaviour in particular situations	Ask people to think about and discuss what they feel when visitors to their home ask if they can smoke, and how they respond
Generate lists	Ask a group to make a list of all the ways they could deal with a toddler who won't settle down to sleep
Answer sheets	A quiz with yes/no or multiple answers on 'How much do you know about sensible drinking?'
Drawing charts or bubble diagrams	Draw a stick-person picture of yourself in a supermarket in the middle of a page. Draw bubble thoughts about all the things which influence what food you buy.
Writing instructions	Ask a group learning about food hygiene to write down instructions for someone else on how to store food safely in a fridge.
Practical skills development	Practise bathing a baby using a doll or a real baby.

Ensure Relevance

When teaching you should ensure that, as far as possible, what you say is relevant to the needs, interests and circumstances of the clients. For example, recommendations about health-promoting activities which cost money may be helpful to a relatively well-off audience, but not of much use to an audience which has no money for 'extras'. A discussion on vaccination may be irrelevant to a pregnant woman whose overwhelming concern is the birth itself; she may not relate to an issue which will not affect her until afterwards.

You will help your clients to see the relevance of your subject if you use concrete examples, practical problems and case studies to explain and illustrate your points. Abstract generalizations and quotations of high figures are difficult to relate to. For example say 'one person in ten' instead of 'X million people in this country', tell the story of a home accident rather than describe a list of risk factors, and describe 'increasing the risk' by saying 'It's like driving a car with faulty brakes – there's no guarantee that you will have an accident, but your chances of having one are greater'.

Identify Realistic Goals and Objectives

We have already discussed (in Chapter 5) the importance of clearly identifying health promotion aims and objectives but it is worth emphasizing again how essential it is to be clear about what you are trying to do (raise awareness of a health issue? give people more health knowledge?) and what you want your clients to know, feel and/or do at the end of your teaching session. As we mentioned above, your clients may be involved in these decisions.

A common mistake is to attempt too much. Three or four key points are all that you can ever expect people to remember from a teaching session. Teaching more than that does not mean that they learn more; it usually means that they forget more. For example, if you are asked to give a talk on a huge theme, such as Food for Health, Avoiding Accidents, First Aid or Pollution, you will need to select what you feel to be the few points most relevant for your audience, and avoid the temptation to give an everything-you-ever-wanted-to-know-about talk. A well-moved molehill is better than an abortive attempt to shift Everest.

Use Learning Contracts

In traditional education the learner is told what objectives to work towards. This conflicts with the adult's psychological need to be self-directing and may induce resistance, apathy, or withdrawal. Learning contracts are an agreement between the learner and teacher about what is to be learnt. Teacher and learner (or group of learners) decide it together. By participating in this process of diagnosing needs, formulating goals, choosing learning methods and evaluating progress, learners develop a sense of ownership of the plan, and feel committed to it.

The stages of developing a learning contract are set out below:

Step 1. Diagnose Learning Needs with the Learners

First decide the competencies required to carry out the actions, or behaviour, or role that the learners want to learn (for example, the competencies required to be the parent of a new baby at an antenatal education class). A competency can be thought of as the ability to do something, and it is a combination of knowledge, understanding, skills, attitudes and values.

For example, 'the ability to ride a bicycle from home to the shops' involves: knowledge of how a bicycle works and of the route from home to the shops; understanding of the dangers inherent in riding a bicycle; skills in mounting, pedalling, steering and stopping. It is useful to analyse competencies in this way, even if it is crude and subjective, because it gives the learners a clearer sense of direction.

Next, assess the gap between where learners are now and where they should be in regard to each competency. Learners may wish to draw on the observations of friends or family or experts to make this assessment. Each learner will then have an idea of the competencies needed, that is, a profile of learning needs.

Step 2. Specify the Learning Objectives of each Learner

Translate the learning needs identified in step one, into objectives which describe what each learner wants to *learn*. Each learner should state the learning objectives in terms most meaningful to them. For example, in order to ride a bicycle from home to the shops, learners may decide that they need knowledge of how to work the bicycle gears and improved skills of steering and stopping safely.

Step 3. Specify Learning Methods

Review the learning objectives of the learner or (if you are working with a group of learners) all the members of the learning group perhaps through listing them on a flip-chart and identifying shared objectives and areas of difference. Now think about how you could go about accomplishing these objectives. Specify the methods you would use. In the bicycle example, you could specify that practical demonstration followed by supervised practice in a traffic-free area would be the way to learn. Ask learners to suggest the methods they prefer.

Step 4. Evaluate Learning

Now describe what evidence you will need to show that these objectives have been achieved. For example, knowledge can be tested through quizzes. Understanding can be tested through solving problems. Skills can be tested through demonstrations of performance. Attitudes can be tested through role play and games. Values can be tested through games and values-clarification exercises.

An example of a learning contract for a group is provided in Box 12.2. Each individual in a group can have their own personal version of the learning contract.

Organize your Material

Whether you are talking to a group or teaching an individual, it helps if you organize your material into a logical framework, and tell your client(s) what this is, both at the beginning and during your teaching session.[3]

For example, with an individual patient, say:
'I am going to tell you:

- what we have found to be wrong with you;
- the treatment I am going to suggest for you;
- how much time you will need off work.

First, what we have found out is that…
Secondly, I think that the best treatment for you is…
Finally, about taking time off work, I think that you will probably need…'

The same principle applies if you are talking to a group. The old adage is: 'Tell 'em what you're going to tell 'em; tell 'em; then tell 'em what you've told 'em'. This is sound advice, because it helps both you and the audience to know where you are and where you are going. 'Flagging' where you are at intervals is helpful: 'That's all I've got to say on the benefits of yoga; now, to move on the how you can get started …', or 'Now I'd like to move on to my third and final point, which you may remember I said was about…'.

Evaluation, Feedback and Assessment

See the section called Stage 5 Plan Evaluation Methods in Chapter Five and the section on Asking Questions and Getting Feedback in Chapter 10.

As emphasized previously, it is important to get feedback on your teaching, so that you can assess how much your client is learning and improve your own performance in the future.

Box 12.2   **Learning Contract for Mary's Young Parent's Group**

Group members said they wanted to know more about how to cook cheap interesting healthy meals for their families, as a change from the usual fish fingers, beans, chips, etc. Mary and group members worked out the following learning contract.

Learning objectives	Learning methods	Evaluation of achievement of objectives
Know what to eat to be healthy	Keep food diaries for 2 days Mary to produce guidelines and members discuss how far their food matches up to guidelines	Be able to say what sort of food each member should aim to eat more or less of
Know where to buy good cheap food	Group members share experience of where they buy food, its price and quality	Two weeks later, members identify changes in where they buy food, and whether it is better quality and value for money
Be able to cook healthy meals that their families enjoy eating	Mary and group members bring recipes, choose some to try out and cook together	Have cooked new healthy meals at home

Three aspects to consider are:

1. how you will assess your own performance as an educator/facilitator (self-assessment) and record how well you feel the session went, and what could be improved;
2. how you will get feedback from your learners on how well they think the session went;
3. how you will assess the extent to which your learners are achieving the planned learning outcomes.

We now consider each of these.

Assessing your own Performance

You need to ask yourself what went well, what didn't, why, and how things could be improved next time. You may find it helpful to use a simple form to record your thoughts. This is especially useful if your session is part of a course with a team of people involved. An example is given in Box 12.3 – a form used by a group facilitator to record issues after a group session on healthy eating and cooking.[4]

Getting Feedback from Learners

You could include oral feedback as part of your session. For example, at the end ask people to do a round of sentence completion:

'The thing I liked best about today's session was…'.
'The most important thing I am taking away from this session is…'.
'The thing I liked least about today's session was…'.

However, people may find this intimidating, and may not feel comfortable with expressing what they feel directly to the educator. You may wish to use a written evaluation form, and we give two examples below (Boxes 12.4 and 12.5).

Box 12.3   **Nutrition and Cooking Project Monitoring Form[4]**

Session no:

Date:

Course leader:

Number of attenders:

Number in crèche:

Activity:

Positive outcomes:

Negative outcomes:

Feedback/comments from participants:

Crèche issues:

Issues needing further action:

Action plan:

Completed by:

Box 12.4   **Evaluation form A**

Title of session:

Date:

Please help me to get the session right for you by completing the following sentences about how you feel. Thank you.

It helps me when   . . . .

It is difficult for me when   . . . .

I would like more of   . . . .

I would like less of   . . . .

Box 12.5   **Evaluation form B**

Title of course:

Date:

We would like your views to help us assess this course and make plans for similar courses in the future. All your comments will be valued and used, and treated confidentially.

	Yes	No	Partly
1. Overall, have you found this course beneficial? (please tick)	☐	☐	☐

2. What did you expect to gain from the course?

	Yes	No	Partly
3. Did the course match up to your expectations?	☐	☐	☐

   Please comment:

4. Which parts of the course have you found most beneficial?

5. Which parts of the course have you found least beneficial?

6. How do you think the course could be improved?

7. Do you have any other comments you would like to make?

Please write your name here (or leave blank if you prefer to remain anonymous)

Thank you very much for filling this in.

Assessing the Learning Outcomes

Assessing learning outcomes is an important aspect of evaluation in teaching and learning situations. It is the process of measuring the extent and quality of your clients' learning: judging how successful they have been in progressing towards goals which they set themselves. It may be carried out very informally through getting apparently casual feedback from clients about how they have applied the learning to real-life situations. Or it may involve setting tests in formal situations. Here are two examples of ways in which health promoters assess how well they are doing:

- Sandra teaches Yoga. She does not feel it appropriate to assess her students formally, so she uses the British Wheel of Yoga standards to check on their performance and give them feedback.

■ Marleen teaches cookery and healthy eating to adults with learning difficulties. She keeps records of their progress in relation to their previous level of competence in choosing healthy menus and cooking healthy meals.

Monitoring students' progress by keeping records of achievements can be valuable for helping them to see what they have achieved. If your teaching is geared towards people learning to change behaviour, it can help to keep diary-type records: of what they ate or drank, or how much physical activity they did. If they are learning practical creative skills, photographic records can help. For example, on a course designed to help people cook and eat healthier food for their families you could give them a single-use camera to make a pictorial record of the dishes they cooked and their family enjoying the meals.

Guidelines for Giving Talks

Giving a talk, or perhaps a formal lecture, is a frequent feature of a health promoter's work. There are considerable disadvantages in this method: a talk is largely a one-way communication process with little opportunity to assess how much people are learning or understanding, with only a small proportion of it likely to be remembered at the end and still less a few days later.

Despite these limitations, talks and lectures can be valuable for several reasons. A talk can be used to introduce a subject by giving a bird's-eye view of it, and this may lead people to take further action. For example, an introductory talk on first aid may lead people to enrol for a first-aid course. A talk may awaken a critical attitude in the audience, for example, by drawing their attention to issues such as pollution or the lack of understandable information on food labels. Many people do not read books and articles or habitually watch documentary programmes on television; for them, a talk may be an important source of health information. Giving talks is also a relatively economical way to use a health promoter's time, since large numbers of people can be addressed at one time.

In addition to the general principles discussed in the last section there now follow some specific points which may help you to plan, and deliver, a successful talk.

Check the Facilities

If possible, visit the place where you are going to give your talk, and check the seating, lighting and audiovisual equipment including electric power points and extension leads. On the day of the talk, arrive in good time so that you can arrange chairs, open windows, put up blackout and check that the equipment is working. Get your video player, overhead projector, or slide projector ready for use, and if you need blackout, check that you can turn the lights on and off quickly so that you do not lose rapport with the audience while they are left in the dark.

Make a Plan

It can be useful to make an outline plan of your whole session, indicating the sections, times and any audiovisual aids you are using. This is particularly useful if you are sharing a teaching session with a colleague, so that you are both clear what you are doing. You can either use this as a skeleton overall plan to guide you when you make detailed notes to speak from (see section below) or you may find that it is enough to enable you to speak from the plan itself (Box 12.6).

Making and Using Notes

It is generally best to give a talk from notes written on paper or cards. The more experienced you are the fewer notes you are likely to need, unless your talk is full of technical detail or likely to be taken down and quoted verbatim (e.g. by the press). However, very few people can give a successful talk with no notes at all, and beginners may find it helpful to write out a talk in full before they transfer the main points to notes.

Box 12.6.	Plan for giving a talk

TALK ON 'SENSE IN THE SUN – PREVENTING SKIN CANCER'
Bloggshire Secondary School Parent-Teachers Meeting
21.5.94 $\frac{3}{4}$ hour at the end of the business meeting, 8.00–8.45 p.m.
Mrs N (school nurse) & Mr DH (deputy head)
AIM: to give parents basic information on risks and prevention of skin cancer

Time	Section	Content	Audiovisual aids (OHT = overhead projector transparency)	Who
8.00	Intros	Intro Mrs N & Mr DH Why we are now concerned about skin cancer–rising incidence	OHT graph showing rise in skin cancer in UK	Mr DH
8.05	What is skin cancer?	Different types of skin cancer How you spot it Who is most at risk (fair skin, sunburn, etc.)	OHT key points	Mrs N
8.15	Prevention	Key message: respect the sun–avoid exposure at hottest times, use good sunscreen, cover up with sun hats and light clothing Be a mole-watcher	Examples of sun hats, light clothing (big, long-sleeved, cotton shirts etc.) Examples of sunscreen creams	Mrs N
8.25	What the school can do	Encourage the use of cover-up and sunscreen creams in outdoor PE Include topic in health education and science teaching	Main points on OHT	Mr DH
8.30	Summary	Aim for school and parents to work together Main points to remember: Care in the sun, Cover up, use sunscreen Creams	OHT: 3 C's to remember: Care in the sun Cover up Creams Leaflets to take away.	Mrs N
8.35	Any questions?			Mrs N

If you are writing out your talk in full to begin with, it is useful to know that a 50 minute lecture consists of about 5000 words, allowing for pauses and an estimated speed of delivery of about 110 words per minute. You can then try transferring the key points as notes to cards or paper.

Never give a talk by writing it out in full and then reading it. Unless you are an exceptional orator who can 'act' the lines, it will sound flat and stilted. Furthermore, you will find difficulty in looking at your audience, because you will need to keep your eyes on the notes, and once you look up you are likely to lose your place.

Prepare Your Introduction

Secure the attention of your audience with your opening words. Some ways of doing this are:

- state a startling fact;
- ask a question which has no easy answer;
- use a visual image to trigger interest;
- get the audience to do something active (some suggestions are discussed in the earlier section on 'Aiming for Maximum Involvement');
- tell a joke, if you have the confidence to do it successfully.

Establish eye contact with your audience and, if necessary, ask them whether they can see and hear you.

State your aim and theme at the beginning of your talk ('Tell'em what you're going to tell 'em'). It should be a brief statement, not a complex summary of the whole talk. For example, say 'I'm going to talk about what to do if someone is unconscious, not breathing, bleeding or in a state of shock' but do not go into detail at this point about what the correct actions should be; save that for the main part of the talk.

By the time you have finished the introduction, you should have:

- established your aim and theme with the audience;
- obtained their interest and commitment;
- ensured that they can hear and see you clearly.

Prepare the Key Points

Identify the three or four main points you wish to make, and prepare your talk around each point in turn. Illustrate and support your points with evidence from your experience or from research, with examples, audiovisual materials, and so on. (See Chapter 11 on using and producing audiovisual materials, including leaflets, handouts, videos and slides.)

Plan a Conclusion

You need to plan how you will end your talk in order to avoid rambling on or trailing off. Some ways of ending are:

- a very brief recapitulation (not a boring repetition) of what you've said – 'We've now covered the basics of life-saving first aid'.

- a statement of what you hope the audience will do with the information you have given them – 'I hope that you can confidently do the right thing next time you have to help someone who's had an accident'.
- a suggestion for further action – 'If you'd like to learn more please come to see me afterwards'.
- a question – 'Don't you think that basic first aid is so simple and so important that it should be taught to every child in school?'
- thanking the audience for their attention and/or participation.

Ask for Questions

If possible, include a question-and-answer session in your talk. It gives you feedback, and gives the audience a chance to participate.

When you ask for questions, allow people time to think; do not assume that there are to be no questions just because one is not instantly forthcoming. When a question is asked, it is often helpful to repeat or summarize it. This gives you a little time to consider the question, and ensures that everyone else in the audience has heard it. Never ignore or refuse to answer a question – if you don't know the answer say so, and ask whether anyone else in the audience does. In any case, this helps to involve the audience; you could also ask for comments on answers 'Does anyone else have suggestions which could help the person who asked that question?'

Work on Your Presentation

Important points about presentation include pace and timing, which usually means having consciously to slow down your rate of speaking; the nervous beginner finds the silence of pauses to be threatening and wants to get the whole thing over! Other factors are looking at the audience and using notes appropriately.

Thorough preparation will help you to feel confident, but however nervous or inexperienced you may feel, do not apologise for being there. For example, if you have been asked to give a talk about your work, *do not* say 'I'm going to talk about the work of health visitors, but I'm afraid I've only been qualified for a year so there's a lot I don't know yet'. Instead, present yourself positively 'I'm going to talk about the work of health visitors. I've been qualified for a year now, and I'd like to share my experience of the work with you'.

The way to improve presentation is by practice. Practise giving your talk out loud, or to friends or colleagues. Ask a trusted colleague to sit in when you give a talk, and to give you feedback afterwards. It is even more helpful to see yourself on videotape, so that you can assess your own strengths and weaknesses.

Plan for Contingencies

A major fear when giving a talk is that you may 'dry up' or lose your place. If this is a possibility, it is better to face it and think beforehand about what you will do if it should happen. It is best to acknowledge that you have a problem rather than leave an embarrassed silence. For example, say 'Sorry, my mind seems to have gone blank' or 'I've lost my place'. Then remember that an audience is likely to be friendly rather than hostile and will probably want to help you. So let them help by asking for time: 'Would you mind if I took a minute to get myself together' or 'Excuse me for a moment while I look through my notes'.

Another fear is that audiovisual equipment will break down. You cannot insure against this, so it is best to have a contingency plan ready. For example, 'As we can't see the sequence on the video as I'd hoped, I'll write the stages up on the blackboard and talk through them instead'.

See also the section on *Dealing with Difficulties* in Chapter 13.

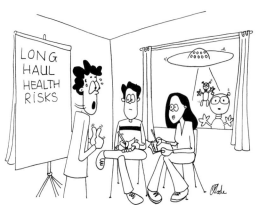

Plan for contingencies.

Improving Patient Education

Research over many years has shown that patients want information but have difficulty in understanding and remembering what they have been told by their doctor, nurse or other health worker.[5] Substantial numbers of patients feel dissatisfied with the communications aspect of their encounters with health professionals, and are reluctant to ask for more information. Furthermore, a large proportion of patients do not comply with the advice and treatment prescribed for them.

There are many reasons for these apparent failures, but certainly some of the cause lies in the way in which information, advice and instructions are given to patients. Often the circumstances are less than ideal, because patients are distressed or feeling unwell, and there may be little time in a busy surgery, out-patient clinic or hospital ward. Therefore, there is all the more reason to ensure that the best possible use is made of the time and opportunities for patient education.

All the basic communication skills discussed in Chapter 10, and the principles of helping people to learn outlined earlier in this Chapter, are important. There has also been considerable research in the field of patient education and information.[6] Some particular principles which have been found helpful in patient education are set out in Box 12.6.[7]

The following exercise is designed to help you practise the skills of patient education we have discussed here, as well as the basic communication skills outlined in Chapter 10. Another useful way of learning to improve communication skills is to video and analyse an interview with a patient.

| Box 12.7. | **Some Principles of Patient Education** |

Say important things first: patients are more likely to remember what was said at the beginning of a session, so give the most important advice and instruction first whenever possible.

Stress and repeat the key points: patients are more likely to remember what they consider to be important, so make sure they realize what the really important points are. For example, say:

'The most important thing for you to remember today is...'

'The one thing it's really essential to do is...'

Repetition of key points also helps people to remember them.

Give specific, precise advice: sometimes it is appropriate to give general guidance, but specific, precise advice is more likely to be remembered than vague guidance. For example, say:

'I advise you to lose five pounds in the next month' rather than 'I advise you to lose weight'

'Try to take an hour's rest with your feet up every afternoon' rather than 'Get more rest' or 'Take things easier'.

See Organise Your Material above.

Structure information into categories: this means telling the patient headings and then categorizing your material under these headings as you present it.

Avoid jargon and long words and sentences: if you need to use medical terms or jargon, make sure the patient understands what they mean. Never use a long word when a short one will do. Use short sentences.

See Chapter 11 on Using Communication Tools.

Use visual aids, leaflets, handouts and written instructions.

Avoid saying too much at once: three or four key points is all that you can expect someone to remember from one session.

See Ensure Relevance above.

Ensure advice is relevant and realistic in the patient's circumstances.

See the section on Asking Questions and Getting Feedback in Chapter 10.

Get feedback from patients to ensure that they understand.

Teaching Practical Skills

Health promoters are often called upon to teach practical skills, such as relaxation or keep-fit exercises, how to bath a baby or change a nappy, and how to give an injection or test urine.

All the communication skills we have discussed are relevant, but a few additional points are useful. Teaching a skill is not just about achieving 'knowing' and 'doing' objectives; that is, it is not *solely* concerned with giving the client information and teaching new practical skills. It is also necessary to pay attention to what clients *feel*. If people are afraid to do something because they are worried about looking foolish or doing it incorrectly, they are unlikely to succeed:

Exercise 12.2   **Skills of patient education**

Work in groups of three, taking each role in turn.

The **first person** takes the role of the health promoter. She selects the topic to be taught, drawing on her own experience, and tells the 'patient' his medical history before roleplay starts.

The **second person** plays the patient. This patient has one of the following sets of characteristics:

- intelligent, but with very limited understanding of spoken English, no ability to read or write English, and no-one available to translate;
- extremely worried, tense and anxious about his medical condition and prognosis;
- has some learning difficulty, finds great difficulty in understanding and remembering instructions although he tries hard to be cooperative.

The **third person** takes the role of the observer, using the observer's checklist below.

Role play the scene in which the health promoter is teaching the patient for ten minutes. The observer keeps time. Then give constructive feedback as follows:

- firstly, the 'health promoter' assesses herself, saying what she felt she did well, and identifying points she feels the need to work on in the future.
- secondly, the 'patient' describes how it felt to be the patient, identifying what the health promoter did or said which made him feel at ease/put down/ anxious/reassured/ more confused, and so on.
- finally, the observer gives feedback using the checklist as a guide.

Communication checklist

1. Non-verbal aspects of communication e.g. tone of voice, posture, gestures, facial expression, use of touch
2. Sequence and structure of key points e.g. important things first, logical sequence, information in categories
3. Choice of language e.g. appropriately simple and short, use of jargon/ idioms, medical terms
4. Two-way communication e.g. encourage patient to talk and express feelings, get feedback about how much is understood, open/closed/biased/multiple questions
5. Amount of information e.g. too much or too little
6. Clarity of objective(s)
7. Use of repetition
8. Use of emphasis to stress important points
9. Any assumptions made but not checked e.g. about previous knowledge, facilities for carrying out instructions, willingness to comply
10. Anything else?

encouragement and step-by-step progress is needed. Confidence-building is as important a part of the health educator's role as developing practical skills.

In order to develop clients' ability to perform a skilled task, a three-stage approach is most effective, namely:

Stage 1. Demonstrate.
Stage 2. Rehearse.
Stage 3. Practise.

Clients will be watching and listening in stage 1, but they become actively involved in *doing* in stages 2 and 3.

It may be useful to begin by using a dummy, for example, when teaching safe lifting techniques, or to use an orange instead of a person when teaching injection techniques. As skills develop, the techniques can be tried in real life situations (lifting people, for example) and perhaps under more difficult circumstances.

Individual learners need to progress at their own pace and build up confidence at each stage. For this reason teaching practical skills needs time and patience, but it is worth the investment to get the right skills programme from the beginning. People who have lost confidence in their ability to do something are even more difficult to help than a new learner.

PRACTICE POINTS

- To be successful in health education with adult clients you need to understand principles of adult learning and factors which help and hinder learning. Key principles include paying attention to planning, involving learners in the learning process as much as possible, ensuring material is relevant and structured into a logical sequence, and having realistic objectives. You may find it helpful to use informal learning contracts.

- If you are giving talks, you need planning, preparation and practice.

- You can help patients to understand and remember more if you take account of some key principles of patient education.

- It is best to use a three stage approach of demonstration, rehearsal and practice when you are teaching practical skills.

Recommended Reading

On Adult Learning

➤ Rogers J (1989) *Adults Learning*, 3rd edn. Buckingham; Open University Press.
➤ Sotto E (1994) *When teaching becomes learning.* London: Cassell.
➤ Castling A (1996) *Competence-based teaching and training.* Basingstoke: City and Guilds/Macmillan.

Guidance on Learning for Adults with Learning Difficulties

➤ Sutcliffe J (1991) *Adults with learning difficulties: education for choice and empowerment.* Leicester: NIACE.

On the Nurse's Role as a Teacher

➤ Hinchcliffe S (ed.) (1992) *The Practitioner as Teacher.* London: Baillière Tindall. (Looks at the nurse's role as a teacher and examines the skills and methods that help the nurse become a more effectiive teacher.)

On giving Talks

➤ Williams D (1997) *Communication Skills in Practice – a practical guide for health professionals.* Part Four: Presentation Skills. London: Jessica Kingsley Publications.
➤ Stevens M (1996) *How to be better at giving presentations.* London: Kogan Page/Industrial Society.
➤ Stanton N (1996) *Mastering Communication*, 3rd edn. Chapter 2. Basingstoke: Macmillan.

On Running Workshops

➤ Bourner T, Martin V & Race P (1993) *Workshops That Work.* London: McGraw-Hill.

On Patient Education

➤ Ley P (1988) *Communicating with patients – improving communication, satisfaction and compliance.* London: Croom Helm.
➤ Redman BK (1993) Patient Education at 25 years: where have we been and where are we going. *Journal of Advanced Nursing* **18** (5), 725–730.
➤ Tones K & Tilford S (1994) *Health Education – Effectiveness, Efficiency and Equity.* Chapter 5. London: Chapman and Hall.

Notes and References

1   A 'classic' text is:

Knowles M (1978) *The Adult Learner: A Neglected Species.* 2nd edn. Gulf: Houston. Texas.

2   Rogers C (1969) *Fredom to Learn.* Merrill: Ohio (This is another classic text.)

3   One study found that the use of this technique improved patients' recall by 17%:

Ley P *et al.* (1973) A method for increasing patients' recall of information presented by doctors *Psychological Medicine* **3**, 217–220.

4   Form used by Hartcliffe Health and Environment Action Group and health visitors from Hartcliffe and Withywood, Bristol, in their 'Feed Your Face' project on nutrition and cooking. Reproduced with their kind permission.

5   Research into patient education by hospital nurses revealed that there was a tendency for education to be disease-orientated and standardized. See:

Macleod Clark J, Wilson-Barnett J, Latter S & Maben J (1992) *Health Education and Health Promotion in Nursing: a study of practice in acute areas.* Report of a research project funded by the Department of Health. Department of Nursing Studies, King's College, University of London.

Bullivent and Reeve asked cancer patients and their carers for their perceptions of cancer services. Communication in the consultation process was the greatest cause for concern. Issues raised included lack of time, lack of consistency in messages, use of jargon by medical staff and the need for privacy. See:

Bullivent D & Reeve J (1996) Consulting with Consumers: back to basics. *Health Service Journal* **106** (5485), 28–29

6   For some further reading on reviews of research, and research in specific areas, see: Arthur V A M (1995) Written patient information: a review of the literature. *Journal of Advanced Nursing* **21**(6), 1081–1086.

Kok G, van den Borne & Mullen P (1997) Effectiveness of health education and health promotion: meta-analyses of effect studies and determinants of effectiveness. *Patient Education and Counselling* **30**(1), 19–27. (Research showing effectiveness of health education and pointers to effective practice.)

Vahabi M & Ferris L (1995) Improving written patient education materials: a review of the evidence. *Health Education Journal* **54**, 99–106. (Discusses evidence on how to improve written patient education material.)

Austoker J, Davey C & Jansen C (1997) *Improving the quality of written information sent to women about cervical screening: guidelines on the presentation and content of letters and leaflets.* NHS Cervical Screening Programme and Cancer Research Campaign, NHSCSP Publication No 5. (Provides guidelines based on research about the presentation and content of written information, and evaluation of exisiting letters and leaflets. Guidelines are in the form of practical checklists for letters and leaflets at all stages on the screening process. Specifically for cervical screening, but the principles could be applied to other situations. Available from NHSCSP Publications, NHS Cervical Screening Programme, The Manor House, 260 Eccleston Road South, Sheffield S11 9PS).

Williams S & McIntosh J (1996) Problems in implementing evidence-based health promotion material in general practice. *Health Education Journal* **55**, 24–30. (An account of developing audiovisual materials with clients on the cervical smear test.)

Wise A *et al.* (1996) The structure and content of nutrition education messages. *Journal of Human Nutrition and Dietetics* **9**(2), 117–126. (Questionnaire study to investigate people's responses to different styles of nutritional messages, including positive and negative commands, medical and technical terms.)

7   This section is based on:

Ewles L & Shipster P (1981) *Education One-to-One Health* East Sussex Area Health Authority, and

Ley P (1988) *Communicating with Patients – improving communication, satisfaction and compliance.* London: Croom Helm.

13   Working with Groups

SUMMARY

This chapter is about working with clients in groups. We begin by considering the range of groups in health promotion, appropriate leadership styles and responsibilities. We then discuss some aspects of group behaviour, before moving on to the practicalities and skills of setting up a group, getting groups going, discussion skills and dealing with difficulties. We include exercises on leadership styles and planning a group meeting.

Health promoters work with many different kinds of groups in a variety of settings. We looked at working with groups of colleagues in Chapter 9; in this chapter, we are focusing on the health promoter's work with groups of clients, but it is worth saying that many of the skills we discussed in Chapter Nine (such as co-ordination, teamwork, making meetings and committees effective) may also apply when working with clients.

See Chapter 9.

Group work can be seen as part of the movement away from clients as passive recipients of services, towards clients as people actively involved with their own health issues and active within their communities. Many of the groups health promoters are involved with will already exist, where members have come together for a common purpose and health issues form part, or the whole, of the agenda. The role of the health promoter may vary widely, from leading a one-off session, to facilitating the development of a new group, or leading a group with a defined lifespan. Whatever the role, competencies in group work are needed, and this chapter sets out some of the basic ones. (We are excluding leading therapeutic groups from our discussions; therapy requires in-depth professional training in a range of possible approaches, outside the scope of this book.)

Specialist training in group work is recommended to develop skills and confidence further.[1] Group work may only be given a brief introduction in basic professional training courses and in-service professional development; consequently many practitioners feel ill-equipped for the task. For further reading, see the suggestions at the end of the chapter.

First, we discuss the kinds of groups which exist for different purposes.

Kinds of Groups

Groups are not random collections of individuals; group members have a sense of shared identity, common objectives, defined membership criteria and their own particular ways of working. Groups are formed for a variety of purposes. The term *group work* can be applied to a range of activities such as group therapy, social action or self-help. We suggest that the main groups in the context of health promotion are formed for one or more of the following purposes:

For awareness raising. To increase members' interest in, and awareness of, health issues through group discussion. This may be a group already in existence, such as a women's group, which may agree to discuss a health issue.

For mutual support. To support members in difficult decision taking, or to help each other to cope with shared problems/disabilities, or to change a health damaging behaviour. Examples are self-help groups such as groups of people living with HIV, patients' associations, tenants' associations and Alcoholics Anonymous.

For social action. To use the collective power of the group to campaign for social change, for example on tackling a local problem of drug misuse, housing standards or community facilities.

For education. To impart skills, offer information and sometimes to prepare members for specific life events, for example becoming a parent.

For group counselling. To help members to find solutions through exploring a shared problem with a counsellor, for example a group of menopausal women.

Being clear about the purpose of a group is important; confusion can result if the tasks of a group are changed, especially if this means that individual members have to adopt different roles. For example, an individual will have difficulty if she attends a group to obtain support, and finds the task is changed to campaigning. A new group is required for the new task.

The type of task will determine the most effective size for the group; for example, educational groups may be larger than support groups.

Different kinds of groups may also require the health promoter to take on different roles, and use different skills. Leading or facilitating groups requires special skills and methods, and the next section is about group leadership.

Group Leadership

Two aspects of group leadership are useful to consider. One is your leadership style and the other is your responsibilities as a group leader.

Leadership Style

It is important that all the members of the group are agreed on who is the leader, and support the leader in this role. The leadership style needs to be compatible with the group members, especially if the group has to work together to complete complex tasks. For example, a group of highly motivated and trained professionals will work best with a leader who encourages participation and shared decision making. It is essential for leaders to be aware of which style members prefer, and to develop the ability to adjust their style if the situation demands it.

A key dimension of leadership style is where the leader stands on a continuum from authoritarian to participative.

authoritarian |_____| *participative*

An **authoritarian** style is directive, with the group leader acting as a 'director', who is a source of expertise. If you adopt this approach, you rely on your status, credibility and expertise to ensure acceptance of your views and leadership role.

The *strength* of this style is that children and vulnerable people (such as those who are sick or handicapped) may feel secure, reassured and protected from harm.

The *weaknesses* of this style are that clients may become fearful, anxious and reluctant to take independent action; it does not develop their ability to take responsibility for their own decisions and actions. Furthermore, clients may respond by rebelling and rejecting your guidance.

A **participative** style involves shifting power from the group leader so that it is shared between the leader and the group members. This means using all the skills and knowledge of the group members as well as the leader, who is more likely to choose the title of 'facilitator'. As a facilitator, you will need to show warmth and empathy, encourage group members to express their feelings, and provide counsel and encouragement. You will need to be tolerant of different viewpoints, showing fairness and impartiality. You will need skills and ability to confront difficult issues and resolve conflict using a problem solving approach.

See the section in Chapter 9 on conflict resolution styles.

The *strength* of this style is that clients learn to trust their own judgements and at the same time to appreciate other people's rights and opinions.

The *weaknesses* of this style may be that strong feelings are uncovered and distress experienced by the client; this may also be distressing for you as the leader and hard for you to cope with. Also, clients who are used to being told what to do may feel confused and dissatisfied because they are not receiving the advice and direction they want. They will need to have the approach explained to them and be given suitable learning experiences to show them that it works.

There is no 'right' or 'wrong' style, and indeed most leaders probably operate somewhere between the two extremes, providing some authoritative leadership while also encouraging a degree of participation.

It is commonly assumed that groups will be more effective with a participative rather than authoritarian leadership style, but research and experience do not always support this conclusion.[2] Rather, we suggest that the reality of leadership is more complex, and that successful group leadership depends on a variety of factors such as:

- the leader's preferred style of operating and personality. For example, if you have been used to being perceived as the 'expert' with the authority of professional knowledge which you want to pass on, you will probably feel (and look) uncomfortable if you try to switch to a 'facilitator' style without sufficient training, and this will produce tension in the group.
- the group members' preferred style of leadership in the specific circumstances of the group. For example, if group members are low in confidence, they may need you to be more authoritarian to start with, so that they feel secure. You can then gradually encourage participation and adopt a more facilitative style as members learn to trust you and each other, and feel confident enough to join in.

- the group's objectives and tasks. For example, a group which has the objective of learning new skills (such as an exercise class) will need a more authoritarian leader who will tell them how to do the exercises properly, whereas a group of parents in a support group which aims to help them recover from the death of a child will need a facilitator to help members to express and work through their grief.
- the wider environment, such as the culture of the group members, and of the organizations they belong to. For example, the culture of some ethnic minorities may be such that members (especially women) are brought up to be passive, and will not only lack confidence about active participation in groups, but may perceive it as 'wrong'.

You need to consider these factors, and how they might be modified, in order to achieve the 'best fit'. The easiest thing to modify in the short term may be your own style, but in the long term it may also be possible to make other changes, for example to develop the group members' confidence so that they are willing to take on more responsibility and participation.

See Chapter 3.   The participative style fits best with the self-empowering client-centred approach to health promotion, as discussed in Chapter 3. However, many health promoters will have been trained by people operating in an authoritarian style and will have modelled themselves on this experience. If this is true in your case, you will need to learn how to work in a participative style and this could be fundamental to becoming more effective in self-empowering your clients.

Finally, a participative style must be distinguished from a permissive style. A permissive style lets clients come to their own conclusions and aims to avoid conflict and keep everyone happy. Helping the clients to enjoy the educational experience is more important to the leader than achieving the goals of the group. Difficulties and conflict are not confronted and the clients may feel neither secure nor cared for. Group leaders may need to build up their own assertiveness skills in order to avoid an overly permissive approach.

Leadership Responsibilities

The responsibilities of group leaders will depend on the role they take; for example, whether they are responsible for the practical organization such as booking a venue. But whatever the role, a leader's responsibilities will probably include:

- helping members to identify and clarify their interests and needs, and what they would like to gain from the group in the short and long term.
- helping to develop a relaxed atmosphere in which members feel able to be open and trusting with each other, and able to participate freely.
- offering her expertise to the group on the understanding that members are free to accept or reject the offer.
- accepting and valuing all contributions from group members.

But it is not only the group leader who has responsibilities: group members have them too. They will probably include:

- participating in clarifying the aims of the group.
- choosing whether and how much to participate.
- identifying their own goals and concerns.

Exercise 13.1   Looking at your leadership style

The following questions aim to help you to examine
your own leadership style. Put a tick in the
appropriate box.

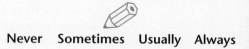

	Never	Sometimes	Usually	Always
1. Do your clients say what they feel?				
2. Do clients finish what they are saying before you respond?				
3. Do you think you are able to see things from your clients' point of view?				
4. Do clients disagree with you?				
5. Do you explore with your clients the consequences of alternative actions?				
6. Do you help clients to discuss painful memories or sensitive issues?				
7. Do you share all the information at your disposal?				
8. Do you help clients to discover their own strengths?				
9. Do you respect your clients' right to reject your advice?				

What leadership style – authoritarian, participative or permissive – do you think you usually use?
What were the influences which led you to develop this style?
Can you identify any advantages in using alternative leadership styles in your work?
Can you identify any aspects of your leadership style that you would like to change?

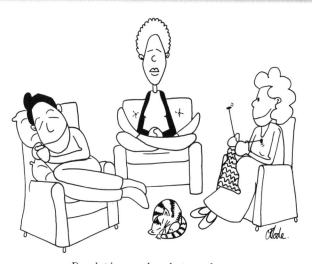

Developing a relaxed atmosphere.

■ deciding which challenges and risks they are prepared to take. For example, how much are they prepared to expose their own weaknesses and vulnerability to other people in the group?

Group Behaviour

Health promoters will be able to work with a group more effectively if they are aware of the ways in which people are likely to behave when they come together in groups (sometimes called 'group dynamics'). We focus on three aspects of group behaviour which you may find particularly useful: the pattern of behaviour which usually develops in a group's life, the different roles group members may perform, and the concept of 'hidden agendas'.

Group development

Groups tend to show a particular pattern of behaviour as they mature and develop. This developmental cycle has been categorized as having four stages:[3]

1. **Forming.** The group is in the process of forming. People meet each other, and get to know one another, with individuals establishing their own identity and role within the group. The group's purpose and way of working is established.
2. **Storming.** Most groups go through a conflict stage when the leadership and ways in which the group is working are challenged. For example, people may question how things are being done, what the leader's role is and may get into heated discussions with each other. This can be a difficult period for both leader and members, but it is a vital stage in the group's maturing process, rather like the period of rebelling and questioning during adolescence. Successful handling of this period leads to the development of open communication, trust and shared responsibility for achieving the purposes of the group.

See the section on Understanding Conflict in Chapter 9.

3. **Norming.** At this stage the group settles down, with the norms and accepted practices of the group established.
4. **Performing.** The group is fully effective at this stage and is able to concentrate on its tasks.

When the developmental process fails in some way, backstage politicking and attempts to sabotage the group may occur. It is thus worth investing time and effort to help new groups to develop successfully.

Many groups have a limited time span, meeting for a set number of sessions or until a particular task has been completed. At the end of a group's life, it is natural for members to feel a sense of loss. It may be helpful to have a final 'rounding up' session, which could give group members an opportunity to express their appreciation of each other, their sadness at parting, and perhaps arrange a follow-up or 'reunion'.

Group Members' Roles

A classic study of the characteristics of members of groups concluded that a mix of eight roles is needed for fully effective groups.[4] These roles are outlined in Box 13.1.

Box 13.1.	**Eight roles needed for effective groups**

The Leader – coordinates the efforts of the group and enables it to work effectively.
The Shaper – is action oriented and encourages the group to get on with its tasks.
The Plant – is the creative source of ideas and proposals.
The Monitor/Evaluator – is good at analysing and criticizing.
The Resource Investigator – has a good network of contacts and liaises with other people and agencies.
The Company Worker – is good at organizing and administration.
The Team Worker – supports the members of the group and is a good listener.
The Finisher – contributes foresight and perseverance to ensure that the group completes its tasks.

Each person may play a variety of these roles in a group and most people have their preferred roles. If one or more of these roles is lacking, a member or leader can help to make a group more successful by consciously adopting a new role herself, or helping someone else to do so.

Hidden Agendas

People will have their own individual reasons for joining a group, which may be in addition to, or instead of, the reason expected. For example, a woman may attend a women's health group because she is lonely and sees the group as way of meeting people; she has not joined because she is particularly interested in health issues. Or a group member may seek a prominent position in a group, such as being the chairperson or secretary, to fulfil her need to be valued and useful; she may or may not also be committed to the work itself and the aims of the group. In these examples, fulfilling these personal objectives are 'hidden agendas'.

Most people bring their own 'hidden agendas' to groups, in addition to the agreed group objectives; these commonly include meeting the need for social contact, or making a particular alliance. Members will work together best when there is communication about individual objectives and agreement about shared objectives. Otherwise members may promote their own interests at the expense of the group's. You will be more effective as a group leader if you are aware of the hidden agendas in the group and can find ways of dealing with them.

Setting Up a Group

See also Chapter 5 on The Basic Planning and Evaluation Process

Planning and preparation are essential for successful group work. The checklist below takes you step-by-step through the thinking and planning you need to do when setting up a group.[5]

Why are you proposing to run the group?

- Are you reacting to a demand from clients, other professionals, a community or your own observations?

- Are you trying to develop your health promotion role and see this group as a way of progressing?
- Are you aiming to provide advice and support, or to supply information, or to help people to change health-related behaviour?
- Are you aiming to satisfy your own needs or your clients' needs? (Your reasons can include both, but it is helpful to distinguish between them.)

Who will the members be?

- Will the members be referred to the group (from their GP, for example); will they be coerced into joining or will membership be entirely voluntary?
- Have you given everyone an equal opportunity to join, e.g. by ensuring facilities for wheelchairs, disabled toilets, signing for those hard of hearing, hearing loops, translation into appropriate minority languages? Have you made provision for people to let you know of any special needs?
- How will you identify the potential members of your group – from individuals requesting a group, from local or national registers, from people with shared characteristics (age, sex, lifestyle, culture, job, health risks, etc.), or by other means?
- How will you recruit your members? Do you need to advertise?
- How many members do you aim to have? What is the ideal number, bearing in mind the purpose of the group and any constraints imposed by your location?

What are the group's aims and objectives?

- Are these within the realistic abilities of yourself and the members?
- Can all the potential membership understand them?
- Are you clear about your own objectives in setting up the group, and whether these are different from the members' objectives?
- Is each member clear about their individual objectives, i.e. the specific outcomes they hope to achieve through attending the group?

Where will the group be held?

- Is the location appropriate? For example, a health centre or hospital may appear clinical and cold and remind people of illness. 'Neutral' territory, such as a room in a pub or community centre, or in someone's house, may be more relaxing and inviting.
- What is the seating like? If you are aiming for participative group work, seating people in a circle is best (Fig. 13.1), with physical barriers to communication such as tables or desks removed. Can you put chairs in a circle, where all group members can see each other?
- What are the facilities like? Is there enough space for the activities you plan? Is the floor covering suitable for the purpose? Is the temperature suitable and adjustable if necessary? Are the facilities adequate for the purpose (for example access for pushchairs, toilets, catering facilities, washing/shower rooms, crèche)? Are there facilities for people with special needs (for example wide access for wheelchairs, disabled toilets, hearing loops, signs in minority languages)?

Fig 13.1   **(a) Seating in a circle – best for group work; (b) traditional seating in rows – not suitable for group work.**

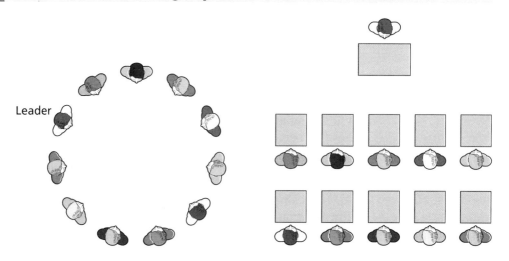

- Is there good access? Is the venue accessible by local transport? Do you have transport for members who cannot manage on public transport? Are parking arrangements satisfactory?
- What are the security arrangements? Where are the fire extinguishers and what is the fire drill? In case of an emergency, who do you contact? Do you need insurance cover?

What resources do you need?

- Do you need any special equipment, for example video equipment, power points? Are you familiar with the equipment and confident you can operate it? Does the equipment have to be booked in advance and if so, are you familiar with the booking system?
- Do you need any additional resources, for example videos, leaflets, posters, books, outside speakers? If so, have you made all the necessary arrangements in advance?
- Do you need money to pay for anything? If so, have you identified a source of funding (for example, a charge to the group members, a trust fund or a sponsor)?

When will the group be held?

- Is the time you have chosen the best one for the clients, or have you chosen it to suit yourself? Does the length of meetings suit members and take into account the other commitments of members? Have you consulted potential members about timing and tried to satisfy the majority?

How will the group be run?

- Will it be a self-help group and directed by the members, or leader-led?
- To what extent will the structure be flexible and the content negotiable?

- Will the group be open (anyone can joint at any time) or will there be restrictions on admitting new members once the group has started?

How will the group be evaluated?

- At the end of each meeting? At the end of the group? Or both?
- Verbally or in writing or both? How will you ask questions in order to obtain accurate feedback from members (for example by providing opportunities for anonymous feedback)?
- How will you know that the agreed group objectives have been achieved? How will you know whether your own objectives have been achieved? How will you know whether each individual has achieved her objectives?
- Were there any unplanned outcomes of the group? Were these desirable or undesirable and what caused them?
- What have you learned? What would you do differently next time?

See also the section on Evaluation, Feedback and Assessment in Chapter 12.

Getting Groups Going

Almost everyone feels nervous about going to a group meeting for the first time, especially if knowing anyone else there is unlikely. The initial task for the group leader is to 'break the ice' and help people to feel at ease.

Before the First Meeting

If you know in advance who is coming to a group, it may be helpful and welcoming to confirm by letter or telephone that you are expecting them, and the time and place. If anyone has let you know they have special needs, it is helpful to contact them in advance to discuss their needs and let them know what facilities will be available.

On Arrival

It helps if clients can be greeted personally and introduced to other people. Giving people something to do also helps: 'Help yourself to a cup of tea', 'There are some books and leaflets on the table if you'd like to look at them till everyone has arrived'. Ensure that anyone with special needs has appropriate facilities and assistance (e.g. with mobility or hearing loops).

Getting to Know Each Other

Knowing each person's name and something about them is the first step towards constructive groupwork because it helps them to feel valued as a member of the group, and is the beginning of openness and trust between members.

There are many ways of going about this, some of which are as follows:[6]

Introduction in pairs. Ask each person to sit next to someone he has not met before – one person in each pair then 'interviews' his partner. After a few minutes (the leader keeps the time) the partners swap roles and the other person is interviewed. Then, in turn, each member of the group introduces his partner by name and says something about him. You may like to remind people that no-one has to answer any questions if he does not wish to.

The leader could also suggest appropriate questions: in groups for prospective parents, that partners find out if this is the first baby, where the mother goes for antenatal check-ups, or where she is booked to have her baby; in a session to help people towards healthy eating and weight loss, that people find out whether their partners have tried slimming or dieting before, what methods they used, and if they found them helpful.

Name games. Group members sit in a circle and you, the leader, take an object, such as a pen, and hand it to the person on your left, saying 'My name is A and this is a pen'. You ask the person who now holds the pen to say 'My name is B and A says that this is a pen'. B then passes the pen to the person on his left, who says 'My name is C and B says that A says that this is a pen'. This continues until the pen gets back to the beginning. If group members forget someone's name, the rest of the group can prompt them. This helps to establish a cooperative and supportive atmosphere as well as helping people to learn each other's names. Any tension and embarrassment are relieved by laughing and ice is effectively broken.

At subsequent group meetings, it is often helpful to do a quick round of names at the beginning, e.g. 'Who would like to have a shot at naming every member of the group?' or 'I'm going to try to see if I can remember everyone's name'.

You may like to set the tone by suggesting how people are addressed, by first names or more formally by Mr, Mrs etc. The important thing is to encourage people to use whatever feels comfortable. 'My name is Ann Jones, and I'm happy for you to call me Ann if you like'.

Sharing initial feelings and expectations. People may be helped to relax if they know that others also feel nervous or shy. So ask 'What did you feel about coming here today? Did anyone feel nervous? Did anyone almost *not* come?' – this can open the way for people to express their anxieties. You can also encourage them to say why they have come to the meeting and what they expect to gain from it. It might help to ask members to complete a checklist, ticking statements that are true for them. Such statements could include:[7]

- I'm afraid I won't have anything to say.
- I'm afraid I'll talk too much.
- I'm worried I'll make a fool of myself.
- I'll be too embarrassed to join in.
- I'm afraid I might get upset.
- I'm afraid I may be bored.
- I want to meet other people in the same boat.
- I enjoy talking to others.
- I enjoy a good argument.
- I want to get out of the house.
- I want to go somewhere different.
- I enjoy listening to other people.

People can then compare their list with that of one or two other people, and then it may be helpful to share what has been discovered with the whole group.

Setting Ground Rules

People joining a group will have different expectations and assumptions about how the group will run. Problems may arise if these are not brought out in the open and clarified at the beginning. For example, people may assume that what they say in a group will be treated confidentially, then be upset if they find that another member did not realize this and had discussed the issue elsewhere. Or some members may expect the group leader to take all the responsibility for organizing the group, and feel let down if they later discover that the leader expects them to do some of the work.

To prevent these difficulties, it is often helpful to establish a clear 'contract' or 'set of ground rules'. So early on in the life of a group members need the opportunity to explore their expectations, and reach agreement, about issues such as:

- How members are expected to behave in the group. For example, is smoking allowed?
- Are any rules and sanctions to be set, for example about non-attendance at group meetings or whether members can join in if they arrive late?
- What is confidential to the group?
- Can new members join at any time? Or is the group 'closed' to new membership?
- How will the leader and the members exercise control in the group?
- Who has responsibility for the practical aspects of running the group, such as bringing the refreshments along or booking the room?

For example, in a self-help group, mutual rights and responsibilities will be agreed on the basis of equality of leader and clients. In reality the power balance will not be completely equal and a contract will help with power sharing. In a counselling group the power of the counsellor is much greater than that of the clients and the leader has a duty to respect the members and to promote their autonomy.

Discussion Skills

It is a fallacy to believe that leading a discussion will just happen by putting a group of people together and saying 'Let's discuss ...'. Discussion needs planning and preparation, and there are many ways of triggering it off and providing structures which will help everyone to participate. Some of these are as follows.

Trigger Materials

Discussion can be triggered by providing a focus, preferably a controversial one. This can simply be a question ('What do you think about the decision to close the cottage hospital?'), or it might be a leaflet, a poster, a videotape, or an item in a newspaper or magazine ('What do you think the makers of this cigarette are trying to convey in this advertisement?'). Choose something that people are likely to have strong views about.

Some health promotion videos are specially made as trigger materials, presenting situations for people to talk about. Helpful notes for group leaders often accompany such videos.

Brainstorms

This is a useful way to open up a subject and collect everyone's ideas. Ask an open question to which there is no single right answer ('Why do people drink?', 'What do you feel you need to know before your baby is born?'). Accept every suggestion, without comment or criticism, and write them down in a list on a flip-chart or blackboard. Ask the group not to start discussing the ideas until everybody has finished. You can make your own suggestions and write them down along with everyone else's.

In this way all members' contributions are equally valued and everyone has a chance to participate. Encourage shy members by asking 'Anything else?' and allowing silent pauses while people think.

Then you can set the group to work by asking them to put the ideas into categories, and to identify the key features of each category. For example, people might categorize reasons for drinking into a 'constructive' category ('It helps me to socialize', 'It helps me to relax, to feel good') and an 'escape' category ('I can forget my problems', 'It stops me from feeling upset').

Rounds

A 'round' is a way of giving everyone an equal chance to participate. You invite each group member, in turn round the circle, to make a brief statement. You may like to start the round yourself or to join in when your turn comes in the circle. For example, ask everyone to make a brief statement about one of the following:

'My first feelings when I knew I was pregnant were . . .'
'What I think about jogging is . . .'
'The main reason why I can't lose weight is . . .'
'The thing which has helped me most is . . .'

There are four essential rules for successful rounds, which must be explained, and gently enforced if necessary. These are:

- no interruptions until each person has finished his statement;
- no comments on anybody's contribution until the full round is completed (i.e. no discussions, praise, interpretation, criticism or I-think-that-too type of remark);
- anyone can choose not to participate. Give permission, clearly and emphatically, that anyone who does not want to make a statement can just say 'pass'. This is very important for reinforcing the principle of voluntary participation.
- it does not matter if two or more people in the round say the same thing. People should stick to saying what they had intended to say even if someone else has said it already; they do not have to think of something different.

Rounds are also useful ways of beginning and ending sessions. For example:

'One thing I've put into practice since last week is . . .'
'The main thing I've got from today's session is . . .'
'One thing I'm going to find out by next time we meet is . . .'

It's also a useful way of getting feedback. For example:

'One thing I really liked about today's session was . . .'
'One thing I didn't like about today's session was . . .'
'One thing I wish we'd done is . . .'

Buzz Groups

Buzz groups are small groups of two to six people who discuss questions or topics for short periods, usually about 10 minutes. It is especially useful for large groups to be divided up in this way, as it gives everyone more chance to talk. Divide the groups first of all, and then say what you would like each one to do ('Make a list of the times when you want a cigarette' or 'Talk about the things which you find helpful when you feel stressed'), and how long they have in which to do it. If you want people to share ideas with the rest of the group as a whole afterwards, it may be helpful to provide large sheets of paper and felt-tip pens, so that 'posters' can be put up for everyone to see and discuss.

Safe Revelations

Sometimes people may hesitate or refuse to say what they really feel for fear of looking silly, being embarrassed or getting upset. One way of overcoming this is to give everyone a piece of paper and ask them to write down, for example, what their biggest worries are, or what they really want to know. All the papers are then folded and put in a receptacle such as a waste-paper basket or a shopping bag. Each person in turn picks out one piece of paper and reads aloud what it says. Tell people not to say if they happen to pick out their own piece of paper, and that, of course, nobody needs to identify themselves as the author of any of the statements.

The aim is to find out the concerns of the group members in the security of anonymity. Make sure that everyone listens and does not comment until all the papers have been read out. Then you can discuss what was discovered.

Dealing with Difficulties

Group workers often find the prospect of group work daunting, and anticipate being unable to cope with problems. A way forward is to acknowledge and face these fears, and work out strategies of coping should the problem actually arise. Some common fears and possible strategies for coping are as follows.

Silence

Are you afraid that you may be left with your group in an awful silence? If so, remember that silence can be useful; it can be time which group members need to think. Silence often does not feel as threatening to group members as it may do to you. However, you may find it helpful to:

- run a group with a partner, so that you can help each other out if either of you gets stuck;

Planning a group meeting

1. **Identify a health promotion opportunity that you have encountered or are likely to encounter, where informal group work would be appropriate.**

   (For example, this could be a group of food handlers, a preretirement group, an antenatal group, a group of patients in hospital recovering from a heart attack, a stop-smoking group or a group for healthy eating and weight control.)

   Assume that your group consists of about 12 people who do not know each other, and that this is the first of several meetings.
   What do you think would be the best place, time and physical features of the meeting room?
   What are your aims for the first meeting?
   What are your objectives for your group members for the first meeting?

   Complete the following:
   At the end of the first meeting, each group member will
   1. . . . . . .
   2. . . . . . .
   3. . . . . . .
   etc. . . . . . .

2. **Make a plan for what you will do**

   - as people start to arrive;
   - to get people to know each other;
   - in the main part of the group meeting;
   - to round off the meeting at the end;
   - to evaluate whether you have achieved the objectives you set above.

- ensure thorough preparation, so that you have planned activities and questions. Write down a plan, and a list of questions to ask (e.g. at the end of a video) and don't be afraid to refer to it in front of the group;
- have a 'spare' activity ready to use if the reason for the discussion 'drying up' is that what you have planned does not seem to be working.

Disasters

Unexpected 'disasters' include such things as getting lost and arriving late, or finding that too few or too many people have turned up. There is no blueprint strategy to cope with the unexpected, but it will help if you acknowledge what has happened and share it with your group ('I'm delighted that so many of you have come along, but I wasn't expecting such a crowd, so we may be a bit squashed this week'). Also share your plans for dealing with the 'disaster' ('I'm going to try to get a bigger room next time' . . . 'I'm going to start 10 minutes late'). Sharing the problem and enlisting cooperation can have the positive benefit of encouraging mutual support; *not* sharing it can leave your group feeling angry.

Distractions

Distractions can take many forms: noises outside the room (e.g. road works), noises inside the room (e.g. crying babies, coughing), people coming in late or leaving early, or interruptions. Distractions can also be caused by group members themselves, for example by becoming very angry or upset.

As a rule, there are three choices for you as group leader:

Ignore them. This is seldom a good idea, as it leaves people wondering whether you are going to do anything, and this in itself is a distraction.

Acknowledge and accept them. This is generally best with things you cannot change ('I know the traffic is really noisy, but there's nothing we can do about it, so I think we'll just have to put up with it').

Do something about them. It is preferable to involve the group in the decision ('As so many of you found it difficult to get here by 2 pm, shall we start at 2.15 next week?' 'Do you think it would be helpful if you took it in turns to look after the babies in the next room?').

If someone is showing emotion, such as crying, acknowledge it ('I can see that you're upset'), offer reassurance that it is OK to show emotion ('there's no need to be embarrassed ... we don't mind if you cry ...'), and offer the opportunity to talk about it ('Would you like to tell us what is upsetting you?') or to take some time away from the group, accompanied by you or someone else ('Shall we go outside for a few minutes?'). Do not put any pressure on people in distress. Help them to do what they want to do, whether it is crying, talking, keeping silent, staying, leaving or being by themselves. But do not ignore a show of emotion; ignoring it will only cause tension and embarrassment.

Difficult behaviour

How group members behave can pose difficulties for the leader. There are two broad categories of difficult behaviour: non-participation and talking too much. The latter category takes many forms, such as the know-all who always chips in with all the 'answers', people who launch into long stories, people who interrupt, people who do not let other people get a word in edgeways, people who talk off the point, people who always disagree and people who always crack jokes.

A starting point for dealing with these difficulties is to try to think *why* people behave like this. Are they nervous, threatened, worried? Are they desperately in need of attention? If you can deal with the underlying cause, the situation is likely to improve. Secondly, note that people often change their behaviour as they get to know others and feel more comfortable in a group. Thirdly, try getting people to work in pairs or small groups, which can help quiet members to join in and give others a break from the constant talker. Fourthly, use structures in your discussion such as 'rounds' or make a point of asking for other people's opinions ('Would someone else like to say what he thinks?' 'Would you like to give us your opinion, Ann?'). Finally, it may be necessary to confront the difficult person (not in front of the rest of the group!). For example, you could say: 'I've noticed that you contribute a great deal to the group discussions. That makes me concerned about whether other people are getting enough chance to talk. I'd like to suggest that you keep your comments to just a couple of sentences. Would you feel OK about doing that?'

When to Use Group Work

See also Stage 3 – Decide the Best Way of Achieving Your Aims in Chapter 5 on The Basic Planning and Evaluation Process)

Health promoters can be unsure about when it is appropriate to use a group work approach to health promotion. The following guidance can help you to decide.

We suggest that group work is appropriate when your plans fulfil the following criteria.

- You have looked critically at what other health promotion opportunities exist, and you have concluded that group work is needed to meet the particular needs of specific groups of people;
- You have evidence that group work is effective for this particular client group, for example there is evidence that group work is an effective approach to the education of young mothers;[8]
- You are going to be working with a defined group of people over a period of time, which will allow the group to build up trust and be able to help each other, for example a group of prospective parents, a 'self-help group' of patients who are recovering after heart attacks, or people who have been diagnosed as HIV positive;
- You have access to a comfortable, private and relaxed environment in which to run the group, for example in a community centre;
- You have access to support and supervision in order to provide you with support when you need it and help you to develop your group work.

In special circumstances group work may be particularly helpful. Examples are:

- you are planning to work with people who are already in a close-knit small group, and possibly already used to group work, for example a group of adolescents who are in a residential drug rehabilitation setting;
- you are starting a long-term relationship with a number of people who have a common interest, and wish to develop an equal and respectful partnership with them, for example a group of mental health patients who have recently moved into a group home as part of 'Care in the Community';
- you want to work with a particular ethnic minority community but you do not come from that group yourself and are faced with issues of differences in culture and language. In this case, it could be helpful to run a group to look at health issues in partnership with a link worker or health advocate who can offer culturally sensitive help and skills in translation and interpretation.

There are times when it may *not* be advisable to embark on group work, or to continue to run an existing group. These may include situations when:

- you have not consulted with prospective clients to establish their needs;
- group members are from such a diverse range of backgrounds that they have little in common and feel uncomfortable with one another;
- the cultural background of the group will make it difficult for them to adapt to group work, for example older people who are uncomfortable with informal group work methods, or groups from ethnic minority communities;

- the group will only meet once or twice, which means that people will not have long enough to get to know and trust one another;
- the membership of a group is not stable and members are constantly leaving or joining;
- your aim is solely to transmit information, so that a talk with questions-and-answers would be better;
- the aim of the group is to encourage a change towards a healthier lifestyle but the people concerned do not have the opportunity to make changes because of lack of money, skills, support or facilities;
- you do not have suitable accommodation for meetings, for example you only have access to a large, tiered lecture theatre;
- you do not yet have the skills or confidence to embark on group work, nor access to training and support.

Case study 13.1	Good practice in group work.

45 Cope Street in Nottingham is a health project which works with mothers between 16 and 25 years. It is complementary to the existing health services which provide antenatal and postnatal education. The aim of the project is to work in partnership with parents to improve the health of the child and the family. It is based on the principle that people learn best from others who have been in the same situation as they are. The group work is designed to be self-empowering and stresses the importance of self-confidence as an outcome. Evaluation of the intervention was to do with increased self-confidence and improved health.

Source: Rowe, J & Mahoney P (1993)[9]

PRACTICE POINTS

- Group work covers a range of activities, and in health promotion groups are useful mainly for raising awareness of health issues, mutual support, social action, education and group counselling.

- You need to develop skills of group leadership, appreciate the range of leadership styles, understand the roles and responsibilities of group leaders and members and the way in which groups develop over time.

- Thorough planning and preparation are essential for successful group work, which includes having a clear rationale and aims, and paying attention to recruitment, venue, facilities, resources, timing and evaluation.

- If you run groups, you will find it helpful to develop a range of skills and strategies for getting groups going, encouraging discussion and dealing with difficulties.

- Group work is not always the most appropriate health promotion method to use; you need to be sure that it is right for your particular clients and circumstances.

Recommended Reading

A Comprehensive Introduction to Group Theory and Practice

➤ Johnson D W & Johnson F P (1991) *Joining Together: Group Theory and Group Skills*. London: Prentice Hall.

On the Working of Groups

➤ Baron R S, Kerr N & Miller N (1991) *Group Process, Group Decision, Group Action*. Buckingham: Open University Press.

An approach to group work practice based on the idea that groups can discover and utilize the resources (current and potential) which exist within the group for the benefit of the members:

➤ Douglas T (1993) *A Theory of Groupwork Practice*. Basingstoke: Macmillan.

Groups from the Viewpoint of the Group Members

➤ Douglas T (1995) *Survival in Groups: The Basics of Group Membership*. Buckingham: Open University Press.

An Introduction to Team Theory and to Activities which will Help Build Teams (Groups of People who Focus on a Task and Accomplish Shared Goals) in Health Promotion Settings:

➤ Rolls L (1992) *Team Development: A Manual of Facilitation for Health Educators and Health Promoters*. London: Health Education Authority.

Notes and References

1 Short courses on working with groups are often run by health promotion departments in health authorities or trusts.

2 Handy C B (1985) *Understanding Organisations*. Chapter 6. Harmondsworth: Penguin Business Library.

3 Tuckman B W (1965) Developmental sequence in small groups. *Psychological Bulletin* **63**, 384–399.

4 Belbin R M (1981) *Management Teams Why They Succeed or Fail*. Oxford: Butterworth Heinemann.

5 We acknowledge, with thanks, that much of the material in this section is derived from a checklist produced by Louise Walker and Margaret Douglas, Health Promotion Officers, Bristol & Weston Health Authority, August 1990.

6 There are many more 'games' for group leaders in:

Brandes D and Phillips H (1978) *Gamesters Handbook*. London: Hutchinson.

Brandes D (1983) *Gamesters Two*. London: Hutchinson.

7 Adapted, with kind permission, from:

Open University (1983) *Community Education Group Notes*, p 10. Buckingham: Open University Press.

8 Mackeith P, Philipson R & Rowe A (1991) *45 Cope Street: Young Mothers Learning through Group Work: an Evaluation Report*. Nottingham Community Health, Old Basford Health Centre, Nottingham.

9 Rowe J & Mahoney P (1993) *Parent Education: Guidance for Purchasers and Providers*. London: Health Education Authority.

14 Helping People Towards Healthier Living

SUMMARY

This chapter is about helping people towards healthier lifestyles and changing their health-related behaviour. In the first section we look at models of the process of changing health-related behaviour. In the next section we discuss how to work towards client self-empowerment before outlining strategies for increasing self-awareness, clarifying values and changing attitudes. Strategies for decision-making and for changing behaviour follow. The chapter ends with principles for using strategies effectively and summarizes key points. It includes exercises, case studies and quizzes.

In this chapter we look at the competencies you need when you are helping people to change their health-related behaviour and lifestyles. Much health behaviour appears to have developed without conscious decision-making; it has 'just happened' in response to individual and group circumstances and external events. Active control of behaviour is different because it involves committing time and effort (yours and your client's) to understanding the factors which influence health choices and behaviour, and to taking considered decisions and actions.

However, it has to be accepted that people may prefer to carry on with behaviour which seems 'unhealthy' to you. To a client, it may not seem 'unhealthy' as the benefits outweigh the risks. Respect for people's right to their own points of view and their right to choose are fundamental to establishing relationships between health promoters and their clients.

See the first section of Chapter 10 on Exploring Relationships with Clients for further discussion.

On the other hand, you also have to consider that people's right to individual freedom of choice has to be balanced against the effect of that choice on other people; for example, choosing to drink and drive could affect many others as well as the driver.

Furthermore, choosing a 'healthy' behaviour does not automatically lead to practising it. Changes such as taking more exercise, practising relaxation, going for screening tests, wearing ear protectors in noisy surroundings, eating different foods and stopping smoking are all hard work, and these changes in themselves may be stressful. Social or economic circumstances may also prevent people from carrying out new health behaviours, even if they would like to.

However, despite these limitations, it can be very rewarding to help people to look at their own motivations, beliefs, values and attitudes, and to make and carry out decisions which will lead to improved health and well-being. We first turn to the theory of behaviour change and how you can use it in your practice.

Models of Behaviour Change

Models are a simplified way of describing reality. Health-related behaviour change is a very complex process involving a web of psychological, social and environmental factors. Models provide frameworks and routes to help you make sense of a situation, know where to start and what to do. So using behaviour change models will help you to clarify your thinking and make your practice more effective. Several models have been used by health promoters[1] and suggestions are made for further reading at the end of the chapter. Here, we describe two useful models: the Health Action Model and the Stages of Change Model.

The Health Action Model

The Health Action Model (HAM) was devised by Tones[2] and emphasizes the important influence of self-esteem on behaviour. It assumes that someone with high self-esteem and a positive self-concept is likely to be more motivated towards ways of healthier living. Furthermore, it suggests that people with low self-esteem may feel that they have limited control over their behaviour and that they are victims of bad luck or fate. Many health promoters, particularly those working in the field of drugs, have used this model, through concentrating on boosting peoples' self-esteem and their skills in resisting peer group pressure. According to this model, learning 'life skills' such as how to be assertive may be essential before someone is ready to change their lifestyle.

The HAM identifies a variety of psychological, social and environmental influences which research and practice have shown to be important determinants of a number of health-related choices. The model offers an explanation about how these influences work. It suggests that health decisions and actions are influenced by our beliefs, our values, our motivation, our expectations of how other people will react to our actions, and our self-concept and self-esteem (Fig. 14.1).

The HAM is concerned with empowerment – with increasing the control people have over their lives. It suggests that health promotion should not just focus on the provision of information and the pros and cons of particular behaviours. More important than this is helping people to feel good about themselves, to value themselves, and to acquire the skills to assert themselves. Equally important is the provision of environmental circumstances which facilitate healthy choices, rather than acting as barriers. And at the macro level, policy needs to address basic environmental determinants of health such as poverty and deprivation.

Stages of Change Model

A helpful way of thinking about how people make health-related decisions and change their behaviour is to consider all the stages in the process, and how people move from one stage to another. A useful model, rooted in extensive research and integrating the understanding drawn from a range of psychological theories has been developed by Prochashka and DiClemente.[4] Research shows that strategies based on this model are effective for changing a range of health-related behaviours, such as alcohol and drug abuse, smoking, taking more exercise, weight control and accepting the offer of various types of screening.

Fig 14.1   **The Health Action Model[3]**

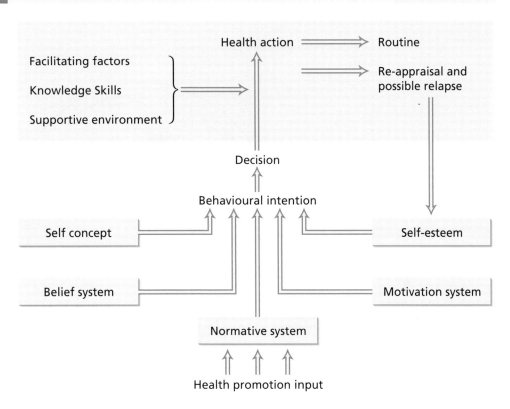

The model identifies a number of stages which a person can go through during the process of behaviour change. It takes a holistic approach, integrating a range of factors such as the role of personal responsibility and choices, and the impact of social and environmental forces that set very real limits on the individual potential for change. It provides a framework for a wide range of potential interventions by health promoters, as well as describing the process through which individuals go when acting as their own agents of change, for example, when someone stops smoking without any professional support. The main stages identified in the model are set out in Fig. 14.2.

The key to the model is to regard the cycle in the centre as a series of stages people go through in the process of changing health behaviour, such as stopping smoking, taking more exercise regularly or adopting healthier eating. A crucial point is that the cycle can be thought of as a 'revolving door', because people usually go round more than once before emerging to a permanently changed state. It is also important to recognize that some people may never get as far as entering the revolving door.

Pre-contemplation stage. The stage which precedes entry into the change cycle is referred to as 'pre-contemplation'. At this stage a person has no awareness of a need for change, or does not accept it, and no motivation to change habits or lifestyle.

Fig 14.2   **Stages of changing health behaviour (Adapted from Neesham C, 1993 and Prochaska J & DiClemente C, 1984)**

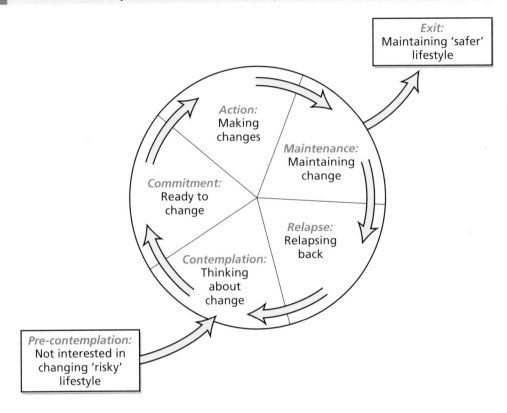

Contemplation stage. This stage is the way in to the 'revolving door' cycle of stages of change. People enter this stage when they have enough motivation to contemplate seriously changing their habits – the entry stage is therefore called 'contemplation'.

Commitment stage. If people continue to progress round the cycle they enter the 'commitment' stage in which they make a serious decision to change the particular habit concerned, such as stopping smoking or taking more exercise.

Action stage. They next enter the 'action' stage as they actively begin to change the habit.

Maintenance stage. At this stage people struggle to maintain the change and may experiment with a variety of coping strategies.

Relapse stage. Although individuals experience the satisfaction of a changed lifestyle for varying amounts of time, most of them cannot exit from the revolving door the first time around. Typically, they relapse back, for example they start smoking again. Of great importance, however, is that they do not stop there, but move back into the contemplation stage, engaging in the cycle all over again. Prochaska and DiClemente have found that on average successful former smokers take three revolutions of change before they find the way to become fully free of the habit, and exit from the revolving door.

Exit stage. This is the stage where people are settled into a changed behaviour, such as stopping smoking permanently.

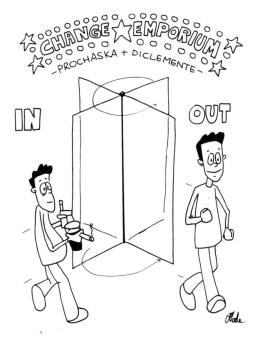

By identifying where clients are in the stages of change, health promoters can tailor their interventions to the particular stage of change a person has reached. For example, behaviour change strategies are appropriate for someone in the 'action' or 'maintenance' stages. Education and awareness-raising is appropriate for someone in the 'pre-contemplation' stage. Working for client self-empowerment is appropriate for someone in the 'contemplation' stage[6] and strategies to help people to make decisions are useful for those in the 'commitment' stage.

This model of change has been used as the basis of the 'Helping People Change' training programme, provided by the Health Education Authority's Primary Health Care Unit, for primary health care workers[7]. The model is particularly useful in primary health care settings, because a patient's needs can be assessed and appropriate advice or information be given, within the constraints of a few minutes consultation. Research, including controlled trials, into the effectiveness of this approach, is currently taking place in England and elsewhere, and the application of the model has been the subject of challenge and debate as it grows in its application to the everyday work of health promoters.[8]

We now turn to the strategies and skills you require to help people to change. These strategies relate to two of the health promotion aims we discussed in See Chapter 5 Chapter 5: 'self-empowering' and 'changing attitudes and behaviour'.

Working for Client Self-empowerment

Making health choices and carrying them out can bring benefits. These are not only the benefits that go with a healthier lifestyle (such as improved health and well-being), but also increased self-esteem from the feeling of taking active control over a part of life, such as being in control of the smoking habit rather than cigarettes being in control: in other words, making a positive choice about health can be a self-empowering process.

There are a number of different ways of working towards self-empowerment. Using the Stages of Change model is empowering, because people can follow their own progress. It encourages them to try to get to the next stage of the cycle, and not to see change as all or nothing. Also the recognition that relapse is not the end of the world helps people to feel better about themselves[9]. Behaviour change messages can be tailor-made for individuals, for example through providing clients with access to specially designed computer programmes[10]. Other methods include group work and experiential learning, individual counselling and therapy, and advocacy. We consider them all in the following sections, except therapy which is beyond the scope of this book. (In any case, unless you are a mental health specialist, most people you work with probably do not need in-depth therapy but could benefit from counselling.)

The process of empowering people involves modifying the way people feel about themselves through improving their self-awareness and self-esteem. It involves helping them to think critically about their values and beliefs and build up their own values and beliefs system. This is in contrast to traditional teaching which operates largely in the hope that the 'right' attitudes and values will be 'caught' by learners. In the next section, we outline some strategies you may find useful for helping clients to become more self-aware (having greater insight into, and understanding of, themselves, their attitudes, motivations and feelings), and to help them clarify their values and attitudes.

Strategies for Increasing Self-awareness, Clarifying Values and Changing Attitudes

See Chapter 13

Many of the strategies which are useful for increasing self-awareness, clarifying values, developing beliefs systems and changing attitudes (i.e. for the 'contemplation' stage of change) are designed for group work. However, some of them can be adapted for health promoters to use in one-to-one situations, to give clients to use by themselves.

See Chapter 12

They all use the principle of experiential learning which emphasizes the importance of personal experience as a source of learning[11]. It encourages 'active' learning through undertaking exercises and other activities designed, for example, to increase self-awareness or aid decision-making. Some experiential learning methods are now described.

Ranking or Categorizing

Ranking is a way of analysing an issue in order to distinguish the relative importance of different aspects. It is therefore useful for clarifying values. (For example, in the exercise in Chapter 1 'What does being healthy mean to you?' readers are asked to rank aspects of 'being healthy'. Health is a value and this exercise is designed to help readers to clarify which aspects of health they value most.)

Another approach to increasing self-awareness and values clarification is to generate a list of items, and then code them into different categories. The following exercise illustrates this approach; it is designed to raise awareness of the link between enjoyment and health.

Exercise 14.1   **Enjoyment and health**

Quickly list as many things as you can think of that you enjoy doing. Write them down the left-hand side of a piece of paper. On the right-hand side, code each item according to the following categories.

£ – any items that involve spending money.
A – any items that you do alone.
P – any items you do with other people.
R – any items that involve some kind of risk.
F – any items that help to keep you fit.
C – any items that involve creativity.
D – any items that involve consumption of drugs (including alcohol and tobacco).
H+ – any items which positively affect your health.
H– – any items which negatively affect your health.

Items may be coded in more than one category. For example, if one of the things you enjoy is going out to the pub for a drink, this may be coded £, P and D, as well as H+ and/or H–.

What have you learned about enjoyment and health through doing this exercise?

Using Polarized Views

This is a way of getting people to clarify their views about a particular issue. Views about the issue are polarized – that is, phrased to reflect extremely different views. For example, if the issue was 'Is jogging good for you?', polarized views could be summed up as 'Jogging kills people and only very fit athletes should do it' or 'Jogging is very beneficial to health and all people would be fitter if they took it up'. Examples of polarized views can be described by the group leader or taken from writings which express opposite views.

The group leader may ask people to work in pairs, with each individual acting as if he fully adopted one of the points of view for the duration of the exercise, whatever his personal opinions may be. First, each person writes down all the arguments he can think of which support his position, without discussing it with his partner at this stage. After a few minutes, the partners are asked to start arguing the case, usually for about 15 minutes. The leader then lists the points in favour of each view by asking each pair in turn to contribute one point, until all the points have been collected. She then asks the group to comment on what they have learnt. In this way, members of the group can consider a whole range of arguments, which helps them to understand other people's points of view, tolerate differences of opinion, clarify their own views, and perhaps see the issue in a new light.

Another example of a values clarification exercise using the polarized arguments approach is the exercise 'Analysing Your Philosophy of Health Promotion' in Chapter 3, where readers are asked to consider arguments for and against two polarized views about the aim of health promotion.

Using a Values Continuum

This is an extension of the polarized argument technique. It helps people to understand the spread of opinion on a particular issue and to clarify where they stand.

The leader describes two extremes of opinion and asks the group to imagine that these can be represented by two points, A and B, joined by a straight line. With a small group this line can be across a room; with a large group it could be drawn on the blackboard. The group members are then asked to mark or place themselves at a point along the line that best reflects their own view. For instance, in the jogging example discussed above, pro-joggers place themselves at one end, with the most extreme at the farthest point, people with moderate views stand around the middle, and the most ardent anti-jogger stands at the other end. The leader asks each person to state his views briefly as he takes up his position. Other people are asked not to interrupt or comment until everyone has taken up a position, or passed if they choose not to participate.

This technique can encourage a more detailed discussion of the range of possible options than the polarised argument technique. On the other hand, if everyone seems moderate, a better discussion may be stimulated by the polarized argument technique. The values continuum technique is used in the last task of the exercise 'Analysing Your Philosophy of Health Promotion' in Chapter 3.

Using Role Play

Role play generally means taking on the role of another person in a specified situation, and acting out what that other person might do and say in that situation. This helps people to understand what it feels like to be in another person's shoes. For example, adults role playing an unemployed young person may be helped to understand feelings of rejection and boredom. Health promoters role playing non-English-speaking patients visiting a clinic may be helped to understand how those patients feel, especially if the role play is given added authenticity by using a foreign language which the health promoters do not speak.

It is also possible to role play oneself in a new situation. This is a useful way of practising a new skill or rehearsing for a future event. For example, patients can role play a consultation with a doctor in order to practise the skills of presenting their health problems to doctors.

For an example of a role-play exercise, see 'Skills of Patient Education' in Chapter 12.

Playing Games

By games we mean structured activities, usually for a group of people, but sometimes for one or two people only. Games are useful for meeting a variety of aims. One is to help people to get to know each other ('ice-breakers'), such as

See Chapter 13 the name games described in the section on Getting Groups Going in Chapter 13. Other games are devised to help people to trust each other, to communicate more openly or to increase self-awareness.[12]

For example, games can be used to help people to identify 'irrational beliefs'. Irrational beliefs are misconceptions which hinder people from achieving their goals. They are usually expressed in terms of 'must', 'should', or 'ought'. There are three major irrational beliefs:[13]

- 'I must win everybody's approval otherwise I am worthless'.
- 'Other people must treat me exactly how I want them to (and if they don't they must be blamed and punished)'.
- 'Life must give me everything I want and nothing I don't want'.

These beliefs lead to self-defeating thinking and this in turn can affect health. It can lead to health-related behaviour with destructive consequences, such as emotional disorders, heavy drinking and physical ailments. The quiz in Exercise 14.2 is an example of a game; this one aims to help you to identify your own irrational beliefs.

Strategies for Decision-Making

As a health promoter, it is likely that you will often be involved in counselling with the aim of helping people to make a choice, such as which treatment to have, whether an elderly person should stay put or move into residential accommodation, whether to have a blood test for HIV or how to select healthy foods in particular circumstances. Research has shown that brief counselling sessions can be an effective way of bringing about health-related behaviour change.[14]

See Chapter 10 Basic skills of counselling to help people to make decisions (the 'commitment' stage of change) are the same ones we discussed in Chapter 10: understanding non-verbal communication, listening, helping people to talk, asking questions and obtaining feedback.[15] We do not discuss counselling in depth here, but include suggestions for further study in at the end of this chapter and in reference[16].

See Chapter 5 There are at least five stages involved[17]. These stages may seem familiar to you because counselling involves a framework of planning and evaluating similar to the one we used in Chapter 5.

Stage 1. Identify the need and create the climate

Carl Rogers (a 'founding father' of counselling) has identified the qualities necessary for a counsellor to establish a climate in which a client can 'open up'.[18] These are warmth, openness, genuineness, empathy and unconditional positive regard. Unconditional positive regard is the quality of totally respecting the worth and dignity of a person, irrespective of whether you like the person or agree with their views or behaviour.

The practical aspects of creating the climate include ensuring that you will not be interrupted and cannot be overheard, that you have sufficient time, and that you are comfortably seated in chairs of the same height, with the counsellor adopting an open posture and making direct eye contact when appropriate.

Exercise 14.2   Beliefs Quiz

Look at the following statements and put a tick in the appropriate column:

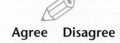

Agree   Disagree

1.   **I believe in the saying that
     'A leopard cannot change his spots'**
2.   **I believe that 'wait and see' is a good philosophy for life**
3.   **I want everyone to like me**
4.   **I usually put off important decisions**

Now identify your rational beliefs and your irrational beliefs (misconceptions):

Q 1. If you agreed with this statement you may believe that the past has a lot to do with determining the present and that people are largely unchangeable. 'I'm made that way.' The idea that you are no good at playing sports, for example, can be used to avoid trying out new behaviour and learning the skills necessary to participate in a sport. The truth is that people who take risks, experiment and work on things, generally find that they can become reasonably competent at most of the things they attempt. (Not necessarily perfect, but good enough.)

Q 2. If you agreed with this statement you may believe that human happiness can be achieved by hoping for the best – and waiting to see what happens. This belief could result in you becoming merely a spectator in life – watching television every night and somnolent on a sun-lounger for the whole of your holidays. Getting more actively involved could be more satisfying and actually provide you with more energy. If you feel too 'burnt out', now may be the time to take a close look at how you are managing your life and make some changes.

Q 3. If you agree with this statement you may only believe you are as good as other people think you are. Because of this you may feel worthless if, despite your efforts, people don't seem to like you. Having the approval of others is pleasant, but in order to run our own lives we shall almost certainly have to do some things which some people do not like. Work on giving yourself the approval you deserve.

Q 4. If you agreed with this statement you may believe that life's problems will go away if you avoid them. Don't waste your time hoping that things will work out – make them.

Stage 2. Explore the needs and the concerns

Through giving full attention and actively listening, by encouraging the client to talk and by asking questions, the counsellor begins to establish trust and to enable the client to move from superficial issues to deeper needs and concerns.

Stage 3. Help the client to set goals and identify options

Having gained a new perspective on the issues and concerns, it becomes possible for the client to identify goals and ways these might be achieved. The counsellor may help the client to identify themes or to get a clearer vision of the future through asking key questions such as:

'How would you feel if …?'
'If things were exactly how you wanted them to be, how would it be different from now …?'
'Have you ever felt like that on other occasions …?'

The counsellor may also provide the client with information in order to establish options:

'If you do X what's likely to happen is …'
'If you do Y the chances are that …'
'You might find it helpful to consider that …' and so on.

Stage 4. Help the client to decide which option to choose

The important thing about this stage is that the choice must be the client's, not the counsellor's. Making decisions – that is, choosing between alternative options – is a highly complex process. It involves:

- weighing up the pros and cons of the alternative options;
- considering the likely consequences of pursuing each alternative;
- deciding which is the best alternative.

If the client is reluctant to commit himself to a decision, then both parties need to consider whether it is worth undertaking further work at stages two and three.

If the client chooses an alternative which the counsellor feels won't work, she should nevertheless back the client's choice and help the client to develop an action plan (knowing that if it doesn't work, the door is still open for exploring other options).

Stage 5. Help the client to develop an action plan

See the next section on Strategies for Changing Behaviour.

Having made a decision, the client now needs to think about turning that decision into action. He may need to identify coping strategies and sources of support. Once an action plan has been agreed, the final details are to set a review date and to clarify how progress will be monitored.

| Example 14.1 | **Counselling about a health choice** |

A health visitor has the task of helping a mother to decide what to do about having her baby vaccinated. The stages could be:

Stages 1 and 2. Identify and explore the need

For example, is the mother worried about having the child vaccinated at all, or is it just the whooping cough vaccination which is worrying? Is it *when* to have the child vaccinated, or *if?*

Stage 3. Help the client to set goals and establish options

For example, the parent may identify the goal of her child having the best possible chance of staying healthy.

The options might be: no vaccinations at all, some vaccinations, or all the vaccinations?

Stage 4. Help the client to decide which option to choose

- Weigh up the pros and cons – the health visitor provides unbiased information on the risks from catching each disease compared with the risks of having the vaccinations.
- Consider the likely consequences of pursuing each alternative: for the child, in terms of health risk; for the parent, in terms of anxiety, guilt and responsibility; for other people, in terms of spreading the diseases.

Stage 5. Help the client to develop an action plan

For example, the mother may decide to go ahead with the vaccination programme, but also to join a mother's group, in order to get support from other mothers facing the same anxieties and decisions. The health visitor suggests to the mother that she keeps a record of the vaccinations for future reference, and provides her with a record card for her child. They set a date for the first vaccination.

Strategies for Changing Behaviour

Having made a choice, people may need considerable help to carry their decision through into the 'action' stage of change. A number of techniques developed from behavioural psychology are useful, and the philosophy behind them (that people are responsible for their own behaviour and are capable of exercising control over it) is as important as the techniques themselves.[19] A variety of material has been developed to help people to change different aspects of their behaviour, such as stopping smoking, controlling drinking, changing eating habits and taking up exercise.[20] Some useful techniques are as follows.

Self-monitoring

Self-monitoring is keeping a detailed and precise account, often in the form of a diary, of behaviour which is to be changed. Its aim is to help people to analyse their pattern of behaviour and become fully aware of what they are doing, which is a starting point for gaining control. Secondly, the 'diary' provides a baseline against which progress can be checked.

Self-monitoring involves answering questions such as:

- how frequently does the problem occur?
- when the problem occurs, what else is happening both externally (in the environment), and internally (in thoughts and feelings)?
- what event leads up to the problem?
- what happens afterwards: the consequences?

Example 14.2 is a Smoker's Diary.

Example 14.2   **A smoker's diary**

Day . . . . (Complete one of these charts every day)

Each time you smoke a cigarette, note down in the columns:

1. The time.
2. How urgent your craving for a cigarette is, on a scale of 1–10 (1, very little craving; 10, extremely high craving).
3. Where you smoke the cigarette.
4. Whether you are alone or who you are with.
5. Do you smoke it with drinks (coffee, tea, alcohol)?
6. Do you smoke it after a meal?
7. What else are you doing at the time (e.g. chatting, reading the paper, working, talking on the phone)?
8. Why did you decide to smoke this cigarette?
9. What do you feel about it afterwards?

Time	Craving	Where	Who with	With drinks	After meal	Doing what	Why	Afterwards

Total number of cigarettes smoked today = _____

Identifying Costs, Benefits and Rewards

The cost of changing behaviour can be considerable, involving deprivation of 'crutches', such as cigarettes, and pleasures, such as eating and drinking, or there may be a heavy price to pay in terms of time, effort and perhaps money. So it is helpful to identify the benefits clearly, and set up a system of rewards to encourage perseverance.

Benefits may be long-term, such as better health or increased life-expectancy. They may be abstract ('It will prove I've got will-power') or in other people's interests ('for the family's sake'). Important though these benefits may be, it is also necessary to find immediate, short-term rewards which people genuinely enjoy, such as small treats.

Setting Targets and Evaluating Progress

Targets should be realistic rather than idealistic. Losing an average of one pound in weight a week is realistic for most people; losing a stone in a month usually is not. People may have unrealistic hopes and expectations about what can be achieved, which lead to disappointment and a sense of failure when the target has not been met.

In order to evaluate progress, it is necessary to keep a record of behaviour so that achievements can be seen clearly. Progress should be assessed once the 'new' behaviour has been given a fair trial perhaps for two or three weeks, although short-term reviews ('How have I done today?') can also be useful.

If the target is not being achieved, possible reasons must be looked for and changes made. For example:

- Is the target too difficult? Should it be lowered?
- Are the rewards too distant? Is there a more immediate reward which could be more encouraging?
- Is there an unforeseen crisis or illness? If so, encouragement to continue self-monitoring and to look on the setback as a learning experience may be needed.
- Are other people unhelpful? More strategies to cope with the negative influence of other people may be needed.
- Are there other problems which require help, such as learning to cope with anxiety or stress?

Devising Coping Strategies

Changing behaviour can mean coping with numerous difficulties, for at least a short period of time, until the new behaviour becomes a normal part of life. Someone who is stopping smoking has to cope with problems such as the craving he feels, the need to put something in his mouth, not knowing what to do with his hands, doing without his accustomed 'tension-reliever' in moments of stress, and resisting the offer of a cigarette.

People adopt a wide variety of coping strategies, and it is often useful to get a group to share their ideas about what helps them to cope.[21] The list of strategies here is certainly not exhaustive:

- finding a substitute, such as substituting chewing gum or herbal cigarettes for the real thing, or eating low-calorie foods instead of high-calorie ones;
- changing some routines and habits which are closely associated with the 'problem' behaviour. Examples are drinking tea or fruit juice instead of coffee, because coffee is closely associated with cigarettes;
- making it difficult to carry on with the 'problem' behaviour, by, for example, keeping cigarettes in an inconvenient place, sitting in a no-smoking compartment, and deciding to restrict eating to mealtimes, not between meals.

What all these strategies have in common is that they require only a small step to achieve a large degree of help for self-control. Other strategies may be:

See Chapter 13 for further reading on self-help groups

■ getting support from other people in the same boat, who might be from a slimming group, an anti-smoking clinic, or a self-help group. Another helpful way of getting support is by linking with another person on the understanding that each may telephone or meet the other if either of them needs help;[22]

■ practising ways of responding to unhelpful social pressures, for example refusing the offer of a cigarette or a drink;

■ adopting a one-day-at-a-time approach. The prospect of the whole of the rest of life without a cigarette may be overwhelming, but the prospect of one day without one is far more tolerable. Even shorter time-spans may be helpful, such as putting off eating, drinking or smoking for just five minutes at a time;

■ learning relaxation techniques and other ways (such as exercise) of relieving stress. Simple relaxation routines which can be practised at any time and place can be helpful in coping with stressful moments when the 'old' reaction would have been to reach for a drink or a cigarette.

Case study 14.1	**Changing behaviour in practice**

Joan is divorced. She has a toddler who constantly wakes her at night. She has used various strategies, including trying to tire him out physically just before bedtime, keeping him up later, leaving toys for him to play with in the night, and playing with him herself in the night. She has started to have a few glasses of sherry in the evenings to help her to relax and now finds that she needs another sherry to help her get back to sleep after getting up in the night.

She goes to her doctor for help. He explains that the strategies she used to try to get her son to sleep do not work because they merely stimulate him and give him rewards (playing and getting attention from his mother) when he wakes up. He suggests that the toddler needs to learn to relax before he goes to bed. The doctor asks Joan if she knows anything which seems to help her child to relax, and using her suggestions they devise a suitable bedtime routine for Joan to try out.

Turning to Joan herself, the doctor asks how she has been coping and Joan responds that a few sherries in the evening helped at first but now she is worried that she may be relying too much on drinking to help her to cope. He then asks about her reasons for drinking. She has already identified that it helps her to cope; it makes her feel less anxious and 'strung up'. She says 'When I've had a hard day I deserve a drink … it helps me relax and forget my problems for a while'.

The doctor asks her to think of reasons why drink may not be the most helpful way to reward herself, help herself to relax or solve her problems. He suggests that she should think about alternatives, such as leisure activities. He tells her about a local mother-and-toddler group where she can meet other mothers in similar circumstances. He suggests that she keeps a drinker's diary so that they can together find out more about her drinking patterns and help her to set limits on her drinking. He shows her an example of a drinker's diary and explains how to count each drink using standard measures. Joan agrees to fill it in every time she has a drink during the next fortnight.

Finally, he asks Joan to come back and see him in two weeks' time to discuss whether the new routines are helping the toddler to sleep and to see what she has discovered from the suggestions he has made. He also arranges for the health visitor to visit Joan in a few days' time.

What strategies does the doctor use to help Joan with her problems? What other strategies could he have used?

Using Strategies Effectively

We have discussed a number of different strategies which you can use when you are trying to help clients to increase their self-awareness, clarify their values and beliefs, change their attitudes and behaviour and to maintain behaviour change, in other words to move them through the stages of change cycle. Research emphasizes that while it may be relatively easy to influence attitudes and behaviour short-term, it can be very difficult for people to sustain behaviour change over the longer term.[22] In order to use these strategies with maximum effect there are a number of principles to bear in mind.

Advocacy and Working in Partnership with Lay People

Some people may need extra help to make health choices. Advocacy is generally taken to mean representing the interests of people who cannot speak up for themselves because of illness, handicap or other disadvantage. In the context of health promotion, it is better seen as a variety of ways of empowering those people who are disempowered in our society. It is concerned with using every possible means to assist people to become independent and self-advocating.

There can be deep conflicts of loyalty for health promoters who take on an advocacy role. There may be a need to challenge employers, or those in authority, about services which fail to meet people's needs.

For example, if a patient complains to a community psychiatric nurse that his drugs are making him feel drowsy and generally unwell, but the doctor insists he should continue to take them, where should the nurse's loyalties lie: to the patient, to the doctor, to the Health Authority (which funds her) or to the profession (which controls her registration)? How can the nurse most effectively act as an advocate in this situation?

Because of these conflicts of loyalties, many advocacy schemes use non-professional workers who come from a similar background to those they are empowering. For example, 'Maternity Links' schemes provide workers as advocates and interpreters for Asian mothers who do not speak English. The workers are Asian themselves, able to speak English as well as their own mother tongues, and the organization may be run with Health Authority funding but managed independently.

In order to reach and influence disadvantaged groups of people successfully, many projects involve professionals working in partnership with lay volunteers. For example, a community mothers programme involved non-professional mothers as volunteers working with disadvantaged first-time mothers to improve their parenting skills.[23] A randomized controlled trial demonstrated that this approach was effective.

Making Healthier Choices Easy Choices

People do not make health choices in a vacuum; they make them in the context of their own environment, subject to all the pressures and influences that surround them. If this environment is conducive to a healthier lifestyle, clients have greater freedom to choose the 'healthier' alternatives and change their behaviour. For example, the provision of cycleways makes it easier to take regular exercise by cycling to work; provision of litter bins, combined with frequent emptying, helps people to Keep Britain Tidy; a no-smoking policy in public places such as restaurants and cinemas helps people not to smoke. National and local policies can create a climate where it is easier to adopt healthier behaviour.

See the section 'What Affects Health'? in Chapter 1 and 'Changing Policy and Practice' in Chapter 16.

Relating to Clients

Research consistently shows that the degree of client change is related to helper empathy; in other words, clients are more likely to change if the health promoter understands the client, sees things from his point of view, and accepts him on his own terms. Achieving this relationship may be the most difficult part of helping people to change. Furthermore, the attitude and behaviour of the health promoter herself is likely to influence the outcome. For example, it has long been known that doctors who themselves smoke are less likely to be effective in helping people to choose to stop smoking.[24]

This has been discussed at more length in the section in Chapter 10 Relationships with Clients

Using Learning Methods Sensitively

People invest a great deal of emotion in their values and attitudes, which means that the exercises we have described here, especially those that are designed to encourage people to explore feelings, such as role play, need to be handled with care and sensitivity. Special training in the use of experiential teaching methods is recommended, but at the very least, group leaders should not attempt to use them unless they have experienced them first themselves. Some points to remember are as follows.

- Explain the activities carefully and thoroughly, and check to ensure that everybody understands what the exercise is for and what they are expected to do.
- Emphasize that participation is entirely voluntary.
- Allow plenty of time for discussion at the end. If people's opinions and cherished ideas have been challenged, they are likely to feel strongly about it. Increased self-awareness may be a very uncomfortable experience, too. The group leader should ensure that people have time to express their feelings and get any support that they need before they leave the group.
- Ensure that there is an atmosphere of confidentiality and trust, so that people feel free to explore their views and feelings in safety. If they feel they may be laughed at or gossiped about, they will not participate fully, if at all.
- Save your own views to the end, after the group members have had a chance to think things through for themselves. Be open and honest about yourself and your values, and if you, too, are confused, say so!

PRACTICE POINTS

- Some individuals will need to feel better about themselves before they can contemplate change. You may need to help them to develop a number of competencies (often called 'life skills') to do with social interaction, assertiveness and time management, and possibly specific psychomotor skills, for example, in order to participate in a physical exercise programme.

- In order to devise the appropriate strategy for each individual you need to start by exploring clients' health knowledge and beliefs related to the issue of concern; the stage they are at in the 'revolving door' of change; and what outcomes they desire.

- You need to tailor an action plan to the specific needs of each client.

- You need to provide positive consequences for desired healthy behaviour (such as praise or rewards) in order to maintain behaviour change.

- You can improve success by combining a number of strategies. (For example, a patient who is being rehabilitated after a heart attack could have an interview with a hospital doctor, backed-up by a home visit from a nurse to encourage family members to support the patient, and small-group self-help sessions to help patients to manage their problems.)

- Records are important for follow-up. These are most effective if they are kept and 'owned' by the individual concerned, for example in the form of a diary.

- Providing a supportive environment can be the key to success, so that people find it easier to make and maintain a healthier lifestyle.

Recommended Reading

An Introduction to the Determinants of Health Behaviour and Modification of Behaviour Through the Public Health Model and the Therapy Model

➤ Stroebe W and Stroebe M S (1995) *Social Psychology and Health*. Buckingham: Open University Press.

On Health Behaviour and Primary Prevention

➤ Taylor S E (1995) Health Psychology, 3rd edn. Part 2. New York: Mcgraw-Hill International Editions.

On Attitudes and their Influence on Behaviour

➤ Jonas J, Ealy A & Stroebe W (1995) Chapter 1 in Argyle M & Colman A M (eds) *Social Psychology*. London: Longman.

On a Range of Theoretical Models and the Role of these in Predicting Health Behaviours

➤ Conner M & Norman P (eds) (1996) *Predicting Health Behaviour*. Buckingham: Open University Press.

On the Importance of Theory in Relation to Health Behaviour Change, and Further Reading on the Health Action Model

➤ Tones K & Tilford S (1994) *Health Education: Effectiveness, efficiency and equity*. Chapter 3. London: Chapman and Hall.

On Models of Behaviour Change

➤ Cole A (1995) A model approach to health promotion *Healthlines*, October, pp 14–16.

➤ Tones K (1995) *Making a Change for the Better. Healthlines,* November, pp 17–19.

➤ Cole A (1995/96) *The Persuaders. Healthlines,* December 1995/January 1996, pp 17–19.

➤ Naidoo J & Wills J (1994) *Health Promotion: Foundations for Practice.* Chapter 10. London: Baillière Tindall.

Detailed Help on How to Work with People to Change Eating and Exercise Behaviour Based on the 'Stages of Change' Model

➤ Hunt P & Hillsdon M (1996) *Changing Eating and Exercise Behaviour.* Oxford: Blackwell.

On Counselling

➤ Burnard P (1994) *Counselling Skills for Health Professionals,* 2nd edn. London: Chapman Hall.

➤ Nelson-Jones R (1993) *Practical Counselling and Helping Skills: How to Use the Lifeskills Helping Model.* 3rd edn. Cassell: London.

➤ Egan G (1994) *The Skilled Helper: A Problem-Management Approach to Helping,* 5th edn. Pacific Grove, California: Brooks/Cole.

Notes and References

1 The Health Belief Model is the oldest and best known. See:

Becker M H (ed.) (1974) *The Health Belief Model and Personal Health Behaviour.* Thorofare New Jersey: Slack. In essence, this model suggests that when people are faced with pressure to change their behaviour, they will weigh up the pros and cons, and what they decide to do will depend on their perceptions of factors such as how serious they think an illness or danger is. However, the Health Belief Model has been criticized because it assumes that people are rational (and we know that they often act irrationally!) and because it ignores powerful influences on behaviour such as family and friends.

The Theory of Reasoned Action is a model which emphasizes the influence of 'significant others'. See:

Ajzen I & Fishbein M (1980) *Understanding Attitudes and Predicting Social Behaviour.* Englewood Cliffs: Prentice Hall.

However, it too, sees human behaviour as essentially rational.

2 Tones B K (1987) Devising Strategies for Preventing Drug Misuse: the role of the Health Action Model. *Health Education Research* **2**, 305–317.

3 Tones K (1995) Making a change for the better. *Healthlines,* November, p. 17. (Reproduced with permission from the Health Education Authority).

4 Prochaska J O & DiClemente C C (1982) Trans-theoretical Therapy: Towards a More Integrative Model of Change. *Psychotherapy: Theory, Research and Practice* **19** (3), 276–288.

5 The stages of change we use are adapted from

Prochaska J & DiClemente C (1984) *The Trans-theoretical Approach: crossing traditional boundaries of therapy.* Harnewood, Illinois: Dow-Jones. and from:

Neesham C (1993) A Model for Change. *Healthlines,* September, pp. 15–17.

6 A technique useful in the 'contemplation' stage is 'motivational interviewing'. The emphasis is on exploring a client's concerns, in order to help him to move to the 'commitment' stage when he is ready to do so. For more information on motivational interviewing, see:

Miller W & Rollnick S (1991) *Motivational Interviewing – preparing people for change.* New York: Guilford Press.

Rollnick S, Heather N & Bell A (1992) Negotiating behaviour change in medical settings: the development of brief motivational interviewing. *Journal of Mental Health* **1**, 25–37.

7 The Health Education Authority Primary Care Unit at Oxford, established in 1989, has assisted delivery of health education in primary care through its programme of team workshops, publications, and research and through the national facilitator network. For more information about the 'Helping People Change' project, contact the Primary Care Project Co-ordinator, Primary Health Care Unit, Block 10, Churchill Hospital, Headington, Oxford OX3 7JL. Tel: 01865 226061.

Other useful resources for use within primary care are:

- A multidisciplinary training programme for primary health care teams, with a package of materials (course notes, a manual on risk factor management, a detailed practice guide on screening techniques and a resource pack of reference material) available from Radcliffe Medical Press Ltd, 15 Kings Meadow, Ferry Hinksey Road, Oxford OX2 0DP. Tel: 01865 790696.

- Training packs from: Anticipatory Care In Practice, Radcliffe Infirmary, Woodstock Road, Oxford OX2 6HE.

8   An example of research is the 'Get Moving' project in Bristol which evaluated how GPs and practice nurses can help patients to take more physical activity, through a trial using an adapted version of the Prochaska and DiClemente model. This was a joint initiative between a multiagency heart disease prevention programme 'Look After Your Heart – Avon' and Bristol University. For further information contact Bristol Area Specialist Health Promotion Service, Henshaw House, Cossham Hospital, Lodge Road, Kingswood, Bristol, BS15 1LF. Tel: 0117 975 8027.

A number of authors have looked at and challenged the application of the 'stages of change' model, including:

Duncan P & Cribb A (1996) Helping people change – an ethical approach? *Health Education Research* **11** (3), 339–348.

Buxton K, Wyse J & Mercer T (1996) How applicable is the Stages of Change model to exercise behaviour? *Health Education Journal* **55**: 239–257.

Ashworth P (1997) Breakthrough or bandwagon? Are interventions tailored to Stage of Change more effective than non-staged interventions? *Health Education Journal* **56**, 166–174.

Whitehead M (1997) Editorial: how useful is the 'stages of change' model? *Health Education Journal* **56**, 111–112.

9   Recent research shows that focusing on the prevention of relapse can be effective. See:

Marlett G & George W (1995) Relapse Prevention: Introduction and overview of the model. *British Journal of Addiction* **79**, 261–273.

10   Kreuter M & Stretcher V (1996) Do tailored behaviour change messages enhance the effectiveness of health risk appraisal? Results from a randomised trial. *Health Education Research* **11** (1): 97–105.

11   Experiential learning has evolved from two sources. One is from the theories of the American philosopher John Dewey. Another is from Humanistic Psychology. Humanistic Psychology sees people as free decision-makers actively controlling their own destinies. We have already discussed some limitations to this viewpoint in Chapter 3, but humanistic psychology has had a huge influence on health care, education and health promotion both in this country and worldwide. The literature is vast. One classic text still worth reading (and available in print) is:

Rogers C R (1967) *On Becoming a Person: A Therapist's View of Psychotherapy*. London: Constable.

12   The games in the 'gamesters handbooks' were devised some years ago, but are still useful. See:

Brandes D & Phillips H (1978) *Gamesters Handbook*. London: Hutchinson.

Brandes D (1983) *Gamesters Two*. London: Hutchinson.

13   Irrational beliefs can be identified and changed through 'Rational Emotive Behaviour Therapy'. For basic introductions to the principles and practice of this, see:

Dryden W (1996) *Inquiries in Rational Emotive Behaviour Therapy*. London: Sage.

Dryden W (1995) *Brief Rational Emotive Behaviour Therapy*. Chichester: Wiley.

14   There are many occasions when a discussion between health promoter and client can only be brief. A technique has been developed which is essentially a brief and effective approach to empowering others, useful for clients who are at the 'commitment' (ready to change) stage of change. It focuses on building the confidence of the client that he has the capacity to change, through focusing on successes (what the client is already doing to reach the goals), rather than focusing on mistakes or failures. See:

Cade B and O'Hanlon W (1993) *A Brief Guide to Brief Therapy*. New York: Norton.

15   For a useful introduction to counselling skills, see:

Burnard P (1994) *Counselling Skills for Health Professionals*. London: Chapman Hall.

16   For guidance on counselling for those working with lesbian, gay or bisexual clients, see:

Davies D & Neal C (eds) (1996) *Pink Therapy: a guide for counsellors and therapists working with lesbian, gay and bisexual clients*. Buckingham: Open University Press.

For guidance on counselling young people, see:

Noonan E (1983) *Counselling Young People*. London: Routledge.

For guidance on counselling in schools, see:

Bovair K & McLaughlin C (1993) *Counselling in Schools: A Reader*. London: David Fulton.

For guidance on counselling older people, see:

O'Leary E (1996) *Counselling Older Adults: Perspectives, approaches and research.* London: Chapman and Hall.

Terry P (1997) *Counselling the Elderly and their Carers.* Basingstoke: Macmillan.

For guidance on counselling in the workplace, see:

Carroll M (1996) *Workplace Counselling.* London: Sage.

For guidance on counselling people with communication problems, see:

Dalton P (1994) *Counselling People with Communications Problems.* London: Sage.

For guidance on counselling people with alcohol problems, see:

Velleman R (1992) *Counselling for Alcohol Problems.* London: Sage.

For guidance on counselling in terminal care and bereavement, see:

Parkes C M, Pelf M & Couldrick A (1996) *Counselling in Terminal Care and Bereavement.* Leicester: British Psychological Society.

For counselling people under stress, see:

Ellis A, Gordon J, Neenan M & Palmer S (1997) *Stress Counselling: A Rational Emotive Behaviour Approach.* London: Cassell.

For an American text with a historical perspective on the origins of counselling, including a chapter on what it means to be psychologically healthy and chapters on counselling special groups such as clients with disabilities, clients from ethnic groups, older people, children and families, see:

Capuzzi D & Gross D R (eds) (1991) *Introduction to Counselling: Perspectives for the 1990s.* Boston: Allyn and Bacon.

17   We have adapted our five stages from:

Burnard P (1985) *Learning Human Skills: A Guide for Nurses.* Oxford: Heinemann Nursing. and:

Inskipp F (1986) *Counselling: The Trainer's Handbook.* Cambridge: National Extension College.

18   Rogers C R (1983) *Freedom to Learn for the Eighties.* Columbus, Ohio: Charles E Merril.

19   For a general introduction to health behaviour and behaviour change, see:

Glanz K, Markus-Lewis F & Rimmer B (1990) *Health Behaviour and Health Education: Theory, Research and Practice.* San Francisco: Jossey-Bass.

20   For examples, see the Health Promotion Department of your local health authority or NHS Trust.

21   Many coping strategies are listed in leaflets from the Health Education Authority and the Health Education Board for Scotland, which deal with the relevant aspect of behaviour change such as stopping smoking or drinking more sensibly.

22   A longitudinal study of self-initiated change by working class mothers in South Wales, shows how difficult it is to sustain long-term change:

Pill R M (1990) Change and stability in health behaviour: a five-year follow-up study of working-class mothers. *Lifestyle, Health and Health Promotion,* pp 63–79. Cambridge: Health Promotion Research Trust.

23   Johnson Z, Howell F & Molloy B (1993) Community mothers programme: randomised controlled trial of non-professional intervention in parenting. *British Medical Journal* **306**, 1449–1452.

24   Pincherle G & Wright H B (1970) Smoking habits of business executives: doctor variations in reducing consumption. *Practitioner* **205**, 209–212.

15 Working with Communities

SUMMARY

We introduce this chapter with an explanation of the term 'community-based work in health promotion' and the range of activities it may include. We discuss some key terms and principles before looking at three particular ways of working with communities: community participation, community development and community health projects. Each of these includes an exercise, and there is also a case study of a community development project. We finish by looking at the competencies health promoters need to develop when working with communities.

See Defining Health Promotion in Chapter 2. As we have discussed in previous chapters, health promotion is the process of enabling people to increase control over, and improve, their health.[1] The challenge this presents is never more apparent than when considering people in the community who may be disadvantaged and discriminated against, and who feel powerless to do anything about their health. This chapter is about taking on that challenge, and working in the community with groups of people in a way which *does* enable them take more control over their health.

Community-based Work in Health Promotion

By 'community-based work in health promotion' we mean work which directly involves the health promoter in working with groups of the public in a sustained way which will enable them to increase control over, and improve, their health. It may involve different kinds of activities, including:

- community development work;
- setting up a group and working with members on health issues (such as a group with learning difficulties addressing issues of sexual health);
- working on projects or campaigns focusing on a particular health issue (such as sickle cell disease or drug misuse);
- outreach work, which means workers going out to meet people where they are, rather than expecting people to come to them (such as community workers on sexual health, who might work with people in the sex industry on the streets or in clubs and massage parlours);
- providing health information services (such as well-women information centres);
- health-related work undertaken by organizations with wider remits (such as health courses for older people run by national older people's organizations);

- advocacy projects (such as organizations undertaking interpreting and/or advocacy for Asian women),
- self-help groups getting together for mutual support on health problems.[2]

This list begins to identify specific tasks health promoters may find themselves tackling, but first we need to clarify some of the key terms and principles involved in community-based work.

Key Terms

Community

A community may be thought of as a network of people. The link between them may be:
- where they live (such as a housing estate or neighbourhood);
- the work they do (such as 'the farming community');
- their ethnic background (such as 'the Jewish community');
- the way they live (such as 'new age' travellers or homeless people)
- or other factors they have in common.

The people in the network come together on the basis of a shared experience or concern, and identify for themselves which communities they feel they belong to. Networks may be formal or informal.

Community Work

This means working with community groups and organizations to overcome the community's problems and improve people's conditions of life. Community work aims to enhance the sense of solidarity and competence in the community. A **community worker** is usually a paid worker undertaking community work.

Community Health Work

This is community work with a focus on health concerns, but generally health is defined broadly to include social and economic aspects, so that community health work may encompass almost as broad a range of activities as community work without a specific health remit.

Community Action

This means activity carried out by people under their own control in order to improve their collective conditions. It may involve campaigning, negotiating with or challenging authorities and those with power.

Community Participation

This is about involving the community in health work which is led by someone outside the community, for example, a worker employed by a statutory agency. The degree of participation may vary enormously.

Community Development

This means working to stimulate and encourage communities to express their needs and to support them in their collective action. It is not about dealing with people's problems on a one-to-one basis; it aims to develop the potential of a community as a whole. A **community development approach to health** involves working with groups of people to identify their own health concerns, and to take appropriate action. **Community development health workers** are essentially facilitators, locally based, whose role is to help people in the community to acquire the skills, knowledge and confidence to act on health issues. They are usually community workers by background, rather than health professionals.

Community Health Projects

This is a loose term applied to programmes of work which are organized by agencies for the improvement of health in a community, or to local organizations aiming to improve health by supporting some combination of community activity, self-help, community action and/or community development.[3]

Finally, it is worth mentioning that in the health service the word community is often used as an adjective to describe anything that is not based in hospital. Examples are **community care**, **community nurses** and **community services**.

Community participation, community development and community health projects will be explored in greater depth later in the chapter, but first we look at some principles of community health work.

Principles of Community-based Work

We identify four key principles, as follows.

1.   The Centrality of the Community

It is the community which defines its own needs, not the health workers. Community-based work is essentially a 'bottom-up' process, rather than a 'top-down' process where those with power and authority make the decisions. Community workers recognize and value the health experience and knowledge that exists in the community, and seek to use it for everyone's benefit.

2.   The Facilitator Role of the Community Health Worker

Community health workers do not perceive themselves as 'experts' in health, but as facilitators whose role is to validate, encourage and empower people to define their own health needs and to meet them. They start where the community is, recognizing and valuing people's own abilities and experiences. They involve people in the community health work from the very beginning, encouraging and supporting them in working together. Knowledge and skills are shared and demystified. Community health workers aim to complement as well as challenge statutory services by making people's access to statutory agencies easier, and making the agencies more accountable to the people they serve.

3.   The Importance of Addressing Inequalities

See the section *Inequalities in Health* in Chapter 1.

A central concern in community-based health work is the need to challenge and change the many forms of disadvantage, oppression and discrimination which people face, and which adversely affect their health. There is acute awareness of the need to address inequalities in health and health services and to focus on the social, environmental and economic determinants of health.

Work therefore focuses particularly on the needs of disadvantaged and oppressed groups, which is why work with women and minority ethnic and black groups is prominent. Another example is people with learning difficulties who need help to empower them to take more control over their own lives. A central way of working is to bring people in such groups together for support and information-sharing, and to enable them to bring about change through collective action. There is no denying that the work is political, because it means working towards greater equality and social justice. It means working with people who experience power-lessness and inequality as part of their everyday lives, and working towards a redistribution of resources and power.

4.   A Broad Perspective on Health

Health is perceived broadly and holistically as positive well-being, including social, emotional, mental and societal aspects as well as physical ones. It is not seen merely as the absence of disease, and is not limited by medical or epidemiological views of what constitutes a health problem or issue. Health is seen to be affected by social, environmental, economic and political factors.

Community Participation

Participation is a word that is used widely to mean a range of activities, from those that are merely tokenistic to those which are firmly rooted in the concept of empowerment. We look at two aspects where you may be involved: first in planning new developments, and then in identifying practical ways of supporting the principle of community participation.

Community Participation in Planning

The amount of community participation in planning health work organized by an agency (such as a health or local authority) can vary along a spectrum of none to high, as shown in Table 15.1.[4]

Health promoters involved in planning initiatives in the community can use this framework to consider the extent to which their agencies invite communities to participate.

Table 15.1	Community participation in planning health work.
No participation	The community is told nothing, and is not involved in any way.
Very low participation	The community is informed. The agency makes a plan and announces it. The community is convened or notified in other ways in order to be informed; compliance is expected.
Low participation	The community is offered 'token' consultation. The agency tries to promote a plan and seeks support or at least sufficient sanction so that the plan can go ahead. It is unwilling to modify the plan unless absolutely necessary.
Moderate participation	The community advises through a consultation process. The agency presents a plan and invites questions, comments and recommendations. It is prepared to modify the plan.
High participation	The community plan jointly. Representatives of the agency and the community sit down together from the beginning to devise a plan.
Very high participation	The community has delegated authority. The agency identifies and presents an issue to the community, defines the limits and asks the community to make a series of decisions which can be embodied in a plan which it will accept.
Highest participation	The community has control. The agency asks the community to identify the issue and make all the key decisions about goals and plans. It is willing to help the community at each step to accomplish its goals, even to the extent of delegating administrative control of the work.

Ways of Developing Community Participation

Community participation can be encouraged and supported in many ways at different levels. We suggest some ways in which you may be able to develop community participation, particularly if you work for a statutory agency.[5]

Be open about policies and plans. Publicize your policies, invite comments and recommendations on your plans, involve representatives on planning and management groups.

Plan for the community's expressed needs. When planning services, help the community to express its own needs as it sees them, and take this into account when planning services.

De-centralize planning. Set up planning and management of health and allied services on a neighbourhood basis, encouraging and enabling the public's involvement.

Develop joint forums. Develop joint forums, such as patient participation groups in doctors' practices, where lay people and professionals can work together in partnerships. Mental health services often have joint forums to involve service users in service development.

Develop networks. Encourage individuals or groups to come together, thus increasing their collective knowledge and power to change things.

Provide support, advice and training for community groups. Provide opportunities for lay people to develop their knowledge, confidence and skills, such as in running groups, speaking in public, or finding their way around bureaucratic statutory organizations. This could be provided through informal discussions, perhaps on a 'drop in' basis, or structured training courses.

Provide information. Provide information about health issues, details of useful local and national organizations, leaflets, posters and books.

Provide help with funding and resources. Help local groups to obtain funding from statutory agencies, and provide other sorts of practical help such as a place to meet or facilities to photocopy materials.

Support advocacy projects. Support projects which enable people who are otherwise excluded to have a voice, such as interpreting/advocacy schemes for Asian patients.

Exercise 15.1   **Developing community participation in your work**

Consider the following list of ways in which you can encourage community participation in working for health.

- Be open about policies and plans
- Plan for the community's expressed needs
- De-centralize planning
- Develop joint forums
- Develop networks
- Provide support, advice and training for community groups
- Provide information
- Provide help with funding and resources
- Support advocacy projects

(If you are not sure what is meant by these, look back at the explanations above.)

To what extent do you think these things are desirable?

To what extent do you do these things already?

From this list, can you identify ways in which you would like to increase community participation in your work?

Can you identify any other ways in which you would like to increase community participation in your work?

Given that there may be some obstacles to doing what you would ideally like to do, can you identify a practical way forward for acting on at least one of the things you would like to do?

Work either individually, in pairs or small groups.

Community Development

However much you might seek people's participation, it may be that they feel so alienated, dissatisfied or overwhelmed with problems that participation is the last thing they want to do. In this situation, it is necessary to develop a climate and culture where participation can happen. You need to encourage, enable and support people, and *community development* is a way of doing this.

Community development is much more than community participation. It means working with people to identify their own health concerns, and to support and facilitate them in their collective action. It means adhering firmly to the principles of community-based work we outlined above, with the community development worker having the role of a facilitator.

The exercise 'Thinking about Community Development' is designed to help you to consider what community development work means in practice.

| Exercise 15.2 | Thinking about community development[6] |

Working individually, or in pairs or small groups, work through the following questionnaire. If you are working with other people, discuss the reasons for the answers you give. You do not have to reach a consensus – after you have listened to each other's views, you can agree to disagree.

Tick whether you think each of the following statements is true or false:

Community development is about: True   False

1.   Fostering a sense of community among people
2.   Helping people to see the root causes of their ill-health
3.   Enabling a statutory authority to show it 'cares'
4.   Getting involved in a political process
5.   Doing away with 'experts' and 'professionals'
6.   Confronting forms of discrimination such as racism and sexism
7.   Saving money on services by helping people to help themselves
8.   Promoting equal access to resources such as health services
9.   Enabling a community worker to become a leader/spokesperson for the community
10. Helping people to develop confidence and become more articulate about their needs
11. Campaigning for a better environment such as improved housing, transport and play facilities
12. Controlling social unrest, e.g. by providing activities for bored young people
13. Helping working class people become more like middle class people in terms of their attitudes and behaviour
14. Recognizing and valuing the skills, knowledge and expertise of individuals and groups in the community
15. Beginning a process of redistributing wealth, power and resources

Now add any other points you think community development is, or is not, about:

Case study 15.1 illustrates community development in practice, demonstrating how the community and the community's own expressed needs were central, the workers acted as facilitators, inequalities in health were addressed and a broad perspective on health was taken. It also shows how local people were empowered to take action.

| Case study 15.1 | The Granton Community Health Project[7] |

A pilot project was funded in Granton, Scotland, to raise awareness of health issues in a deprived area and to find ways whereby people in the community could communicate their health needs and concerns. The project was staffed by a community development worker and a health visitor, with a research worker at a later date.

The community development worker started by getting to know and documenting all the local resources provided by statutory and voluntary agencies in the area as well as community-based groups. A small survey of local residents and professionals was then carried out to provide information on concepts of health, health needs and so on, and this highlighted interesting differences in the views of residents and professionals.

To encourage local people to give their opinions and become more involved, a larger survey was planned with suggestions from the residents. Eighteen local people were trained and paid as interviewers. The survey helped to build up a picture of health needs in the area, but it was also part of a process of education for the interviewers themselves, who were found to have improved self-image and a raised awareness of conditions in the area. Their desire to discuss some of the issues in greater depth led to setting up a group which then drew in more residents by personal contact. Several groups were initiated in the same way, as people came up with problems and issues they wanted to address. These groups were gradually taken over and run by local residents as they gained confidence.

Some groups remained small and short-lived, but others had far-reaching effects. One example was a women's health discussion group, which started by looking at topics such as stress, childbirth and talking to doctors, and then focused on the problem of damp housing. The group prepared a tape-slide presentation showing the problem and how it affected their lives. This was shown at a seminar at Edinburgh University, and stimulated a research project to investigate the effects of damp housing on health. The process of putting forward their concerns helped group members to gain confidence and demonstrated that residents from a deprived area could stimulate academic research on their own chosen priorities.

Other long-term outcomes included a tranquillizer support group, a drop-in stress centre, and an elderly people's forum which secured funding for a mini-bus, an information worker on pensioners' issues and a visiting scheme for frail elderly people.

The evaluation of the project by the University of Aberdeen concluded that it had been successful in meeting most of its objectives. It had opened up channels of communication between professionals and residents, it had developed ways of fostering the skills of some of the residents in dealing with health issues and had shown how some of these issues could be tackled by lay people in new ways.

Some Implications of the Community Development Approach

If you choose to adopt a community development approach, it is important to appreciate the implications. The experience of community development projects around the country has shown that five areas of tension are likely to surface.[8] We identify these below, and some ways of trying to prevent them.

1. **Different priorities.** Priorities chosen by communities may not be the same as those of local statutory agencies or indeed the body who is funding the work. A common difference is that health problems as defined by health workers are likely to be about physical health problems, risk factors for major illnesses and low uptake of health services, such as low birthweight babies, heavy drinking and poor immunization rates. Community priorities, on the other hand, are often about social conditions, such as housing, poor childcare provision and lack of good public transport. This must be clearly understood and accepted at the outset of any community development work.

2. **A threat to local health workers.** If local people gain confidence and become more articulate through the process of community development, they are likely to voice concern and criticism about local health services. Furthermore, the prospect of members of the community taking an active role in policy-making and planning may be alien to many managers and field-workers in statutory agencies. A thorough educational grounding in the rationale and principles of community-based work is required, although setting this up and getting people to listen may in itself be a daunting task.

3. **No instant results.** Community development work is slow. It takes time to get to know a community and to build up trust with local people, and it may be years before there is any tangible outcome. A common problem is that projects with fixed-term funding for a year or two are often expected to achieve substantial outcomes in these short time-scales, which is unrealistic. Secure funding for several years, with achievable objectives, is fundamental to success.

4. **A token gesture or an easy option.** Well-meaning authorities who want to 'do something' (or be seen to be doing something) about inequalities in health may set up a community health project as a way of addressing the issue. Clearly it cannot be 'the answer' to complex and deeply-rooted causes of poor health; at best it can make a valuable contribution, but at worst it can divert attention from the real political solutions to the problems.

5. **Evaluation conflicts.** Outside agencies may expect to see results in terms of traditional 'outcomes' such as improved immunization rates, a measurable change in community behaviour (less drunkenness, vandalism or crime, for example) or lower rates of hospital admission. However, the objectives of a community development project are rarely couched in such terms, and are more likely to be concerned with far less easily measured results such as increased self-confidence, increased public participation in health planning or better communication between the community and statutory agencies. Once again, education in the process, principles, aims and likely outcomes are essential for all concerned.

Community Health Projects

We now turn from thinking about community development to considering how you might be involved in a community health project. (We defined this earlier as a programme of work organized by an agency or a local organization with the aim of improving health by some combination of community activity, self-help, community action and/or community development.) For example, you might want to set up a project to work with young parents on a housing estate with the aim of improving their confidence, skills and mutual support in parenting, or with older people in a particular area to encourage social activities with a health benefit, such as relaxation and exercise groups, tea dances or lunch clubs.

See Chapter 5 The Basic Planning and Evaluation Process

In order to think systematically about setting up and running a community health project, we suggest using the Planning and Evaluation Flowchart from Chapter 5. Additional help can be gained from reading the growing number of community health projects which have been written up so that the processes, successes and failures, and lessons learnt, can be shared.[9]

The experience of community health workers has highlighted specific issues which it is helpful to consider. These points are discussed below, set out within the Planning and Evaluation framework.[10] Figure 15.1 summarizes the planning and evaluation flowchart, highlighting issues particularly relevant to community health project work. This is not a comprehensive guide to setting up and running community health projects; it is intended to be complementary to the information in Chapter 5.

Stage 1. Identifying needs and priorities

At this stage, two particular issues are: how do you get to know the community and who do you consult?

Getting to know the community and its needs. Get all the relevant information you can about the health of the community. Search out data from the health authority and local authority.

Try contacting neighbourhood centres, community groups, voluntary organizations and tenants associations. People who might be able to put you in touch with these include local workers in health and social services, local churches and schools, the local Council for Voluntary Service, the Community Health Council and the local Council for Racial Equality. Talk to members of the public, perhaps at local markets and festivals. It might be useful to hold public meetings or conduct a small survey.

Talk to local professionals, but bear in mind that professional perceptions will often stem from a problem-centred view of a locality; for example, police may talk about crime, social workers about the numbers of children on the 'at-risk' register.

Local newspapers may be a useful source of information about the needs, interests and activities of a locality, and may even have a library service to select material on a particular issue for you. Another approach is to walk – not drive – around the neighbourhood. Groups of young people on street corners, smells

Fig 15.1　　　**Flowchart for planning and evaluating health promotion, with special reference to community health work.**

1. Identify needs and priorities
Consider how you will get to know the community and who you will consult

⇓

2. Set aims and objectives
Work with the community to define aims and objectives.
Be flexible: community work is developmental, and you will need to review and possibly change your objectives as you go along.
Be realistic about what you can reasonably expect to achieve.

⇓

3. Decide the best way of achieving the aims
Consult, be flexible and realistic.

⇓

4. Identify resources
Think about people as a resource: their collective energy, ideas and expertise.
Think about their development needs.
Think about appropriate premises.

⇓

5. Plan evaluation methods
Think this through carefully: what, why, who and how are you going to evaluate?
What will you do with the findings?
Look at both process and outcome.
Recognize that you may be assessing small changes over a long period of time.

⇓

6. Set an action plan
Do this step by achievable step, in a realistic time frame.
You need to consider consultation, and project/project worker management.

⇓

7. ACTION! Implement your plan, including your evaluation
You may need to consider ways of keeping going if interest flags, how to keep on course if you feel you've lost your way, and how to wind up when the work is finished

from fast-food shops, and the range and price of goods in shop windows can reveal a lot about local lifestyle and socioeconomic conditions.

Consulting before setting up. Consult with local health and social service workers at a very early stage. Consult with the community only if you are sure the project is going to happen: consultation before funding is secure, for example, could raise people's expectations falsely, waste their time and diminish their trust.

Stages 2 and 3. Setting Aims and Objectives, and deciding the best way of achieving them

Key issues here are about being flexible and realistic. It is helpful to consult the people you have already made contact with, and the management group/steering group of the project (if there is one). These people may help you to set realistic, achievable aims and objectives, and to work out the best means of achieving them.

Flexibility is vital because community work is essentially a developmental process, so you need to review and modify your objectives regularly. Objectives may change, and indeed should change, if new opportunities arise and/or previous objectives no longer seem achievable or compatible with changing needs.

Being realistic: this applies to identifying what you plan to achieve, and by when. For example, if you are planning a community development approach, ensure that you have a realistic time scale; three years is suggested as a reasonable minimum.

Stage 4. Identifying resources

People and premises are two key resources.

People. By bringing people with a common interest or experience together, you may find that the collective energy of the group generates ideas for future action and you can begin to share the work. This means that your role may also begin to change, from being an initiator to being a supporter.

It is also important to think about the training and development needs of the people who are the key resource of the project. Not only project workers, but also the project management committee (if there is one) and local health professionals may need help in understanding what this type of work is all about. What training is needed, who will do it and how will it be funded?

Premises. You need to consider what premises you need: rooms for meeting in (large and small meetings), a room for a crèche, a place to keep and use equipment such as video equipment and photocopiers, a library/place where people can look up information? Access for wheelchairs, pushchairs and prams? Running water and toilets? Facilities for making refreshments or meals? Good access by public transport? Well-lit premises so that people feel safe going there after dark?

You also need to consider the 'image' of possible premises: if you are offered space in a clinic, for example, this may mean that people perceive the project to be part of the statutory health services.

Case study 15.2   **A checklist for charting changes in a community**[12]

A 3-year project ran on a housing estate where residents were identified as high risk for heart disease. Using a community development approach, a community health worker worked with local residents on issues which residents identified as important. Over the life of the project, changes were noted, many of which became embedded as permanent features in the community. These changes were charted by the project worker in a systematic way, using the following **outcomes measures checklist**.

Outcome measures checklist

Type of change	Information recorded	Examples
Participation of target population in health-related action	Numbers and characteristics (age range, sex, etc.) of people who attend groups and community activities	Number and age range of young parents attending a new parent and toddler group
Perceived changes in knowledge, attitude and behaviour of target population	Changes in attitude towards participation in group and community activity; change in beliefs about ability to have control over one's own life and the power of group action; changes in the subjective experience of belonging to a community; changes in the capacity of local groups to identify problems and collaborate to solve these.	Action group set up by local people to get better play facilities on the estate. Led to establishment of local play group run by local women. Many members stopped smoking.
Changes in demand for health-related services	Changes in demand or requests for services or facilities	Groups requested talks from health visitors on health issues. Request for more accessible primary health care facilities on the estate.
Changes in the availability of support, facilities and resources for people wanting to change lifestyle	Changes in group and community activities, informal social and support networks within the community	New groups to support young single parents. 'Get Cooking' group to help people learn to cook healthier food for their family. Exercise group for older people.
Other physical changes to the environment	Any changes to the built or natural environment	Playground built. Traffic calming schemes introduced
Changes in knowledge, attitudes, skills and practices of local health and allied workers	Changes in attitudes towards local residents to exercise choice and control over the services they receive, or changes in ways of working	Local health visitors use experienced local mothers to support young new parents
Changes in policy and procedures by local statutory and voluntary organizations	Changes that enable local people to have more say in decisions about local services	Consultation with local residents about location and design of new GP surgery on the estate
Dissemination of good practice	What information was sent out and why, talks, presentations, papers published and any evidence that good practice elsewhere has been affected.	Article in community health journal. Community health projects featured in health authority Public Health Report.
Any other outcomes	Any other outcomes, expected or unexpected, which do fall into the above categories	

Stage 5. Planning Evaluation Methods

It is vital that evaluation is planned before any work starts, as this will avoid mis-understandings and false expectations. All parties (funders, managers, workers, participants) need to agree together on key issues:[11]

- Why are you undertaking an evaluation? Who and what is it for?
- What will you be evaluating?
- How will you do it? What methods will you use?
- Who will do it? Will you evaluate yourselves or will you use someone who is not involved in the work as an external evaluator?
- Who will be involved in the evaluation process? Will it involve the community, the workers, the funders, the steering group?
- What will you do with your evaluation findings? Will you publish a report? Who will be responsible for publication? Who will the evaluation report be distributed to? Who will own it? Will findings be widely disseminated, e.g. in journal articles?

Bear in mind the possibility of evaluation conflicts which we discussed in the previous section, and make sure that your evaluation looks at both process and outcome, and identifies realistic ways of assessing what may be very small changes over long periods of time.

It may be helpful to think in terms of charting changes as they occur, using a framework to record these systematically. An example of this approach is the 'Outcome Measures Checklist' used in a community health project described in the case study below.

Stage 6. Setting an Action Plan

There are many things to consider here, but the main one is to identify what you plan to do, step by achievable step.

You may need to build the following activities into your action plan:

Reviewing aims and priorities. It is necessary to review continuously the aims and priorities originally set down for the project, and compare them with those of the people who are now involved. You may need to modify your original aims, and constantly check out whose agenda you are working to – your own or the community's?

Consulting and being accountable to the community. We recommended consultation before you set up, but this needs to continue all through. Once established, you have a continuing responsibility to tell the community about what the project's role is and what work is going on. This could be through meetings, newsletters and open days, for example.

Arranging a management committee or steering group. A management committee or steering group should provide a secure foundation for the project, taking responsibility for its continued development, its policies and management tasks such as fund-raising and recruiting. It should also provide support for the workers. Usually the workers are members of the group; they should not be expected to run the management committee themselves, but sometimes this is the case. This is not desirable because it leads to confusion about who is managing who, and puts an unreasonable burden on the workers.

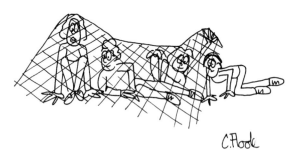

Networking fosters a vital sense of 'not going it alone'.

A management group could consist of both local workers such as health visitors and social workers, and local people, perhaps representing groups with whom the project is in contact.

It may be helpful to get the members of a management committee/steering committee together for a day, to talk through the issues, clarify aims and foster a sense of teamwork.

Writing job descriptions. Paid project workers need clear job descriptions, specifying what is included. For example, does the job include fundraising, doing your own typing, servicing or even running the management committee meetings, keeping the accounts, evaluating, writing progress reports?

Ensuring support for the project workers. Recognize the value of networking as a means of informal training and support. By 'networking' we mean making time and resources available to meet other people doing similar work and to link with other community health projects in different parts of the country. This enables information and ideas to be shared, problems discussed and encouragement given. It fosters a vital sense of not 'going it alone'. The need to ensure that project workers are not isolated in what may be very slow and, at times, discouraging work cannot be over-stressed.

Networking also means that more people will know about your project and you may get more support. Other people, too, may benefit if they have also been experiencing isolation.

Formalizing your project group. It may be helpful at some stage to look at the costs and benefits of formalizing a project group which started off as a loose collection of interested people. The advantages of having a formal organization are that it can apply for financial help and for recognition as a legitimate body; the disadvantages might be that control could be exercised from outside, or that members are attracted who turn out to be more of a hindrance than a help. The local Council for Voluntary Service can be extremely useful since it provides a helpful service for newly-formed groups, and affiliation to the Council brings credibility in itself.

Dealing with friends and enemies. The issues your project is concerned with will probably have a local history, and be likely to have both lost and won support in the past. You need to identify other interest groups, and decide how to tackle them. Study the tactics and arguments of any 'opposition' and plan your strategy.

Stage 7. Implementing Your Plan

As you implement your plan, you may run into difficulties because of flagging interest, a feeling of losing your way, and, finally, that the project has to come to an end. Some suggestions about these three issues are as follows.

Keeping going. With the passage of time, people may lose their enthusiasm. You may be able to provide additional impetus by having the advantage of being involved as a whole or part of your paid work. You need to be sensitive to the many ways by which a project can lose its way, and in such circumstances you may be able to help by:

- discovering what similar activities are taking place elsewhere and circulating details;
- drawing the issue to the attention of relevant statutory agencies, and conveying the response to the group;
- helping the group to produce their own health promotion materials such as posters, leaflets or even a video, and distributing them;
- looking at other health promotion material on topics of interest;
- encouraging members of the project to talk about their work to other people, such as groups of interested professionals and students;
- sending memos to everyone to remind them of meetings;
- providing practical support such as photocopying or typing;
- introducing new members.

Working out what to do next. If you feel that you have lost your way, it can help to write down what information you have found, what contacts you have made, what needs and aims you have identified and what you have done so far. Then seek the views of your management/steering group (if there is one) or the impartial views of someone who has not been involved. The exercise below – Planning Community Health Work – may help to provide a focus for working out what to do next.

Leavings and endings. There comes a point when your involvement has to stop, maybe because you change your job or the priorities of your work, or because the project work has been taken on by local people. Occasionally, you may need to recognize that you have done all you could do, and there is no potential in the project any more. Ending your involvement provides the opportunity for a final evaluation of what has been achieved, what your own contribution has been and making recommendations for future action.

Developing Competence in Community Work

To be a successful community health worker, you need to develop a range of knowledge and skills, and have certain crucial values and attitudes.[13]

In terms of values and attitudes, you will need to be committed to the principles and ideals of community based work which we outlined earlier in this chapter: the centrality of the community, your own role as a facilitator rather than an 'expert', the importance of addressing inequalities and a broad perspective on health.

Exercise 15.3   **Planning Community Health Work**

The following exercise may be useful when you are starting community health work or taking stock part way through a piece of work.

Complete the following statements as far as you can:
The key issue is . . .
The people I need to talk to are . . .
The documents I need to read are . . .
I can get to know more about the community by . . .
The information that is likely to be available is . . .
I intend to look for this information by . . .
Work done on this issue elsewhere is . . .
The people who are likely to be supportive are . . .
The people I should avoid offending are . . .
The period of time I can spend on this issue is . . .
The amount of time I can give it during this period is . . .
The person/people I will talk to in order to work out what to do next is . . .

See Chapter 1 on Inequalities and Chapter 3 on Values.

See the section above on Getting to Know the Community and its Needs, Chapter 4 for agents and agencies of health promotion Chapter 6 for finding information.

See Chapter 1 on inequalities.

In order to hold these values and attitudes with depth and conviction, you will need knowledge of key issues, such as the extent and cause of inequalities in health, the effects of racism, sexism and other forms of oppression on health, and awareness of the structures, policies and powers which influence the lives and health of communities. You will also need to be clear about your own particular political ideologies.

Other areas of knowledge include knowledge of local health resources: who and where to go to for information, advice and materials on health issues. Knowledge of local health services and social services is vital; so is understanding how local statutory and voluntary agencies work, and how to use 'the system' effectively. An understanding of the community itself is of course vital too.

A range of skills is required. It is important to have skills of raising awareness of inequalities and discrimination, and being able to counter these by taking positive action when appropriate and working in an anti-discriminatory way.

See Chapters 5, 7, 8 for planning and managing, Chapter 10 for communication, Chapter 11 for using communication tools, 13 on working with groups.

Other skills are to do with working with people: being able to communicate well, facilitate groups and have effective meetings, for example. You also need skills of planning and management, using and producing health promotion materials, and working for political change.

A list of useful agencies is given at the end of this chapter.[14]

PRACTICE POINTS

- Community based work means working with communities (rather than individuals) over a period of time which will enable them to increase control over, and improve their health. It may involve you in community development work, specific community health projects and group work.

- A key principle is that community work is 'bottom-up' not 'top-down'. This means that you respond to issues which the community identifies, rather than working on issues identified by people outside the community, such as health workers from statutory agencies.

- Community health workers are facilitators rather than health experts, whose role is to develop the community's capacity to identify health needs and meet them.

- Work is often focused on addressing inequalities and working with people who are disadvantaged.

- Health is interpreted widely to encompass social, emotional and societal well-being.

- It is important for you to encourage community participation as much as possible in health planning and health promotion activity, and to consider all the ways of doing this.

- You need particular skills and processes for successful community development work and community health projects. You need to be aware of the potential conflicts and difficulties inherent in this kind of work.

Recommended reading

On Community Health Work

➤ *Community Health Action* is the journal of Community Health UK. Each issue contains reports and articles on community health work, with a focus on a specific themes in each issue. (Address see Note 14.)

➤ Twelvetrees A (1991) *Community Work*, 2nd edn. British Association of Social Workers Practical Social Work series. Basingstoke: Macmillan. (A practical guide to the community development process for community workers.)

➤ Jones L & Sidell M (eds) (1997) *The Challenge of Promoting Health – exploration and action*. Basingstoke: Macmillan/Open University. (Part 1, *Promoting Health at the Local Level – the collective approach*, has chapters dealing with working with primary health care teams; local communities; community action; participation; evaluation of community action.)

➤ Tones K & Tilford S (1994) *Health education: effectiveness, efficiency and equity*, 2nd edn. Chapter 8, the community and health promotion. London: Chapman & Hall. (Discusses theoretical and practical aspects of working both with the community as a setting for health promotion, and with the community in a community development approach, with UK and international examples.)

➤ Bruce N *et al.* (eds) (1996) *Research and Change in Urban Community Health*. Aldershot: Avebury. (An edited collection of contributions to a global conference held in Liverpool in 1994 entitled *Health in Cities: research and change in Urban Community Health*. Chapters cover research and evaluation, community needs assessment, and many examples of community health work.)

➤ Laughlin S & Black D (eds) (1995) *Poverty and Health – Tools for Change*. A Public Health Trust Project, funded by the Baring Foundation and the Joseph Rowntree Charitable Trust. Copies available from: The Public Health Alliance, BVSC, 138 Digbeth, Birmingham B5 6DR. (Ideas, analysis, information and examples of action to tackle poverty, including community health action.)

➤ Burton P & Harrison L (1996) (eds) *Identifying Local Health Needs*. Bristol: The Policy Press. (Looks at needs assessment and community health profiling; includes case studies.)

On Evaluation of Community Health Work

➤ *Community Health Action* is the journal of Community Health UK. Issue 41, Journal 4: 1996 contains useful articles on the theme of evaluation. (Address see Note 14)

➤ Luck M & Jesson J (1996) *Evaluation of Community Health Development*. Community Health UK (Address see Note 14). An overview of community health development and evaluation, with particular reference to a project in Corby.

➤ Charities Evaluation Service *Evaluating Ourselves* series: titles include *Monitoring Ourselves, Managing Evaluation*, and *Developing Aims and Objectives*. (Address see Note 14.)

➤ Graessle L & Kingsley S (1988) *Measuring Change, Making Changes*. London: Community Health Resource. (Available from Community Health UK, address see Note 14.)

➤ Beattie A (1995) Evaluation in community development for health: an opportunity for dialogue. *Health Education Journal* **54**, 465–472. (Discusses the wide range of ways of evaluating community development for health.)

On Working with Voluntary Organizations:

➤ Hanvey C & Philpot T (eds) (1996) *Sweet Charity – the role and workings of voluntary organisations*. London: Routledge. (Covers a range of aspects of voluntary organization work, including campaigning, fund-raising, marketing and management.)

Notes and References

1 Definition in:

World Health Organization (1984) Health promotion: a WHO discussion document on the concepts and principles. Reprinted in: *Journal of the Institute of Health Education*, **23**(1), 1985. (For discussion of this definition, see Chapter 2.)

2 London Community Health Resource & National Council for Voluntary Organisations (1987) *Guide to Community Health Projects*. London: National Community Health Resource.

3 These definitions draw on the work of:

Channon G, in Adams L & Smithies J (1990) *Community Participation and Health Promotion*. London: Health Education Authority.

The definition of community development also draws on:

Association of Metropolitan Authorities (1989) *Community Development, the Local Authority Role*. London: Association of Metropolitan Authorities.

4 This framework is adapted from:

Brager C & Sprecht H (1973) *Community Organising*. Columbia: Columbia University Press.

5 These suggestions are adapted from:

Adams L & Smithies J (1990) *Community Participation and Health Promotion*. London: Health Education Authority.

6 Adapted from a questionnaire by Lee Adams and David Hawkins and reproduced by kind permission.

7 This account is taken from:

Whitehead M (1989) *Swimming Upstream: trends and prospects in education for health*. London: King's Fund Institute.

Whitehead's summary refers to a fuller account in:

Research Unit in Health and Behavioural Change, University of Edinburgh (1989) *Changing the Public Health*. Chichester: John Wiley (Chapter 8, Jones J, Promoting Health Through Community Development.)

See also:

Hunt S (1989) *Community Development and Health Promotion in a Deprived Area*: final report Working Paper. Edinburgh: Research Unit in Health and Behavioural Change.

Drummond N (1989) Evaluation of a Community Health Project: the experience from West Granton, Edinburgh, in Martin C & McQueen D (eds) *Readings for a New Public Health*. Edinburgh: University Press.

8   Whitehead M (1989) *Swimming Upstream: trends and prospects in education for health*, p. 34. London: King's Fund Institute.

9   Examples of community health projects can be found in:

Laughlin S & Black D (eds) (1995) *Poverty and Health – Tools for Change*. A Public Health Trust Project, funded by the Baring Foundation and the Joseph Rowntree Charitable Trust. (Copies available from: The Public Health Alliance, BVSC, 138 Digbeth, Birmingham B5 6DR. Chapter 3 contains 16 case studies of community health work.)

Bruce N *et al.* (eds) (1996) *Research and Change in Urban Community Health*. Aldershot: Avebury. (An edited collection of conference contributions including many chapters describing specific community health projects.)

10   This section draws extensively on material in:

'Guidelines for setting up projects' in:

Community Health Initiatives Resource Unit & London Community Health Resource (1987) *Guide to Community Health Projects*, Chapter 4. (This is a useful guide for fuller details.) and

Henderson P & Thomas D N (1980) *Skills in Neighbourhood Work*. National Institute of Social Services Library, no. 39. London: George Allen & Unwin.

11   Based on ideas in:

De Groot R (1996) Much is written, but little is read. *Community Health Action*, issue 41, p. 3.

12   Based on the 'Outcome Measures Checklist' developed for the Health Education Authority/Look After Your Heart – Avon Localities Project, which included a 3-year community development project in an estate of high health need in Weston-super-Mare, Avon. More about the project, and the checklist, can be found in:

Bruce N *et al.* (eds.) (1996) *Research and Change in Urban Community Health*. Aldershot: Avebury. (Chapter 18 is on the HEA/LAYH-Avon Localities project on the Bournville Estate, Weston-Super-Mare.)

Ewles L, Miles U & Velleman G (1995) Promoting Heart Health on an Urban Housing Estate *Community Health Action*, Issue 35, pp. 12–14.

Ewles L, Miles U & Velleman G (1996) Lessons Learnt from a Community Heart Disease Prevention Project. *Journal of the Institute of Health Education* **34**(1), 15–19.

13   This section is derived from:

Smithies J (1987) *Training Needs of Community Health Workers* National Community Health Resource. Unpublished report on community health workers training project.

14   Useful agencies are:

Community Health UK, PO Box 2248, Bath BA3 6YW. Tel 01225 462680.

This organization exists to promote and support community health development in the UK. It acts as a source of information and advice; supports projects and provides forums for community health groups; enables community health workers to share experiences through publications, conferences and other events; creates links and fosters partnerships between the voluntary sector and statutory services; promotes collaborative work by linking groups and individuals sharing common interests and concerns. It has a membership subscription scheme. (Community Health UK's predecessor organizations were the London Community Health Resource and the Community Health Initiatives Resource Unit which merged in 1986 to form the National Community Health Resource; this is now Community Health UK).

Two agencies which can help with evaluation of community health work are: Charities Evaluation Service, 4 Coldbath Square, London EC1R 5HL. Tel: 0171 713 5722. Provides training, external evaluation, consultancy, advice, information and publications.

The Association for Research in the Voluntary and Community Sector (ARVAC), 60 Highbury Grove, London N5 2AG. Tel: 0171 704 2315. ARVAC is a research network with members from academic, voluntary, community and statutory organizations. It provides training, publications and information.

16 Changing Policy and Practice

SUMMARY

We consider how health policy at local and national level is made, how it can be influenced, and discuss how health promoters can challenge health-damaging policies. We look at the characteristics of power and influence and the politics of influence, illustrated with a case study. We follow with sections on developing and implementing policies, a case study exercise on policy implementation, and end with a section on campaigning.

Health promoters are engaged in influencing policies and practices which affect health. (By 'policies' we mean broad plans of action, which set the direction for detailed planning.) These can be at any level, from national (such as policies set by government or political parties, about, for example, housing, transport and future directions for the NHS) to the level of day-to-day work of a health promoter (such as what sort of health promotion programmes will be run in a GP practice, or what resources will be devoted to specific health promotion activities in an environmental health department.)

In order to influence policy and practice, you need to understand how power is distributed and exercised between people at any level, from a group of colleagues to those in positions of great authority or influence. You need to be able to use that knowledge to affect decisions. (This process of understanding the distribution of power and how it used, and using that knowledge to further your work, is what we mean by 'being political'.)

Changing policy and practice includes working with statutory, voluntary and commercial organizations to influence them to develop health promoting policies for their staff and to produce health enhancing products and services. It also includes working for healthy public policies and economic and regulatory changes requiring campaigning, lobbying and taking political action.

Another relevant and important aspect, that of implementing change, is discussed in the section on Managing Change in Chapter 8.

In this chapter, we look first at local and national health policy and the contribution of health promoters to making and influencing policies. We then focus on three practical aspects of changing policy and practice, which we see as especially relevant in health promotion: understanding the politics of influence, developing and implementing health promotion policies, and campaigning.

Making and Influencing Local and National Health Policy

First we consider who makes health policy at local and national level, the mechanism for implementation, and opportunities for influence.

The importance of making policy changes as an integral part of health promotion is increasingly recognized. We are concerned here with both local policies and national policies, because health promoters working at a local level can press for the introduction of policies at both levels and have an influence on how they are implemented. Furthermore, the development of local policies cannot be divorced from government policies. The nature of, and the resources for, health service, local authority and voluntary organization work are shaped by central government's policy and by the allocation of funds. The evolution of national policy is in turn influenced by representations from health and local authorities, voluntary agencies and other bodies.

Local Health Policy

At a local level, many policies and priorities are now jointly agreed, and this can improve their effectiveness.[1] For example, policies can be agreed by the Local Authority, the Health Authority, and other relevant community organizations such as the Council for Racial Equality, trade unions, housing associations and voluntary organizations.

Some Local Authorities undertake health and/or environmental audits of their services. This involves examining the impact on health and/or the environment of all current and planned activities of each department of the Council. The purpose is to develop practical ways in which the current health and environmental impact of services could be improved and to inform the development of a corporate approach to new health and environmental policies.

Health Promotion Policy in the NHS

There are now formal national strategies for health. The NHS contribution to these health strategies needs to be seen in the context of the NHS reforms brought about by the 1990 NHS and Community Care Act, which set up an internal market, described in the Working for Patients White Paper.[2] We discussed the role of health authorities in commissioning (often also called 'purchasing') health services in Chapter 4 (section on The National Health Service), but we now develop this by discussing how national health policy, and national strategies for health, are implemented in the NHS.

Formal national strategies for health are discussed in detail in Chapter 7, and also in Chapters 1 and 4.

Health authorities are responsible for commissioning strategically in order to improve the health status of the population. This improved health status is often referred to as **health gain**, which can be defined as:

> *A measurable improvement in health status, in an individual or population, attributable to earlier intervention.*[3]

Measurable means that it should be possible to put a value, usually a numerical value, onto health status, in order to demonstrate that a change has occurred.

Attributable means proving that the change in health status is the result of the intervention. It is very difficult to do with complete confidence. For example, it can be difficult to be certain that a particular programme to reduce smoking has been effective, because there are so many other influences which can affect smoking habits.

The links between health promotion and health gain are discussed in Chapter 2.

An **intervention** means a planned activity which is designed to improve health. It could be treatment, a care service or a health promotion activity.

The role of purchasers in assessing health needs, deciding on priorities, setting objectives and targets, allocating resources, and monitoring and reviewing outcomes, has given a much clearer focus to health policy. This may be referred to as the **health gain cycle** (Fig. 16.1).[4]

Fig 16.1   **Health gain cycle**

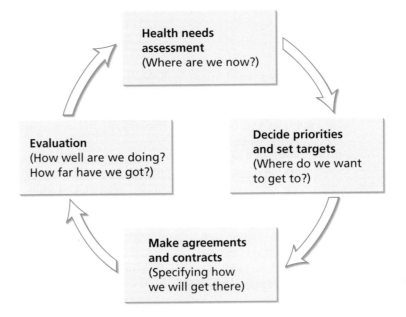

The internal market reforms of the 1990s enabled new ways of planning and managing health improvement to emerge. They have, however, been criticized for the amount of effort necessary to agree and monitor annual contracts, and for making the cooperation so essential to health promotion more difficult.

The Labour government, elected in May 1997, is committed to abolishing the internal market and to replacing annual contracts with long-term agreements. It is expected that GP fundholding will be replaced with GP commissioning, and there may be some mergers of smaller trusts and health authorities. But we do not expect this to mean major reorganization on the scale experienced in the early 1990s. The strategic focus on improving the health of populations, which includes prevention and health promotion, will be retained by health authorities.[5] A further change is the establishment of a Minister for Public Health, signalling a welcome interest in public health as distinct from health service provision.

Health Authorities are public bodies, who offer an opportunity to the public to comment on proposals for purchasing plans. This is a chance for individuals, groups, professional associations and others to express their views on, for example, the balance of resource allocation between treatment/care and health promotion/disease prevention.

Implementing National Health Policies at Local Level

There is more about national strategies for health in Chapter 7.

National strategies for health set national targets for health, which are ways of expressing specific health outcomes. These national targets are translated into, and supplemented with, local targets by local health authorities.

These targets, and the priorities and objectives they are derived from, are an important influence on the content of the contracts or agreements between purchasers and providers. These include agreements to provide specialist health promotion services and programmes, and for health promotion activities as part of general health service requirements. For example, if national strategies have reduction of coronary heart disease (CHD) and stroke as a priority, there are national targets on reduced mortality from CHD and stroke, and targets which focus on changes in risk behaviour, such as smoking. These targets can be translated into requirements in health authority agreements with health service providers for health promotion programmes on smoking prevention, and (for example) to provide smoking cessation help as part of maternity services, and to ensure that hospitals are smoke-free environments. In this way, national strategies become part of local health service provision.

Of course, it is not only the NHS which has a part to play in formulating and implementing national policy which affects health. All the agencies we referred to in Chapter 4 have a role.

Local Agenda 21 Strategies

One important way in which health services and local authorities can work together at local level is through cooperating in implementing Local Agenda 21 strategies. **Agenda 21** is the agreement forged by governments at the Earth Summit in Rio de Janeiro in 1992.[6] All local authorities have now developed Local Agenda 21 strategies (sometimes referred to as 'green plans') which focus on ways of achieving **sustainable development**. This means development that meets the needs of the present without compromising the ability of future generations to meet their own needs. (The 21 in *Local Agenda 21* refers to the 21st century.)

Local Agenda 21 is a process which strives to engage all sectors of the community to work together for a cleaner, healthier environment and better quality of life in the next century. It is about the life we experience as individuals and communities in our local environment, but also about the far-reaching effects of our lifestyles on other parts of the world. Many local authorities have adopted the Local Authority Eco Management and Audit Scheme (LA-EMAS) to ensure that they consider the impact of their activities on sustainable development. Many have started 'green plans'. So, for example, Glasgow launched a regeneration alliance in 1993, and this is now developing a light railway system, bringing derelict land into use, improving the landscape and investing in skills and manufacturing industries.[7] Local authorities are often working with each other and consulting with their communities about the shape of future developments. Health authorities can form part of such alliances – cooperating, for example, on cycleways and the use of public land for people to pursue healthy activities in a safe environment.

See the section on community participation in Chapter 15.
Public participation in Local Agenda 21 is an important part of the process. Health promoters, both in their working role and their role as private citizens, can play their part.

The Voice of the Consumer in the NHS

The 1989 White Paper *Working for Patients* made it clear that the 'needs and wishes' of patients themselves would have a much bigger voice in health policy. How is this voice elicited? Ultimately, it is through the democratic process and the right to vote for the elected government. However, the government in the early and mid 1990s took a number of steps to enable consumers to express their views on health services more directly. One of the most obvious examples is The Patient's Charter.[8] The Patient's Charter sets out patients' rights and what standards of service patients can expect from the NHS. These rights and standards throughout the NHS notably include:

- access to services: to receive health care on the basis of need, including GP services, emergency and hospital treatment;
- personal consideration and respect: such as the right to choose whether to take part in research and student training, respect for privacy, dignity, religious and cultural beliefs;
- information: to have treatments explained, access to your health records, complaints dealt with, 'league tables' on service performance available.

Areas of the health service where rights and standards are spelt out in detail in the Patient's Charter include:

- GP services;
- hospital services (including waiting times to go into hospital, and to receive an out-patient appointment);
- services in the community from nurses, health visitors and midwives;
- ambulance services (including how quickly you can expect an ambulance to arrive following a 999 call);
- services from dentists, opticians and pharmacists.

However, despite the Patient's Charter, many health service users continue to be unhappy with the information they get.[9] The Labour government has promised a review and overhaul of the Patient's Charter.

In addition, health authorities have been charged with setting and publicizing Local Charter Standards, including a named person who can be contacted for further information or comments.

Health promoters can ensure that they, and their clients, know their rights and what standards they can expect, and make positive comments about good standards and appropriate complaints when standards fail to be met. They can also make positive comments when they are particularly pleased with a service.

Future Direction for National Health Policy

In the 1980s and early 1990s the government began to develop a more strategic approach to health policy through coordinating policy across all government departments, although many would argue that this never went far enough. The establishment of a Minister for Public Health in the 1997 government may help.

National health promotion agencies and alliances are also active in the field of policy development.[10] An example is The Association for Public Health which aims to widen the focus of health policy in the UK towards creating a healthy environment, reducing inequalities and improving quality of life. In 1997 it launched a manifesto, *Sustaining the Public's Health* in which it pledged to work with other organizations to create a healthy, sustainable and equitable environment, through eliminating poverty, discrimination, environmental hazards and other threats to health and well-being.[11]

As we head towards the year 2000, it is possible that UK health policies may develop in three main ways:[12]

- We can expect the internal market to lose its competitive features, though not its purchaser–provider structure. Health Authorities may take on more responsibility for coordination, which will enhance the effectiveness of health promotion and continuity of care.
- The Minister for Public Health may seek a shift in emphasis from cure to prevention, with health promotion playing a bigger part in the role of all the health, social welfare and teaching professions. National strategies for health are being reviewed and revised.
- The health dimension may feature more in public policy debate at both central and local government and health authority levels, with the development of more 'healthy public policies'.

Challenging Health-Damaging Policy[13]

A question which health promoters often pose is: what can you do when you are faced with policies which you perceive as health damaging?

This question often induces feelings of helplessness and frustration because such policies come from 'high places' such as national government or (closer to home) your own employing authority or even your own direct manager. To protest may seem a futile waste of energy and can cause a conflict of loyalty between wanting to press for what you see as right and what is decreed to be right by your employing authority. To protest or take action may be seen as 'trouble-making' or 'too political'.

There is no easy answer to this issue, but there are some positive steps worth considering.

- **Use your vote**. At the next general or local election, look at the health implications in the policy manifestos. Raise questions about health policy with doorstep canvassers, at public meetings and by writing to candidates. All this can be done in your capacity as a private citizen rather than a health worker.
- **Use your professional association or trade union**. These groups can raise issues at a national and local level, and can be a powerful voice. You can play your part by joining and supporting their activities, and raising the issues you feel strongly about.

■ **Use your representative**. There are many people whose job is to represent your interests. At European Union or national level, it is your Member of the European Parliament ('Euro MP' or MEP) or your MP. So if you want to raise an issue at these levels, lobby your MEP or MP: send letters, telephone, attend 'surgeries'. At local level, do the same with your local councillor.[14] You could also contact your professional association or union local branch representative.

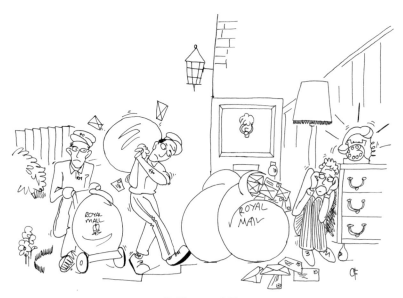

Lobby your MP.

■ **Use your collective power**. If you are concerned about an issue at your place of work, it may help to find out if colleagues feel the same. If they do, join together so that you raise the issue collectively, which is likely to give it more impact and take the heat off any one individual.

However, many areas of policy development are not controversial, and indeed can be a positive and rewarding part of the day-to-day work of health promoters. The main thrust is likely to be in developing, changing and implementing local policies. To do this you need to understand the characteristics of power and influence and to be competent at exerting influence, when necessary. We look at this in the next sections.

Characteristics of Power and Influence

Power is the ability to influence others. There are four generally recognized types of power which are relevant to health promotion work:

■ **Position power** is the power vested in someone because of their position in an organization. For example, the Chief Executive of a Local Authority has position power.
■ **Resource power** is the power to allocate, or limit, resources, including money and staff. It often goes hand-in-hand with position power. For example a senior manager in the health service has both position power and the power to regulate the use of resources.

If you have the power to control the allocation of any resources that people want, then you have a real source of power. Every health promoter will have some power because there will be people who want the skills or services on offer.

- **Expert power** is power related to special expertise. Consultants in the health service will have the expert power associated with their clinical speciality.
- **Personal power** is the power that comes from the personal attributes of a person – including strong personality, charisma and ability to inspire. It is closely related to leadership qualities, such as above average intelligence, initiative, self-confidence and the ability to rise above a situation and see it in perspective (the 'helicopter' trait). However, effective leaders are not always charismatic, and what makes a leader effective in one situation may cause them to be less effective in changed circumstances. The classic example of this is Sir Winston Churchill: the attributes which made him effective in wartime were not so appropriate in peacetime.

You may sometimes be in the position of wishing to exert influence on people who have a stronger power base. For example, a health visitor may wish to influence a general practitioner to adopt a policy of supporting the running of antenatal clinics in the local minority ethnic group's community centre. Or a community worker may want to lobby local councillors about the need for more recreational facilities for young people on a housing estate. To do this requires skills in influencing.

Before embarking on an attempt to influence someone who is more powerful, first consider (as always) the basic questions in the planning process, such as: what are your aims? What resources do you need? Is the investment going to be worth it? Could the aim be achieved more easily another way?

See Chapter 5 The Basic Planning and Evaluation Process.

The Politics of Influence[15]

The elements of any strategy aiming to change policy and practice could include:

- key aspects of planning;
- making allies;
- networking;
- making deals and negotiating;

We now consider each of these in turn.

Planning

Three particular aspects of planning are useful to consider: undertaking a force field analysis, identifying stakeholders, and considering your timing.

There is an example of a force field analysis in the Exercise 'What helps and hinders your health promotion work' at the end of Chapter 4.

Undertake a force field analysis. A force field analysis identifies the helping and hindering forces in your situation and helps to pinpoint how you can influence the process to make progress towards change. You identify how you can increase the power of the helping forces and decrease the power of the hindering forces.

Identify the stakeholders. The stakeholders are those people with a vested interest in the issue, who wish to influence what is done and how it is done. They are obviously powerful forces in the situation. It may be difficult to identify all the stakeholders, because some of them may not wish to be visible and try to work covertly through others.

Time your action. It is also important to consider when to introduce a proposal or when to delay. If people are already preoccupied with other major issues, it may not be the right time to make a new proposal. On the other hand, if a proposal will help other people to attain their own objectives, now may be a good time.

Making Allies

Identify which of the stakeholders could be allies, and gain their trust and confidence in order to establish and maintain an alliance. It helps to pay attention to their concerns, values, beliefs and behaviour patterns, and see what you need to do in order to form an effective working alliance.

For example, if you are concerned about the way in which disabled people may be treated in an organization, you might identify a personnel officer as a key stakeholder. So find out: is she concerned about it? Does she think it is important for her organization? What kind of way does she work: is she likely to respond best to a lively discussion on the subject or to a well-argued paper on the need for policy, backed up with facts and figures? Does she like time to make decisions? Will she be happy to leave you to take the lead, or will she want to feel that the initiative lies with her?

Networking

Many people working in organizations belong to one or more interest groups which meet to discuss, debate and exchange information on issues that concern the members. These interest groups are networks. By playing an active role in networks, people can extend their influence. Networks provide access to information to help with making a case, to people with experience of successful influencing, and to other resources. There are different types of networks:

Professional networks. Members of the same profession. Professional networks may attempt to influence employers and organizations to reconsider their policies or to develop new policies for the future. Professional networks institute criteria for professional practice and are active in the professional development of their members.

Elitist networks. Members of an elitist group who can join by invitation only. The network operates by personal contact and personal introduction, such as 'old boy' links. Members of such networks may have considerable power and influence, often through their position in organizations.

Pressure groups. Members wish to pursue certain objectives which may be environmental, social or political. An example is the UK Health For All Network, whose members are committed to pursuing the WHO HFA 2000 strategy.[16]

In order to enter a particular network it may be necessary to identify the 'gatekeepers' who control entry, and other people who are influential in the network and could act as a sponsor for someone seeking to join. Having entered a network it is important to support the values and established ways of working. Later, having been accepted, it may be possible to challenge accepted practices.

Making Deals and Negotiating

Making deals is common practice in most organizations. Individuals or groups agree to support a proposal in return for agreement on something which benefits them. In order to make deals successfully, it pays to know the person with whom you are dealing, paying careful attention to the values and intentions of the other party and what you could realistically expect from them.

Negotiation is the art of creating agreement on a specific issue between two or more parties with different views. Successful negotiation takes place when there is a desire to solve problems and the parties genuinely commit to going through a number of stages or steps.

For detailed descriptions of these stages and how best to approach negotiations, see the suggestions for further reading at the end of this chapter.

On Being 'Political' . . .

A final point is about 'political' behaviour, by which we mean finding out about who holds power, and working to use this information to change a situation. When is it acceptable and when is it unethical?

Being 'political' can smack of being devious and manipulative. Many people view political behaviour with suspicion and will therefore not be easily influenced by it. Most people mistrust those who seek to manipulate covertly, or who coerce, lie, or deliberately withhold information which affects others. We do not support any of these tactics.

But to ignore the politics within organizations is unwise, because it results in failure to make a realistic appraisal of situations, and failure to make the best of the opportunities for positive health promotion. Furthermore, we contend that it is possible to be 'political' without losing professional integrity. For example, we suggest that deals are best made as the outcome of open negotiations, and that relationships should be based on genuineness, trust, goodwill and mutual respect.

Case study 16.1   **The politics of influence – health and safety at work**

Bob is an environmental health officer working for Midshire City Council. His aim is to improve the implementation of the health and safety at work policy of the council. He makes a list of the *helping* forces and the *hindering* forces:

Helping:

- the existing safety officers;
- existing codes of practice, for example, sight checks for VDU operators;
- a councillor who is a health lecturer at the University;

- a personnel officer interested in improving the working environment for staff;
- an existing commitment to appoint an occupational health nurse.

Hindering:

- the cost of any improvements (the council has severe financial constraints);
- staff time to attend health and safety training;
- problems with recruiting an occupational health nurse;
- deficiencies in the structure of council buildings

(poor ventilation, open plan offices, lack of showers for those staff wishing to take physical exercise during the day);

- lack of councillors' commitment to improve health and safety conditions for staff;
- lack of access to council buildings for disabled people.

He identifies the stakeholders as:

- the staff themselves;
- the trade unions;
- departmental managers, senior and chief officers;
- the councillors;
- the public health medicine department and the health promotion officer of the local district health authority.

He further identifies key stakeholders as:

- officers in the department of engineering because they enforce building regulations;
- council members on the health committee;
- the director of personnel.

He then identifies ways of increasing the helping forces and decreasing the hindering forces. Through making an ally of the interested personnel officer he is able to increase the commitment of the director of personnel, who is also a chief officer.

One short-term outcome is that an occupational health nurse is recruited. Another outcome is a plan agreed by the personnel department and the trade unions for training staff in health and safety.

By joining a local network of people interested in health promotion he is able to find out what is going on elsewhere and this gives him some useful ideas, including sources of help in stress management training which he incorporates into the training plan.

He makes a deal with the engineering department by agreeing to assist with monitoring construction sites of new buildings in order to prevent accidents on the site. In return, they agree to assist with a plan for improving soundproofing and modifications to open plan offices. Their commitment grows after a report shows that accidents on construction sites are reduced. He discusses with them the issue of raising with council members the plan for modifying council buildings.

Finally, he makes an ally of the councillor at the University by offering to provide an input to some of the courses. This councillor is on the health committee and provides him with useful advice on how to approach the committee and how to prepare documents for its consideration.

Developing and Implementing Policies

In this section, we look first at the range of health promotion policies, and then at practical guidelines on how to develop and implement polices.

First, what kind of health promotion policies are there? Many are about health issues which relate to workplaces or other settings. (**Settings** is a term commonly used since its introduction with the *Health of the Nation* strategy.[17] It means locations where people live and work, and therefore can be reached with health promotion programmes. Common examples are workplaces, schools and hospitals.) Other policies can be about health issues in a range of contexts, such as a national policy on HIV prevention which would cover action across many different population groups and settings. For some health issues, such as smoking at work, it is common practice to have a policy, and there are practical guidelines and model policies available.[18] Other examples of health issues where there are often policies are HIV/AIDS, mental health, healthy eating, alcohol and exercise.[19]

We now look in more detail at policies in specific settings.

Policies on Promoting Health in Workplaces

The benefits of health promotion at work are well established in the USA and Canada, and reviews of the literature identify the major benefits as a significant decrease in absenteeism and staff turnover, and significant increases on productivity and morale.[20] Oxford Regional Health Authority has produced a comprehensive review of the literature on workplace health promotion with a particular focus on smoking and stress.[21] This review suggests that health promotion programmes may not be reaching all sectors of the workforce, and that those in least need of health promotion are the most likely to use facilities and programmes. For general workplace policies, WHO has provided policy guidance.[22] WHO has adopted a broad concept of well-being in the workplace, which includes how work is organized, managerial styles and communication at work, working conditions, job design and type of work.

It is clear that health promotion in the workplace could result in considerable improvements in health. However, there is scope for improving the quality of workplace health promotion programmes, particularly related to their evaluation. Leading employers and trade unions have begun to take on a wider concept of health at work, including giving priority to issues such as smoking, alcohol, and stress.

WHO guidance is in line with the recommendations of a Health Education Authority report,[23] which included:

- setting targets for the reduction of illness in the working population;
- changes in workplace policies, working practices and individual lifestyles to reduce the risk of ill-health and promote well-being of workers;
- systematic elimination of hazardous exposures and sources of unhealthy stress in the workplace.

'Health at Work in the NHS' is an initiative launched in 1992 by the Secretary of State as part of the national strategy for health.[24] It aims to:

- introduce a systematic healthy workplace programme throughout the NHS;
- engage all NHS staff in health promoting activities.

This initiative aims to build on previous good practice. Many Health Authorities, NHS Trusts, GP practices and other NHS workplaces have been active over more than two decades in implementing policies for smoking, healthy eating, and sensible drinking.

Health at Work in the NHS is a long-term project. The aim is that the NHS becomes an exemplary employer, demonstrating to others that a healthy workforce benefits both individual staff members and the organization as a whole. This will help the NHS to provide better services, because healthy staff are more able to care for others.

In 1995 the HEA produced a *Health at Work in the NHS* report which set out a new approach to stress in the NHS.[25] Unlike traditional approaches which tended to focus on individuals, this report set out a method for addressing the problem of stress in the NHS in organizational terms. It provided a practical instrument for carrying out an audit into the organizational causes and sources of distress in order that organizational solutions could be found. This was followed up, in 1996, by a document giving practical guidance on how to plan and implement a programme to tackle organizational stress in the NHS.[26]

Finally, the Health and Safety Executive is a source of information on all regulations governing health and safety in the workplace.[27]

Policies on Promoting Health in Hospitals

'Health Promoting Hospitals' is a WHO initiative designed to improve health and environmental conditions for both staff and patients by reviewing and implementing a range of health promoting policies and activities.[28] The first phase of a WHO Europe pilot hospital project, which in England is based at Preston Hospitals Acute NHS Trust, finished at the end of 1996. Preston Acute Hospitals NHS Trust is committed to supporting the development of an English network of *Health Promoting Hospitals*.[29] Many hospitals have taken up the idea of being a health promoting hospital, but it can be difficult in practice to get everyone informed and involved in an institution as large and complex as a hospital. For example, a survey of cardiology departments in the West Midlands of England found that medical and even nursing staff were not always aware of their hospital's commitment to the Health Promoting Hospital (HPH) movement.[30] Furthermore, some hospitals had a number of HPH-type initiatives, although they had no HPH commitment. For example, one such hospital had a drive to encourage healthy eating involving dietitians, hospital canteens and the catering staff of local schools. One development welcomed by medical staff and other health professionals is the appointment of a named person within a hospital to co-ordinate and facilitate a 'healthy hospital'.

Promoting Health in Urban Settings: 'Healthy Cities'

See the section on the principles of community-based work in Chapter 15 for more about this

See Chapter 1 section on 'addressing the determinants of health' for more about 'healthy cities'

A number of other settings have also been the focus of WHO initiatives. In 1987 the WHO's regional office for Europe initiated a 'Healthy Cities' project, aiming to work from the bottom up, not from the top down, and to involve collaborative work between local government, health authorities, local businesses, community organizations and, of course, individual citizens. The Health for All (UK) Network is the coordinating body for action on *Healthy Cities* within the UK.[31] The Healthy Cities work in Liverpool is a good example of what can be achieved.[32] Liverpool was the first city in the UK to produce a City Health Plan (April 1996) which aims to get everyone moving in the same direction to take action on the underlying causes of ill-health. Priority areas include the environment, the economy, housing, crime, education and transport. Work on *The Health of the Nation* targets is being undertaken through a series of specific, focused strategies.

Policies on Promoting Health in Schools

See section on *Local Authorities* in Chapter 4.

Schools have long been regarded as an important setting for health promotion.[33]
   The European Network of Health Promoting Schools (ENHPS) is a collaborative research and development initiative funded by the WHO (Regional Office for Europe), the European Commission (EC), and the Council of Europe (CE).[34] It involves nearly 40 European countries, each supporting a network of pilot schools. The aim is to develop the effectiveness of schools as settings for the promotion of the physical, social, spiritual, mental and emotional health of young people. The HEA acts as the national support centre within the UK, and both the

Department of Health and the Department for Education and Employment (DfEE) have provided funding and support for the initiative in England. The National Foundation for Educational Research (NFER) is conducting an evaluation of the English dimension of the UK project.

Policies on Promoting Health in Prisons

All prisons are required to develop health promotion programmes. The Home Office has recently been designated a WHO collaborating centre for health promotion in prisons and they are working to develop an award scheme for health promoting prisons.

Guidelines on Developing and Implementing a Policy

Many health promoters have a role in developing and implementing polices. The process of developing and implementing a health promotion policy involves four aspects – preparation, implementation, education and training, and evaluation.[35] We shall now consider each of these in turn.

1.   Preparation of the Policy

The formulation of a policy by any organization is a corporate matter, so the usual starting point is to convene a working group. This group:

- clarifies its terms of reference and elects a chairperson;
- identifies the need for a policy;
- identifies the committee, department or senior officer who has overall responsibility for taking the policy forward;
- identifies key personnel to consult with and convince of the need for a policy;
- establishes a timescale for policy development;
- prepares a draft policy and consults widely;
- prepares the final draft policy for approval.

In the case of a workplace policy, it is important to involve trade unions. This can be achieved either by including trade union representatives on the working group or by setting up an effective framework for consultation and negotiation. This may be crucial in persuading the workforce to look positively on the new policy.

It is also important that an identified senior officer or manager, with political 'clout', acts as a 'champion' for the policy. This person will be crucial in getting the commitment of other managers to the policy.

2.   Implementation of the Policy

This starts with planning, which will include:

- setting aims and objectives;
- setting up a system for monitoring and evaluation;
- identifying resources and defining key implementation tasks;
- defining the role of key personnel;
- developing an action plan.

Key personnel should be encouraged to participate actively in identifying their roles and in discussing boundaries and overlap in roles, so that the potential for conflict and confusion are reduced. For example, managers have the primary responsibility for ensuring that their staff are fully conversant with workplace policies and understand what is expected of them. Nevertheless, the trade unions also have a role in informing the workforce of the policy. These sources of information hopefully will be complementary and spell out the same, not contradictory, messages. The open discussion of these issues will help to increase commitment to making the policy work.

Any policy which is not the subject of regular review risks becoming obsolete. So the working group must reconvene at intervals to consider issues such as:

- does the workforce know about and understand the policy?
- have attitudes to the health issue covered by the policy changed and if so how? How do staff feel about the policy?
- has the behaviour of individual staff changed? Does this include changes in working practices and/or individual lifestyles?
- are staff getting any help they need?
- are managers and trade unions supporting the policy?
- are indicators showing that the policy is making progress towards the attainment of its aims and objectives? For example, in the case of a workplace policy, has absenteeism and sickness reduced? Or have accident rates decreased? Has work performance improved? Is morale better?
- how can we improve the effectiveness of the policy?

3.   Education and Training

This is a continuous process not a one-off event. Wherever possible it should be integrated into existing provision for professional and managerial staff development. The purposes of education and training include:

- securing the commitment of management, for example of elected members, chief officers and senior management in the case of a local authority;
- obtaining the commitment of the whole workforce or group the policy is aimed at (e.g. the prison population);
- providing those responsible for implementing the policy with the necessary skills;
- overcoming prejudices, discrimination and stereotyping where relevant (for example in policies on alcohol and HIV/AIDS);
- encouraging and assisting the workforce/target groups in making choices and individual lifestyle changes.

4.   Evaluation

See the section Plan Evaluation Methods in Chapter 5 for further suggestions.

This should include evaluation of both process and outcomes. It will require the collection of information, both baseline and on-going.

Exercise 16.1   **A workplace alcohol policy**

Westshire NHS Trust is looking at Health at Work in the NHS national initiative. As part of this programme, NHS organizations are encouraged to develop policies on alcohol for their workforces.

A Senior Health Promotion Specialist working with Westshire Trust convenes a working group to develop a policy, which includes representatives of personnel officers, general management, consultant psychiatrists, trade unions and the local voluntary organization on alcohol.

The working group meets four times, and produces a draft policy. The policy specifies that the Trust sees sensible drinking as everyone's responsibility and that all employees will receive basic information about sensible drinking. It also covers the Trust's responsibility to develop an environment conducive to self-referral by anyone with an alcohol problem, early identification of alcohol-related problems and the provision of expert confidential help. It looks at the provision of alcohol on Trust premises, and specifies that non-alcoholic drink should be provided as an alternative at all social functions where alcohol is served, and that alcohol consumption should be discouraged at non-social functions.

This draft policy goes to the Trust Board. It receives a lukewarm reception, and there is much concern that it will interfere with personnel policies on dealing with people who drink on duty. There is also discussion and disagreement about what constitutes 'social' and 'non-social' functions, and resistance to the idea of curtailing 'social' drinking, i.e. selling alcohol at the doctors' bar, and serving it at working lunches, publicity events such as the opening of new clinics, and leaving parties.

Nevertheless, it is passed for consultation, and comes back to the Board for final approval. The Board members are still unenthusiastic, and one major change they make alters the working group's recommendations on implementation. These were that many different staff groups had a key role, including personnel, health promotion, general management and the training department. This is changed so that responsibility for implementation rests entirely with the Trust Director of Personnel. The Alcohol Policy is finally approved formally by the Trust Board.

In the meantime, the Trust has been engaged in a major strategic review which has affected many of its services, and there follows a long period of substantial organizational change. Two years after the Alcohol Policy was approved, it had still not been implemented. There had been no education of the workforce about 'sensible drinking' and no change in the way alcohol was served and sold on Trust premises.

Looking at the stages for developing and implementing a workplace policy in the section above, and the section on 'The politics of influence', consider these questions:

- What steps were taken which helped the policy development?
- What else could have been done?
- Why did the policy receive such a lukewarm reception by the Trust Board? Could anything have been done to prevent this?
- Why was the policy never implemented? Could anything have been done to ensure that the implementation stage actually happened?
- Are there any other significant points to note about the lessons learnt from this case study?

Campaigning

You, or clients with whom you work, may feel strongly about changing policy or practice about a health issue, and decide that the way forward is to mount a campaign.

Campaigns can range from short-lived local ones with the objective of making a single change ('save our local cottage hospital') to long-term national ones such as 'Keep Britain Tidy' or annual 'drinking and driving' campaigns. Pressure groups are made up of the people who are running the campaign, such as the 'Save our Cottage Hospital Campaign Group'. Examples of national pressure groups are 'Shelter' (on homelessness) or 'Friends of the Earth' (on environmental issues). Some pressure groups (such as 'Shelter') may also provide direct services as well as acting as a pressure group.

Principles of Campaigning

Some important principles to keep in mind if you are setting up a campaign are:[36]

- **be persistent:** success requires persistent effort, so you must be committed and prepared to put in a lot of time and energy over as long a period as necessary – which may be a very long time.
- **be professional:** give care and attention to details (such as well-written letters, preferably typed, with the name of the campaign clearly evident) and ensure activities such as keeping records are undertaken properly.
- **keep a sense of perspective:** your campaign may be vitally important to you, but being perceived as a fanatical crank (or even being a fanatical crank!) will do your cause no good.
- **reflect your ideals in your behaviour:** it is no good, for example, campaigning to clean up your neighbourhood if your own front garden looks like a tip. Neither is it helpful to campaign for equal opportunities if the place where your own organization meets.does not enable access for the disabled.
- **be positive:** for example, call yourselves the 'Save the Cottage Hospital Campaign Group' rather than 'Group Against Closing the Cottage Hospital'. 'Shelter' is called the 'National Campaign for the Homeless', not the 'Campaign against Bad Housing'.
- **join with others:** rival pressure groups campaigning on similar (or even identical) issues waste a lot of time and effort. If someone is already campaigning on 'your' issue, join them rather than setting up a rival organization. Or if there is more than one organisation working on similar issues, form a coalition. For example, the 'Save the Cottage Hospital Campaign Group' could link with the local Community Health Council if its members are also concerned about the issue.
- **where you can, do something as you go along:** for example, if you are campaigning to clean up your neighbourhood, you could organize a one-off 'litter collection day' as well as lobbying your local council for better refuse collection and more litter bins.
- **involve as many people as possible:** this is not only to harness their support but so that people can see for themselves what is wrong and what needs to change.

Planning a Campaign

See also Chapter Five The Basic Planning and Evaluation Process.

When you plan a campaign, it helps to go through the same planning process as you would with any other kind of health promotion activity:

- identify your aims clearly;
- decide the best way of achieving them (e.g. public meetings? press coverage? lobbying MPs and local councillors? getting up a petition?)
- identify your resources (do you need to fundraise?)
- clarify how you will know if your aim is achieved (e.g. when the local health authority promises to reconsider the closure of the hospital or when the authority has formally agreed to keep it open for a specified length of time?)
- set an action plan of who is going to what and when.

PRACTICE POINTS

- Recognize that you and all health promoters are in the business of influencing policy and practice at many levels, from national to local and day-to-day.

- If you want to influence policy and practice, you require careful and long-term planning and timing. Know how national and local health promotion policy is created, developed and changed, and how you can have a voice by commenting on proposals and plans.

- Know the rights and standards you can expect from NHS services, and comment on those which you and your clients receive.

- Challenge health damaging policy by working with others, using your vote and by collective action.

- Identify how you could be more effective in influencing policy through reviewing your skills in planning, networking, negotiating and joint working.

- Start policy change by identifying key stakeholders and looking at issues from each of their viewpoints; use techniques such as force-field analysis to establish how to move forward.

- When campaigning on health issues, pay attention to careful planning and be persistent, professional and positive; involve as many other people as possible.

- Keep the ethical aspects of activities in mind when campaigning, lobbying and working towards changing health policy and practice; work with other people to build up trust and mutual respect.

Recommended Reading

On Public Policy and the Politics of Health

➤ Jones L & Sidell M (eds) (1997) *The Challenge of Promoting Health – exploration and action.* Basingstoke: Macmillan/Open University. (Part 2, *Promoting Health through Public Policy* includes chapters on making and changing public policy; and politics of health.)

➤ Naidoo J & Wills J (1994) *Health promotion: Foundations for Practice.* Chapter 7, The politics of health promotion. London: Baillière Tindall.

On Power and Influence

➤ Mintzberg H (1983) *Power In and Around Organisations.* New York: Prentice-Hall. (A classic text on power and the relationship between power, influence and authority.)

➤ Handy C B (1994) *The Empty Raincoat: Making Sense of the Future.* London: Hutchinson.

On Negotiating Agreements

➤ Simnett I (1995) *Managing Health Promotion: Developing Healthy Organisations and Communities,* pp. 160–161. Chichester: Wiley.

➤ Hodgson J (1994) *Thinking on Your Feet in Negotiations: Rapid Response Tactics.* London: Pitman.

➤ Cane S (1994) *Ready Made Activities for Negotiating Skills.* London: Pitman.

On Developing and Implementing Policy

See the list of guidance documents in Note 10.

On Campaigning

➤ Wilson D (1984) *Pressure: the A to Z of campaigning in Britain.* London: Heinemann. (Although this book was published in 1984, its sound advice is still useful.)

Notes and References

1   Two examples of policies developed by partnerships including local councils, health authorities and other bodies are:

Sheffield – see *Healthy Sheffield Information Pack* April 1997. Available from Healthy Sheffield Development Unit, Town Hall Chambers, 1 Barkers Pool, Sheffield S1 1EN.

Glasgow – Greater Glasgow Health Board *Local Health Strategy 1996–2001,* August 1996.

Available from Head of Administration, Greater Glasgow Health Board, 112 Ingram Street, Glasgow G1 1ET.

See also:

Simnett I (1991) *Promoting Health – Local Authorities in Action.* London: Health Education Authority.

2   Secretaries of State for Health (1989) *Working for Patients.* London: HMSO.

3   This definition originates from Dr Peter Brambleby, and is quoted in:

Simnett I (1995) *Managing Health Promotion – Developing healthy organisations and communities,* p. 4. Chichester: Wiley.

4   The health gain cycle is adapted from the leaflet:

Health Gain, Glaxo Pharmaceuticals UK Ltd (1993)

For a description of the approach to purchasing for health gain in Wales, see:

Felvus J, Patterson T, Riley C & Warner M (1991) Lessons in Protocol. *Health Service Journal,* 7 February, pp. 20–21.

5   (1997) News focus: Great Expectations. *The Health Service Journal* **107** (5553), 15 May, p. 11.

6   For a basic guide to Local Agenda 21 see:

Local Government Management Board (1994) *Local Agenda 21 Principles and Process: a step-by-step guide.* London: L G M B.

For detailed information on the UK response to Agenda 21, see:

HM Government White Paper (1994) *Sustainable Development: The UK Strategy.* London: HMSO (CMD 2426).

7   'Global justice begins at home.' A report by David Donnison in *The Guardian,* Society pull-out, p. 3, 23 November 1994.

8   Department of Health (1992) *The Patient's Charter.* London: HMSO. (This was updated in 1995: *The Patient's Charter and You.* London: Department of Health.)

9 See, for example:

Contraceptive Choices: supporting effective use of methods. Available from Healthwise, 2 Pentonville Road, London N1 9FP. This report shows that in 1996 over a quarter of women in a Contraceptive Education Survey were unhappy with NHS information on contraceptive methods.

10 Examples of policy development and guidance by national agencies on health promotion issues and/or health promotion settings are:

UK Health Departments:

UK Health Departments (1995) *HIV & AIDS Health Promotion: an evolving strategy.* London: Department of Health.

Department of Health:

Department of Health (1995) *Policy Appraisal and Health.* London: Department of Health. (A guide from the Department of Health on identifying and quantifying the health impact of policies – for example, policy on housing conditions or alcohol consumption.)

The Health of the Nation (1995) *ABC of Mental Health in the Workplace: A resource pack for employers.* London: Department of Health. (Available from: Department of Health, PO Box 410, Wetherby, LS23 7LN.)

Health Education Authority:

Health Education Authority (1992) *Alcohol Policy Guidelines for Health Authorities*, 3rd edn. London: HEA.

Health Education Authority (1993) *A Survey of Health Education Policies in Schools*, London: HEA.

Health Education Authority (1993) *Smoking policies in schools: guidelines for policy development.* London: HEA.

Bostock Y (1994) *A workplace smoking policy.* London: HEA. (guidelines on how to plan and implement a no-smoking policy in the workplace.)

Health Education Authority (1994) *Contracts for smoking prevention; current practice in the NHS.* London: HEA. (Reviews progress in implementing HoN policy which relates to smoking prevention.)

Stockley L (1993) *The Promotion of Healthier Eating – a basis for action.* London: HEA.

Health at Work in the NHS (1995) *Working for Health: A practical guide to developing a healthy workplace in the NHS.* London: HEA.

Health Education Authority (1995) *Promoting Physical Activity: guidance for commissioners, purchasers and providers.* London: HEA.

Health Education Authority (1996) *Promoting Physical Activity through Primary Health Care.* London: HEA.

Health Education Authority (1997) *Helping smokers to give up: a purchaser's guide to cost effectiveness.* London: HEA.

Health Education Authority (1994) *Young people and physical activity: promoting better practice.* London: HEA.

Health Promotion Wales:

Has produced a number of booklets aimed at helping to develop health policy, including: a series of booklets *Healthy Schools for Wales*, including *Alcohol, Smoking, Implementing food policies in schools*, and *Sex education.*

Youth work and health: developing a strategy for your organisation gives guidelines for developing a strategy on health issues in the youth service.

Mental health promotion: options for Wales sets out proposals for developing a coordinated programme of mental health promotion.

Mental health: a guide for commissioners provides guidance for commissioners of health promotion services on purchasing mental health promotion.

Alcohol Concern:

Has called for a national strategy to tackle alcohol dependence, as twice as many people are dependent on alcohol as on all other drugs:

Alcohol Concern (1997) *Measures for Measures.* Available from: Alcohol Concern, 32–36 Loman Street, London SE1 0EE.

National Forum for Coronary Heart Disease Prevention:

National Forum for Coronary Heart Disease Prevention (1995) *Physical Activity: an agenda for action.* Proposes ideas for coordinated strategy to promote physical activity. Available from National Forum for Coronary Heart Disease Prevention at Trevelyan House, 30 Great Peter Street, London SW1P 2HW, Tel: 0171 222 5300.

Child Accident Prevention Trust:

Hogg C (1996) *Preventing Children's Accidents: a guide for health authorities and boards.* Child Accident Prevention Trust, 18–20 Farringdon Lane, London EC1R 3AU.

11 Association for Public Health (1997) Sustaining the Public's Health: the manifesto of the Association for Public Health. The full manifesto can be obtained from:

Association for Public Health, Trevelyan House, 30 Great Peter Street, London SW1P 2HW, Tel: 0171 222 5300.

12   See, for example:

Paton C (1997) The future in your hands. *Health Service Journal*, 8 May, p. 18.

Crail M (1997) Great Expectations. News Focus. *Health Service Journal*, 8 May, p. 11.

Hudson B (1997) Waiting in the Wings. *Health Service Journal*, 20 March, p 34–35. (A discussion of the controversial question of whether local authorities should take over health authority responsibility for commissioning health care.)

13   For an article which highlights the relationship between politics and health, see:

Munro J & Rayner G (1997) Frank Talking on Health Inequality. *Health Matters* **29**, pp. 6–7.

For case studies of politics and power in health promotion, see:

Rodmell S & Watt A (eds) (1986) *The Politics of Health Education – Raising the Issues*, London: Routledge and Kegan Paul.

Cannon G (1987) *The Politics of Food*. London: Century.

Jacobson B (1988) *Beating the Ladykillers*. London: Gollanz. (On the politics of tobacco with reference to women smoking.)

Davis A (1997) An 'insider' looking out: the politics of physical activity in England. Chapter 30 in Sidell M, Jones L, Katz J & Peberdy A (eds) *Debates and Dilemmas in Promoting Health*. Basingstoke: Macmillan/Open University Press. (Examines the politics and policy issues in relation to sport, physical activity, transport and health policy.)

14   You can find out who your MP and local councillor are, and details of their 'surgeries', from libraries and Citizens Advice Bureaux. You can write to your MP at:

The House of Commons, Westminster, London SW1A OAA Tel: 0171 219 3000.

15   This section is partly based on:

Kakabadse A P (1982) The politics of interpersonal influence, in *Leadership and Organisation Development*, **3** (3). Bradford: MCB University Press.

16   For further information on the UK Health For All Network, contact:

UK Health For All Network, PO Box 101, Liverpool, L69 5BE.
Tel./Fax: 0151 207 0919.

Other health promotion networks include:

The Public Health Alliance, 138 Digbeth, Birmingham, B5 6DR.
Tel: 0121 643 4343.

Association for Public Health, Trevelyan House, 30 Great Peter Street, London SW1P 2HW, Tel: 0171 222 5300.

The Local Authorities Health Network, PO Box 103, Chesterfield, Derbyshire, S44 5UB. Tel: 01246 851143.

17   Secretary of State for Health (1992) *The Health of the Nation: A Strategy for Health in England*. London: HMSO. (Page 26 discusses 'action in different settings' listing healthy cities, healthy schools, healthy hospitals, healthy workplaces, healthy homes, healthy prisons and healthy environments.)

18   Health Education Authority (1993) *Smoking policies in schools: guidelines for policy development*. London: HEA.

Bostock Y (1994) *A workplace smoking policy*. London: Health Education Authority. (Guidelines on how to plan and implement a no-smoking policy in the workplace.)

19   For the results of a survey of a cross-section of workplaces in England, providing information about policies and practice with regard to smoking, nutrition, HIV/AIDS, stress and alcohol, see:

Health Education Authority (1993) *Health Promotion in the Workplace: a summary*. London: HEA.

For other examples of policies and policy guidance see Note 10 above.

20   See, for example:

Bertera R I (1990) The effects of workplace health promotion on absenteeism and employment costs in a large industrial population. *American Journal of Public Health* **80** (9), 307–327.

Of the research studies that have looked at the economic benefits to be derived from health promotion programmes, most have shown them to have reduced staff turnover, reduced absenteeism, improved productivity, reduced frequency of accidents and injuries, and reduced recruitment costs and improved corporate image. For a review of the literature on workplace health promotion, see:

Department of Health (1994) *The Health of the Nation Workplace Task Force Report*. London: Department of Health.

21   Directorate of Health Policy and Public Health (1993) *Workplace Health Promotion: A Review of the Literature*. Oxford: Regional Health Authority.

22 World Health Organization (1988) *Health Promotion for Working Populations* Report of a WHO Expert Committee, Technical Report Series No. 765, WHO: Geneva.

WHO have also published the results of a survey of health promotion in European organizations:

Malzon R A and Lindsay G B (1992) *Health Promotion at the Worksite: A Survey of Large Organisations in Europe*. Copenhagen: European Occupational Health Series No. 4.

23 Webb A *et al.* (1988) *Health at Work? A report on health promotion in the workplace*, Research Report No. 22. London: Health Education Authority.

24 Health Education Authority/NHS Management Executive (1992) *Health At Work in the NHS: Action Pack*. London: HEA.

25 Health at Work in the NHS (1995) *Organisational Stress in the National Health Service: An intervention designed to enable staff to address organisational sources of work-related stress*. London: HEA.

26 Health at Work in the NHS (1996) *Organisational Stress: Planning and implementing a programme to address organisational stress in the NHS*. London: OPUS/Health Education Authority.

27 Health and Safety Executive, Baynards House, 1 Chepstow Place, Westbourne Grove, London W2 4TF. Tel: 0171 221 0870.

28 See: Health Education Authority (1993) *Health Promoting Hospitals: principles and practice*. London: HEA, and:

NHS Executive (1994) *The Health of the Nation: Health Promoting Hospitals*. London: Department of Health.

29 For more information, contact the WHO HPH Project Co-ordinator, North West Lancashire HP Unit, Sharoe Green Hospital, Sharoe Green Lane, Fulwood, Preston, PR2 8DU. Tel: 01772 711223.

30 Perkins E, Jones L & Simnett I (1996) *Hospital Doctors and Prevention: A study of the views of cardiologists in the West Midlands*. Birmingham: West Midlands Board of Postgraduate Medical and Dental Education/West Midlands Regional Health Authority.

31 For further information contact the Network Co-ordinator, Health for All (UK) Network, PO Box 101, Liverpool L69 5BE. Tel./Fax 0151 207 0919.

32 For more information contact: Liverpool Healthy City, PO Box 88, Municipal Buildings, Dale Street, Liverpool LS69 2DH. Tel: 0151 225 2881. Fax 0151 225 2408. See also: Costongs C & Springett J (1997) Joint working and the production of a City Health Plan: the Liverpool experience. *Health Promotion International* **12** (1), pp. 9–19.

33 See for example: *Opportunities for Health and Education to Work Together: Linking the Health of the Nation targets to the National Curriculum*. Available from: Outset Publishing, Saffron House, 59 High Street, Battle, East Sussex TN33 0EN.

On school health education, arguing that school health education is not in good health, and must fight for its survival and growth in a rapidly changing educational climate:

Cale L (1997) Health education in schools: in a state of good health? *International Journal of Health Education* **35** (2), 59–62.

34 Articles on The European Network of Health Promoting Schools (ENHPS): a series of articles on ENHPS and its development and evaluation in Scotland, Wales, England and Northern Ireland can be found in *The Health Education Journal* **55** (4), December 1996, pp. 447–478.

For information about published accounts of work resulting from the ENHPS project, contact:

The Administrator, Young People and Schools Account, Health Education Authority, Trevelyan House, 30 Great Peter Street, London SW1P 2HW, Tel: 0171 222 5300. Fax: 0171 413 8900.

35 This is based on:

Simnett I & Chiles M (1989) *A Practical Guide to Developing and Implementing Alcohol Policies*. Bristol: Frenchay Health Authority.

and:

Health and Consumer Services, Sheffield City Council (1989) *Guidelines for Local Authorities on the Development, Implementation and Evaluation of an Alcohol Policy for their Staff*. London: Health Education Authority.

36 This section is adapted from some material in Chapter 2 of:

Wilson D (1984) *Pressure: the A to Z of campaigning in Britain*. London: Heinemann.

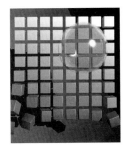

INDEX